Arrhythmogenic RV Cardiomyopathy/Dysplasia
Recent Advances

Frank I. Markus
Andrea Nava
Gaetano Thiene

Frank I. Marcus • Andrea Nava • Gaetano Thiene (Eds)

Arrhythmogenic RV Cardiomyopathy/ Dysplasia

Recent Advances

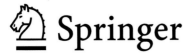

Springer

FRANK I. MARCUS
Section of Cardiology
Department of Medicine
Sarver Heart Center
University of Arizona
Tucson (AZ), USA

ANDREA NAVA
Department of Cardiological, Thoracic
and Vascular Sciences
University of Padua, Italy

GAETANO THIENE
Department of Medical Diagnostic Sciences
University of Padua, Italy

Library of Congress Control Number: 2007922495

ISBN 978-88-470-0489-4 Springer Milan Berlin Heidelberg New York

Springer is a part of Springer Science+Business Media
springer.com
© Springer-Verlag Italia 2007

Cover design: Simona Colombo, Milan, Italy
Typesetting: C & G di Cerri e Galassi, Cremona, Italy
Printer: Arti Grafiche Nidasio, Assago, Italy
Printed in Italy

Springer-Verlag Italia S.r.l.,Via Decembrio 28, I-20137 Milan

PREFACE

This book covers all the recent research highlights of arrhythmogenic right ventricular cardiomyopathy/dysplasia (ARVC/D), a recently discovered heart muscle disease which is a major threat to the life of affected young people. It summarizes nearly 25 years of investigation on the etiology, genetics, pathology, clinical features, diagnosis, and treatment of ARVC/D. In particular, a 5-year research program supported by grants from both the European Community and the National Heart, Lung and Blood Institutes has contributed to the discovery of seven disease-causing genes, thus opening new avenues for the early identification of affected patients and prevention of sudden death.

A Workshop was held in Venice, Italy, October 3, 2005, as part of the Venice Arrhythmia Meeting, where the European and American investigators presented and discussed several major achievements which are now reported in this book. As a result of these coordinated efforts, great advances have been made in the recognition and understanding of the disease, which are summarized in this book.

Molecular genetics has established this cardiomyopathy as a familial disorder caused by mutation of the genes that encode cell junction proteins, resulting in defective cellular adhesion with specific immunohistochemical and ultrastructural alterations. Remodelling at the intercalated disk may trigger a cascade of events including apoptotic cell death, fibrofatty replacement, and electrical instability. The left ventricle may be involved early in the course of some genetic types of this disease. This finding alters the traditional concept of a disease confined to the right ventricle.

Genetic screening can detect symptomatic carriers in the early stage of the disease. Magnetic resonance imaging with gadolinium permits in vivo identification of fibrous tissue. Electroanatomic mapping can reveal areas of fibrofatty replacement of the right ventricular myocardium. The implantable cardioverter defibrillator has been shown to prevent sudden cardiac death. Whether it should be implanted for secondary as well as for primary prevention is still controversial.

Screening prior to participation in competitive sports has been found to be effective for the identification of subjects at risk and is life-saving by disqualifying affected individuals and avoiding competitive type effort. Sudden death of young athletes declined fivefold after implementation of preparticipation screening, mainly due to identification of ARVC/D.

A panel of experts have contributed to writing this monograph, which will be an essential reference for clinicians and scholars in human genetics, pathology, cardiology, and radiology as well as in forensic and sports medicine.

We would like to express our gratitude to the European Commission, Brussels, CARIPARO Foundation, Padua, and Veneto Region, Venice, for their financial support, which made this publication possible. A special thanks is given to Chiara Carturan and Kathy Gear for their continuous, outstanding collaboration over the years of these investigations.

The Editors

LIST OF CONTRIBUTORS

CRISTINA BASSO, MD, PhD
Department of Medical Diagnostic Sciences
University of Padua, Italy

BARBARA BAUCE, MD, PhD
Department of Cardiological, Thoracic
and Vascular Sciences
University of Padua, Italy

DAVID A. BLUEMKE, MD, PhD
Russel H. Morgan Department
of Radiology and Radiological Science
Johns Hopkins Medical Institutions
Baltimore (MD), USA

GIANFRANCO BUJA, MD
Department of Cardiological, Thoracic
and Vascular Sciences
University of Padua, Italy

FIORELLA CALABRESE, MD
Department of Medical Diagnostic Sciences
University of Padua, Italy

HUGH CALKINS, MD
Division of Cardiology
Johns Hopkins Medical Institutions
Baltimore (MD), USA

ELISA CARTURAN
Department of Medical Diagnostic Sciences
University of Padua, Italy

DOMENICO CORRADO, MD, PhD
Department of Cardiological, Thoracic
and Vascular Sciences
University of Padua, Italy

ELZBIETA CZARNOWSKA, PhD
Department of Pathology
The Children's Memorial Health Institute
Warzaw, Poland

LUCIANO DALIENTO, MD
Department of Cardiological, Thoracic
and Vascular Sciences
University of Padua, Italy

GIAN ANTONIO DANIELI, BSc
Department of Biology
University of Padua, Italy

JAMES DAUBERT, MD
Division of Cardiology
Department of Internal Medicine
Strong Memorial Hospital
University of Rochester
Rochester (NY), USA

MILA DELLA BARBERA
Department of Medical Diagnostic Sciences
University of Padua, Italy

N.A. MARK III ESTES, MD
Tufts University School of Medicine
New England Cardiac Arrhythmia Center
Tufts-New England Medical Center
Boston (MA), USA

GUY FONTAINE, MD, PhD
Department of Cardiac Arrhythmias
Institute of Cardiology
University Hospital and School
of Medicine Pitié-Salpêtrière
Paris, France

PHILIP R. FOX, DVM
Caspary Institute
The Animal Medical Center
New York (NY), USA

ROBERT FRANK, MD
Department of Cardiac Arrhythmias
Institute of Cardiology
University Hospital and School
of Medicine Pitié-Salpêtrière
Paris, France

OLAF HEDRICH, MD
Tufts-New England Medical Center
Cardiac Arrhythmia Service
Boston (MA), USA

FRANÇOISE HIDDEN-LUCET, MD
Department of Cardiac Arrhythmias
Institute of Cardiology
University Hospital and School
of Medicine Pitié-Salpêtrière
Paris, France

BARBARA IGNATIUK, MD, PhD
Department of Cardiological, Thoracic
and Vascular Sciences
University of Padua, Italy

JULIA INDIK, MD
Department of Cardiology
Sarver Heart Center
University of Arizona College of Medicine
Tucson (AZ), USA

MAREK KONKA, MD, PhD
Department of Congenital Heart Disease
Institute of Cardiology
Warsaw, Poland

JÉRÔME LACOTTE, MD
Department of Cardiac Arrhythmias
Institute of Cardiology
University Hospital and School of
Medicine Pitié-Salpêtrière
Paris, France

MARK S. LINK, MD
Tufts-New England Medical Center
Cardiac Arrhythmia Service
Boston (MA), USA

FRANK I. MARCUS, MD
Section of Cardiology
Department of Medicine
Sarver Heart Center
University of Arizona
Tucson (AZ), USA

BARRY J. MARON, MD
Hypertrophic Cardiomyopathy Center
Minneapolis Heart Institute Foundation
Minneapolis (MN), USA

WILLIAM J. MCKENNA, MD, DSc, FRCP
Department of Medicine
University College London and
University College London Hospitals Trust
London, UK

ANDREA NAVA, MD
Department of Cardiological, Thoracic
and Vascular Sciences
University of Padua, Italy

MATTHIAS PAUL, MD
Department of Cardiology and Angiology
University Hospital of Münster
Münster, Germany

MICHAEL H. PICARD, MD
Cardiac Ultrasound Laboratory
Massachusetts General Hospital
Boston (MA), USA

KATARZYNA PIOTROWICZ, MD
Heart Research Follow-up Program
Division of Cardiology
University of Rochester Medical Center
Rochester (NY), USA

NIKOS PROTONOTARIOS, MD
Yannis Protonotarios Medical Centre
Hora Naxos, Naxos, Greece

ALESSANDRA RAMPAZZO, BSc, PhD
Department of Biology
University of Padua, Italy

JEFFREY SAFFITZ, MD, PhD
Harvard Medical School
and Department of Pathology
Beth Israel Deaconess Medical Center
Boston (MA), USA

SRIJITA SEN-CHOWDHRY, MA, MBBS, MRCP
Department of Medicine
University College London and
University College London Hospitals Trust
London, UK

DUANE SHERRILL, PhD
Mel and Enid Zuckerman College of
Public Health
University of Arizona
Tucson (AZ), USA

PETROS SYRRIS, PhD
Department of Medicine
University College London and
University College London Hospitals Trust
London, UK

HARIKRISHNA TANDRI, MD
Division of Cardiology
Johns Hopkins Medical Institutions
Baltimore (MD), USA

GAETANO THIENE, MD
Department of Medical Diagnostic Sciences
University of Padua, Italy

JEFFREY A. TOWBIN, MD
Pediatric Cardiology
Texas Children's Hospital
Baylor College of Medicine
Houston (TX), USA

ADALENA TSATSOPOULOU, MD
Yannis Protonotarios Medical Centre
Hora Naxos, Naxos, Greece

PIETRO TURRINI, MD, PhD
Department of Cardiology
Civil Hospital of Camposampiero
Camposampiero (PD), Italy

MARIALUISA VALENTE, MD
Department of Medical Diagnostic Sciences
University of Padua, Italy

MATTEO VATTA, PhD
Pediatric Cardiology
Texas Children's Hospital
Baylor College of Medicine
Houston (TX), USA

DEIRDRE WARD, MRCPI
Department of Medicine
University College London and
University College London Hospitals Trust
London, UK

THOMAS WICHTER, MD, FESC
Department of Cardiology and Angiology
University Hospital of Münster
Münster, Germany

ELZBIETA KATARZYNA WLODARSKA, MD, PhD
Department of Congenital Heart Disease
Institute of Cardiology
Warsaw, Poland

ZHAO YANG, MD
Pediatric Cardiology
Texas Children's Hospital
Baylor College of Medicine
Houston (TX), USA

DANITA YOERGER-SANBORN, MD, MMSc
Cardiac Ultrasound Laboratory
Cardiology Division
Massachusetts General Hospital
Harvard Medical School
Boston (MA), USA

WOJCIECH ZAREBA, MD, PhD
Heart Research Follow-up Program
and Clinical Cardiology Research
Division of Cardiology
University of Rochester Medical Center
Rochester (NY), USA

ABOUT THE EDITORS

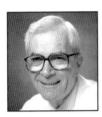

FRANK I. MARCUS, MD
Frank Marcus is Professor of Medicine at the Sarver Heart Center, University of Arizona, Tucson, USA. He reported the first clinical series of ARVC/D patients and continues to contribute to the understanding of the diagnosis and treatment of this disease. He is the principal investigator of the North American Multidisciplinary study of ARVC/D supported by the NHLBI, that consists of a registry, a data coordination center, a genetic laboratory and several international core laboratories.

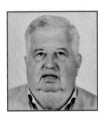

ANDREA NAVA, MD
Andrea Nava is Professor of Cardiology at the University of Padua, Italy. He first recognized the familial occurrence of ARVC/D in the Veneto Region and has made major contributions to the early identification, discovery of defective genes and phenotypic expression of the disease. He is in charge of the family screening program that consists of clinical and genetic investigations.

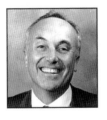

GAETANO THIENE, MD
Gaetano Thiene is Professor of Cardiovascular Pathology and Director of the Institute of Pathological Anatomy at the University of Padua, Italy. He was trained both in Cardiology and Pathology. He first reported ARVC/D as a major cause of sudden, unexpected death in the young and in athletes and established diagnostic criteria for endomyocardial biopsy. He coordinates the European study and has implemented the European Registry of ARVC/D supported by the European Commission.

Introduction: ARRHYTHMOGENIC RIGHT VENTRICULAR CARDIOMYOPATHY/ DYSPLASIA CLARIFIED

Gaetano Thiene, Andrea Nava, Frank I. Marcus

The first monograph on arrhythmogenic right ventricular cardiomyopathy/dysplasia (ARVC/D) was published 10 years ago [1]. Since then, there have been major advancements in the basic knowledge of the disease as well as a better understanding of the diagnosis and treatment. A workshop was held in Venice, Italy on October 3, 2005, where research on various aspects of this disease, both biological and clinical was presented.

This book has assembled contributions in the form of a monograph rather than as the publication of Proceedings. In addition, some topics were added in a similar format to that of the first monograph [1], which followed a meeting on ARVC/D held in Paris in 1996.

In the last 10 years our understanding of this disease has been impressive. This is the logical consequence of a research strategy with clear goals.

At the turn of the millennium, following a series of meetings of experts from both sides of the Atlantic, it became evident that we had to merge the expertise of scientists and clinicians attracted by the mystery of ARVC/D and its devastating physical and social consequences into an "army" for the fight against the disease.

An International Registry was considered mandatory in order to collect study material and concentrate efforts on this rare disease [2].

It was then decided to apply for grants to the European Commission (EC) and to the National Institute of Health (NIH). Two teams were created, one in Europe coordinated by Gaetano Thiene [3] and one in North America coordinated by Frank Marcus [4]. Utilizing a similar database and having some Core Laboratories in common, the two projects were initiated. The structure was somewhat different: the European Registry enrolled patients who were both previously diagnosed as well as those with the recent onset of symptoms, whereas the North American Registry enrolled only newly diagnosed patients. Guidelines for diagnostic criteria and protocols were implemented. Genetic investigation was an integral part of both studies. Fortunately, the two projects were approved and funded for 5 years, thus allowing the start of a major interdisciplinary study of ARVC/D. The results exceeded our best expectations, resulting in numerous important publications in well-recognized cardiovascular journals. In this monograph the advances in our knowledge will be summarized in didactic presentations.

A brief overview of the major advances is as follows:

1. The genetic background of this hereditary-familial, monogenic disease has been clarified. Despite genetic heterogeneity with rare variants, it has been demonstrated that both autosomal and recessive forms are due to defects of genes encoding desmosomal proteins of the intercalated disc: plakoglobin [5], desmoplakin, [6] plakophilin [7], desmoglein [8], and desmocollin [9]. This explains why the disease is now called a desmosomal cardiomyopathy [10, 11]. To date, seven disease genes have been identified during the course of the EC and NIH research projects – an unbelievable achievement. Genetic screening is now feasible for the detection of gene carriers and early clinical diagnosis [12].

2. The pathological substrate of the disease has been clarified at the ultrastructural level with evidence of remodeling of intercalated disc (widening of intercellular space with abnormal desmosomes) [13]. These structural abnormalities can potentially trigger a cascade of events following parietal stretch (apoptotic cell death, fibrofatty replacement, electrical instability). There is now evidence that the left ventricle is also involved. In some variants of the disease it has been shown that the left ventricle is primarily affected, thus expanding the previous concept that the disease is confined to the right ventricle [14-16]. The diagnostic role of endomyocardial biopsy has been improved by updating morphometric parameters.

3. Both the advantages and limitations of imaging modalities have been clarified and are beginning to be subjected to quantitative analysis. Magnetic resonance imaging is being expanded in scope not only to study the morphology and dysfunction of the ventricles, but also to identify tissue composition, particularly fibrosis utilizing gadolinium late enhancement.

4. With regard to advances in the invasive diagnostic techniques, electroanatomic mapping is being evaluated to detect areas of decreased electrical activity, which has been found to correspond to diffuse segmental fibrofatty atrophy [17]. This may be important not only for the diagnosis of the disease, but also for the identification of areas that may be the target for catheter ablation. Nevertheless, the precise diagnostic role of electroanatomic mapping needs further clarification. Also the role of ablation for treatment of ventricular arrhythmias needs to be reinvestigated utilizing the technique of electroanatomic mapping.

5. It is indisputable that the implantable cardioverter defibrillator (ICD) has been lifesaving in patients with ARVC/D who have malignant ventricular arrhythmias including hemodynamically unstable ventricular tachycardia [18, 19]. The efficacy of the ICD in this setting is astonishing and recalls the miracle of the resuscitation of Lazarus, friend of Jesus Christ, from the tomb, painted by Giotto in the Scrovegni Chapel in Padua, where Jesus said "*veni foras, Lazare*" (John's Gospel chapter 11, line 43-44) (Fig. 1). Whether the ICD should be employed as primary as well as for secondary prevention is still controversial.

6. Primary prevention of sudden death in the young and in athletes from ARVC/D may be possible by lifestyle changes, particularly avoiding participation in vigorous and certainly in competitive sports. Preparticipation screening for those who engage in competitive sports has been shown to be highly effective for identification of the individuals at risk, including those with ARVC/D. In Italy, sudden death of young athletes declined five fold after the implementation of preparticipation screening primarily due to identification of cardiomyopathies [20]. The recognition of ARVC/D as a disease entity, as well as the utilization of strict diagnostic criteria [21], accounts for this important achievement.

7. Recent developments from in vitro and in vivo analyses of mutated proteins in transgenic mice are providing mechanistic explanations, with targeted therapies on the horizon for affected patients [22-25].

These studies suggest that sudden cardiac death in patients with ARVC/D may be prevented by different approaches (Fig. 2):

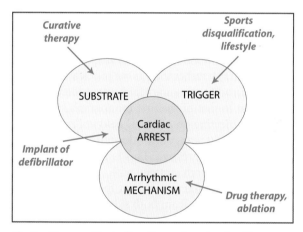

Fig. 2 • Diagram illustrating the various levels of interventions for sudden death prevention in ARVC/D

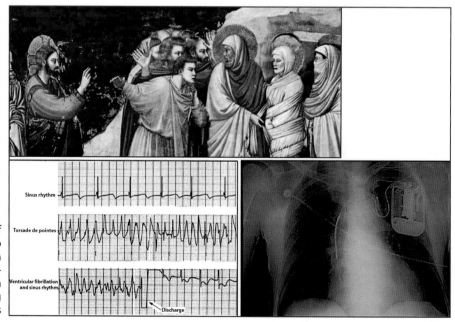

Fig. 1 • The resuscitation of Lazarus, painted by Giotto in the Scrovegni Chapel in Padua (C. 1304), is compared to the rescue from cardiac arrest by ICD; ecg tracing, courtesy of Dr. Moss

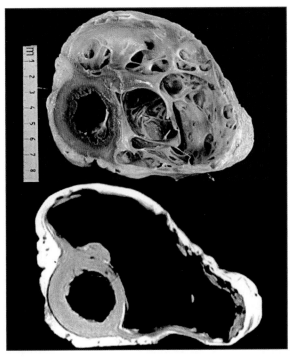

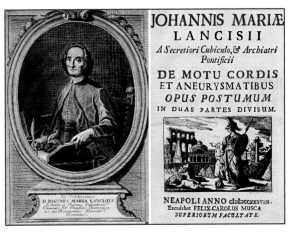

Fig. 4 • The first description of ARVC/D was reported in this book of Giovanni Maria Lancisi, Professor of Anatomy in Rome, 1736

Fig. 3 • The heart specimen with ARVC/D of the original patient reported by Professor Dalla Volta in 1961. The patient underwent cardiac transplantation 35 years later because of right ventricular failure: note the massive dilatation of the right ventricle and the small, normal left ventricle

1. Avoiding the trigger, such as strenuous exercise in patients who are identified as having the disease by clinical or genetic screening;
2. Preventing life-threatening arrhythmias using drug therapy or ablation;
3. ICD implantation, an extremely effective therapy to treat life-threatening ventricular arrhythmias that can result in cardiac arrest.

The selection of appropriate therapy for the individual patient awaits further investigation.

All the above-mentioned therapeutic and preventive measures are palliative, not curative. The definitive cure of the disease is still elusive. Cardiac transplantation is employed to treat end-stage cardiac failure or for refractory electrical instability, but this therapy is not without problems, particularly the need to prevent acute rejection as well as allograft vasculopathy. Prevention of myocyte apoptotic death, inflammation, and fibrofatty replacement, the basic mechanisms of myocardial injury and repair, will require understanding the pathogenetic mechanisms of ARVC/D. At present, replacement of the defective genes (gene therapy) is theoretically possible only by disease identification at the early embryonic stage, with preimplantation genetic diagnosis, an issue that raises major ethical questions [26].

Thus, although the genetic basis of ARVC/D has been largely clarified, there is much work to be done to better understand the cell biology of the disease, to know how to slow disease progression, and ultimately to prevent disease transmission.

Finally, some historical notes. It was in 1961 that Professor Sergio Dalla Volta from the University of Padua reported cases with "auricularization of the right ventricular pressure" with an amazing fibrofatty, nonischemic pathology of the right ventricle [27]. One of those patients survived until 1995, and underwent transplantation due to end-stage cardiac failure. Interestingly, the heart specimen showed severe right ventricular enlargement with a nearly normal left ventricle (Fig. 3).

Attention was focused on the disease following the clinical description of ARVC/D by Marcus et al. in 1982 [28]. In 1988 Nava et al. elucidated the pattern of transmission in family members [29], and Thiene et al. discovered the disease as a previously unrecognized and important cause of sudden death in the young [30]. However, the first description of the disease can be traced to the book *De Motu Cordis et Aneurismatibus* by Giovanni Maria Lancisi, published in 1736. (Dr. Arnold Katz, personal communication) (Fig. 4). In the 5th chapter of this book, paragraph 47, Lancisi reported a family with disease recurrence in four generations. Signs and symptoms were palpitations, heart failure, dilatation and aneurysms of the right ventricle, and sudden death, all features consistent with the current diagnostic criteria of the disease. Thus, we know that the disease is not new, only newly investigated. Nevertheless, tremendous strides have been made in recognition and understanding of the disease which are summarized in this monograph.

References

1. Nava A, Rossi L, Thiene G (1997) Arrhythmogenic right ventricular cardiomyopathy/dysplasia. Elsevier, Amsterdam

2. Corrado D, Fontaine G, Marcus FI et al (2000) Arrhythmogenic right ventricular dysplasia/cardiomyopathy: Need for an international registry. Study Group on Arrhythmogenic Right Ventricular Dysplasia/Cardiomyopathy of the Working Groups on Myocardial and Pericardial Disease and Arrhythmias of the European Society of Cardiology and of the Scientific Council on Cardiomyopathies of the World Heart Federation. Circulation 101:E101-106

3. Basso C, Wichter T, Danieli GA et al (2004) Arrhythmogenic right ventricular cardiomyopathy: Clinical registry and database, evaluation of therapies, pathology registry, DNA banking. Eur Heart J 25:531-534

4. Marcus F, Towbin JA, Zareba W et al (2003) ARVD/C Investigators. Arrhythmogenic right ventricular dysplasia/cardiomyopathy (ARVD/C): A multidisciplinary study: Design and protocol. Circulation 107:2975-2978

5. McKoy G, Protonotarios N, Crosby A et al (2000) Identification of a deletion in plakoglobin in arrhythmogenic right ventricular cardiomyopathy with palmoplantar keratoderma and woolly hair (Naxos disease). Lancet 355:2119-2124

6. Rampazzo A, Nava A, Malacrida S et al (2002) Mutation in human desmoplakin domain binding to plakoglobin causes a dominant form of arrhythmogenic right ventricular cardiomyopathy. Am J Hum Genet 71:1200-1206

7. Gerull B, Heuser A, Wichter T et al (2004) Mutations in the desmosomal protein plakophilin-2 are common in arrhythmogenic right ventricular cardiomyopathy. Nat Genet 36:1162-1164

8. Pilichou K, Nava A, Basso C et al (2006) Mutations in desmoglein-2 gene are associated with arrhythmogenic right ventricular cardiomyopathy. Circulation 113:1171-1179

9. Syrris P, Ward D, Evans A et al (2006) Arrhythmogenic right ventricular dysplasia/cardiomyopathy associated with mutations in the desmosomal gene desmocollin-2. Am J Hum Genet 79:978-984

10. Thiene G, Basso C, Corrado D (2004) Cardiomyopathies: Is it time for a molecular classification? Eur Heart J 25:1772-1775

11. Maron BJ, Towbin JA, Thiene G et al (2006) Contemporary definitions and classification of the cardiomyopathies: An American Heart Association Scientific Statement from the Council on Clinical Cardiology, Heart Failure and Transplantation Committee; Quality of Care and Outcomes Research and Functional Genomics and Translational Biology Interdisciplinary Working Groups; and Council on Epidemiology and Prevention. Circulation 113:1807-1816

12. Corrado D, Thiene G (2006) Arrhythmogenic right ventricular cardiomyopathy/dysplasia: Clinical impact of molecular genetic studies. Circulation 113:1634-1637

13. Basso C, Czarnowska E, Della Barbera M et al (2006) Ultrastructural evidence of intercalated disc remodelling in arrhythmogenic right ventricular cardiomyopathy: An electron microscopy investigation on endomyocardial biopsies. Eur Heart J 27:1847-1854

14. Bauce B, Basso C, Rampazzo A et al (2005) Clinical profile of four families with arrhythmogenic right ventricular cardiomyopathy caused by dominant desmoplakin mutations. Eur Heart J 26:1666-1675

15. Norman M, Simpson M, Mogensen J et al (2005) Novel mutation in desmoplakin causes arrhythmogenic left ventricular cardiomyopathy. Circulation 112:636-642

16. Sen-Chowdry S, Prasad SK, Syrris P et al (2006) Cardiovascular magnetic resonance in arrhythmogenic right ventricular cardiomyopathy revisited: Comparison with task force criteria and genotype. J Am Coll Cardiol 48:2132-2140

17. Corrado D, Basso C, Leoni L et al (2005) Three-dimensional electroanatomic voltage mapping increases accuracy of diagnosing arrhythmogenic right ventricular cardiomyopathy/dysplasia. Circulation 111:3042-3050

18. Corrado D, Leoni L, Link MS et al (2003) Implantable cardioverter-defibrillator therapy for prevention of sudden death in patients with arrhythmogenic right ventricular cardiomyopathy/dysplasia. Circulation 108:3084-3091

19. Wichter T, Paul M, Wollmann C et al (2004) Implantable cardioverter/defibrillator therapy in arrhythmogenic right ventricular cardiomyopathy. Single-center experience of long-term follow-up and complications in 60 patients. Circulation 109:1503-1508

20. Corrado D, Basso C, Pavei A et al (2006) Trends in sudden cardiovascular death in young competitive athletes after implementation of a preparticipation screening program. JAMA 296:1593-1601

21. McKenna WJ, Thiene G, Nava A et al (1994) Diagnosis of arrhythmogenic right ventricular dysplasia/cardiomyopathy. Task Force of the Working Group Myocardial and Pericardial Disease of the European Society of Cardiology and of the Scientific Council on Cardiomyopathies of the International Society and Federation of Cardiology. Br Heart J 71:215-218

22. Garcia-Gras E, Lombardi R, Giocondo MJ et al (2006) Suppression of canonical Wnt/beta-catenin signaling by nuclear plakoglobin recapitulates phenotype of arrhythmogenic right ventricular cardiomyopathy. J Clin Invest 116:1825-1828

23. Yang Z, Bowles NE, Scherer SE et al (2006) Desmosomal dysfunction due to mutations in desmoplakin causes arrhythmogenic right ventricular dysplasia/cardiomyopathy. Circ Res 99:646-655

24. Kirchhof P, Fabritz L, Zwiener M et al (2006) Age and training dependent development of arrhythmogenic right ventricular cardiomyopathy in heterozygous plakoglobin deficient mice. Circulation 114:1799-1806

25. Marcus F, Towbin JA (2006) The mystery of arrhythmogenic right ventricular dysplasia/cardiomyopathy. From observation to mechanistic explanation. Circulation 114:1794-1795

26. Sermon K, Van Steirteghem A, Liebaers I (2004) Preimplantation genetic diagnosis. Lancet 363:1633-1641

27. Dalla Volta S, Battaglia G, Zerbini E (1961) "Auricularization" of right ventricular pressure curve. Am Heart J 61:25-33

28. Marcus FI, Fontaine GH, Guiraudon G et al (1982) Right ventricular dysplasia: A report of 24 adult cases. Circulation 65:384-398

29. Nava A, Thiene G, Canciani B et al (1988) Familial occurrence of right ventricular dysplasia: A study involving nine families. J Am Coll Cardiol 12:1222-1228

30. Thiene G, Nava A, Corrado D et al (1988) Right ventricular cardiomyopathy and sudden death in young people. N Engl J Med 318:129-133

CHAPTER 7

ADVANCES IN GENETICS: DOMINANT FORMS

Alessandra Rampazzo, Gian Antonio Danieli

Introduction

Arrhythmogenic right ventricular cardiomyopathy/ dysplasia (ARVC/D) is a progressive cardiomyopathy with different clinical-pathological patterns: (a) "silent" cardiomyopathic abnormalities localized in the right ventricle in asymptomatic victims of sudden death; (b) "overt" disease characterized by segmental or global right ventricular structural changes, often associated with histological evidence of left ventricular involvement and underlying symptomatic ventricular arrhythmias; and (c) "end-stage" biventricular cardiomyopathy mimicking dilated cardiomyopathy, leading to progressive heart failure and eventually requiring heart transplantation [1]. A scoring system to establish the diagnosis of ARVC/D has been developed on the basis of the presence of major and minor criteria encompassing structural, histological, electrocardiographic, arrhythmic, and genetic features of the disease [2].

The clinical manifestations of the disease mostly occur between the second and fourth decade of life; they include electrocardiographic depolarization/repolarization changes, arrhythmias of right ventricular origin, and structural and functional abnormalities of the right ventricle. In ARVC/D, the myocardium of right ventricular free wall is partially or almost entirely replaced by fibro-fatty tissue [3-5], and involves the epicardium, midmyocardium, and usually spares the subendocardium. The anterior right ventricular outflow tract, the apex, and the inferiorposterior wall are primarily involved [6]. Ventricular tachycardias are thought to be due to re-entrant mechanism, due to slow conduction within the myocardiocytes embedded in fibrous tissue and fat.

Familial occurrence of ARVC/D is rather common. Evidence has been found for autosomal dominant inheritance with variable penetrance in about 50% of cases [7].

ARVC/D has been reported in different human populations [8-10], although it is not known if the disease is equally prevalent in different geographical areas.

Ten years ago, we estimated that prevalence rate of ARVC/D in the Veneto region (northeast Italy) is about 6:10000 [11]. This figure is probably low, because many cases escape diagnosis. In Italy, 12.5%-25% of sudden deaths in athletes under the age of 35 are due to undiagnosed ARVC/D [12].

Two international registries have been established; one in North America and one in Europe, to determine the clinical, pathological, and genetic features of ARVC/D, to validate diagnostic criteria, and to define strategies for disease management and sudden death prevention [13-15].

Since identification of the first ARVC/D locus in 1994 by Rampazzo et al. [11], ten loci have been detected [11, 16-24], but only five disease genes have been identified [22-26] (Table 1.1).

Disease Genes

The first identified ARVC/D gene in a dominant form was ryanodine receptor-2, involved in ARVD2 [25]. In ARVD2, there is fibro-fatty substitution of the myocardial tissue, though much less pronounced than in the typical ARVC/D. The distinctive feature of this form is the presence of polymorphic, effort-induced arrhythmias. RYR2 is one of the largest human genes (105 exons), encoding a 565Kda protein located in the membrane of smooth sarcoplasmic reticulum. The homo-tetrameric structure known as cardiac ryanodine receptor plays a pivotal role in intracellular calcium homeostasis and excitation-contraction coupling in cardiomyocytes [27, 28]. All RYR2 mutations detected in ARVD2 patients were missense resulting in substitutions involving amino acids highly conserved through evolution in critical domains of the protein [25, 29].

Mutations in the human RYR2 gene have also been associated with catecholaminergic polymorphic ventricular tachycardia (CPVT; OMIM 604772) [30, 31] and familial polymorphic ventricular tachycardia (FPVT; OMIM 604772) [32, 33]. Putative pathogenic mutations in RYR2 have been reported in

Table 1.1 • Known ARVC/D loci and disease-genes.

Locus	Chromosome	Gene	Function	Mutations	References
ARVD1	14q24.3	TGFb3	Cytokine stimulating fibrosis and modulating cell adhesion	Regulatory mutations in 5' and 3' UTRs	11, 26
ARVD2	1q42-q43	RYR2	Calcium homeostasis	Missense mutations	16, 25
ARVD3	14q12-q22	unknown	–	–	17
ARVD4	2q32.1-q32.2	unknown	–	–	18
ARVD5	3p23	unknown	–	–	19
ARVD6	10p12-p14	unknown	–	–	20
ARVD7	10q22.3	unknown	–	–	21
ARVD8	6p24	DSP	Cell-cell adhesion	Missense, nonsense and splice site mutations	22
ARVD9	12p11.2	PKP2	Cell-cell adhesion	Missense, nonsense, insertion/deletion and splice site mutations	23
ARVD10	18q12.1	DSG2	Cell-cell adhesion	Missense, nonsense, insertion/deletion and splice site mutations	24

20 out 240 patients referred for long-QT syndrome genetic testing [34].

All RYR2 mutations described to date cluster in three specific domains: the N-terminal amino-acid residues 176-433, the centrally located residues 2246-2504, and the C-terminal residues 3778-4959. Detection of RYR2 mutations in both ARVD2 and CPVT patients raises the question of the possible existence of a single genetic defect, different phenotypes of which might be simply due to variable expression and incomplete penetrance. Both ARVD2 and CPVT-RyR2 missense mutations would alter the ability of the calcium channel to remain closed. Intense adrenergic stimulation due to emotional or physical stress can lead to calcium overload, thus triggering severe arrhythmias. The functional role of mutations R176Q, L433P, N2386I, and T2504M, previously detected in ARVD2 patients [25], was recently investigated [35]. RyR2 mutants N2386I and R176Q/T2504M exhibited enhanced sensitivity to caffeine activation and increased Ca^{2+} release, in agreement with the current hypothesis that defective RyR2 causes Ca^{2+} leak. In contrast, RyR2 L433P mutation showed reduced response to caffeine activation. This mutation might be interpreted as a "loss-of-function." Therefore, RyR2 mutations might be either "gain-of-function" or "loss-of-function," thus suggesting heterogeneity in functional consequences of RyR2 mutations. Even with this additional information, the question of whether ARVD2 and CPVT are different diseases due to different mutations of the RYR2 gene still remains unsettled.

The first disease gene linked to autosomal dominant ARVC/D showing typical right ventricular phenotype was Desmoplakin (DSP) [22]. In 2002, genome scan in a family with ARVC/D indicated a linkage with a region of chromosome 6 short arm including DSP gene. DNA sequencing of all DSP exons in the affected persons of this family revealed a missense mutation in exon 7 (C1176G; AGC→AGG) (Fig. 1.1). The involved amino acid (Ser299Arg) is at the center of a coiled, charged region, separating the two short helices of DSP subdomain Z. The amino acid substitution suppresses a putative phosphorylation site, which, on the other hand, is fully conserved in related proteins belonging to the same family. This mutation is thought to disrupt a protein kinase C phosphorylation site which is involved in plakoglobin binding and in clustering of desmosomal cadherin-plakoglobin complexes.

Desmoplakin, together with plakoglobin, anchors to desmosomal cadherins, forming an ordered array of nontransmembrane proteins, which bind to keratin intermediate filaments (Fig. 1.2) [36]. The primary structure of desmoplakin contains three functional domains: the N-terminal, which binds to the desmosome via connection with plakoglobin and plakophilin; the rod segment, which is predicted to form a dimeric coil; and the C-terminal domain, which binds intermediate filaments [37]. Alternative splicing of the protein produces two isoforms, desmoplakin I and desmoplakin II. The cDNAs encoding these two highly related proteins differ in a 1.8 Kbase sequence that is missing in DSPII, most likely due to differential splicing of a longer transcript [38].

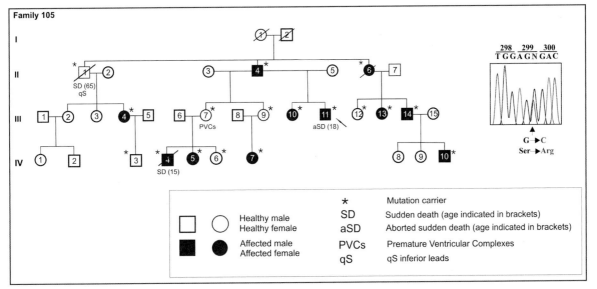

Fig. 1.1 • Family pedigree of the ARVC/D index case carrying the S299R DSP mutation and sequence electropherogram showing the heterozygous missense mutation

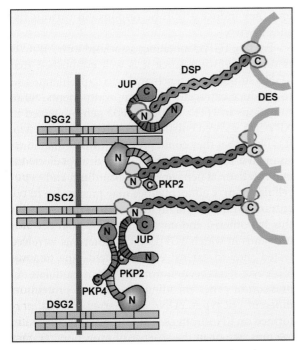

Fig. 1.2 • Schematic representation of relationships between desmosomal proteins in myocardiocytes. DSC2: desmocollin-2; DSG2: desmoglein-2; DSP: desmoplakin; PKP2: plakophilin-2; PKP4: plakophilin-4; JUP: plakoglobin; DES: desmin

Mutations in the desmoplakin gene have been shown to be responsible for some cases of an autosomal dominant skin disorder (striate palmoplantar keratoderma) without cardiac involvement [39-41]; a dominant form of ARVC/D without skin disease

[22]; an autosomal recessive condition characterized by dilated cardiomyopathy, woolly hair, and keratoderma (so-called Carvajal syndrome) [42], an autosomal recessive condition characterized by ARVC/D, woolly hair, and keratoderma [43] and a left-sided ARVC/D named arrhythmogenic left ventricular cardiomyopathy (ALVC) [44].

Mutations in DSP gene were detected in different families: they include twelve missense, two nonsense, and two splice-site mutations. In our experience, DSP mutations may account for a considerable number of ARVC/D cases.

In 2004, Gerull et al. [23] selected plakophilin-2 (PKP2) as candidate gene because a homozygous deletion caused a lethal cardiac defect in mice [45]. PKP2 gene encodes plakophilin-2, an essential protein of the cardiac desmosome. By sequencing all 14 exons of the PKP2 gene, including flanking intronic splice sequences, the authors identified 25 different heterozygous mutations (twelve insertion-deletion, six nonsense, four missense, and three splice site mutations) in 32 of 120 unrelated ARVC/D probands [23]. Plakophilin-2 is an armadillo-related protein, located in the outer dense plaque of desmosomes. It links desmosomal cadherins to desmoplakin and the intermediate filament system (Fig. 1.2). Plakophilins are also present in the nucleus, where they may play a role in transcriptional regulation [46]. Gerull et al. [23] speculated that lack of plakophilin-2 or incorporation of mutant plakophilin-2 in the cardiac desmosomes might impair cell-cell contacts and, as a consequence, might disrupt association between adjacent cardiomyocytes.

The frequency of PKP2 mutations among ARVC/D cases ranged from 11% to 43% in different studies [47-49]. These differences might be attributed to different geographical origin of cases or simply to selection bias.

Recently, we decided to shift from linkage studies in ARVC/D families to a candidate gene approach. Thus, we screened different genes encoding desmosomal proteins. When analyzing DSG2 gene (Desmoglein-2, the only isoform expressed in cardiac myocytes), we detected nine heterozygous mutations in eight of 50 unrelated individuals with ARVC/D which proved negative for mutations of DSP, PKP2, and TGFβ3 genes [24]. Among these, five were missense mutations, two were insertion-deletions, one was a nonsense and one was a splice site mutation; one patient had two different DSG2 mutations (compound heterozygote). Endomyocardial biopsy, obtained from five patients, showed extensive loss of myocytes with fibro-fatty tissue replacement. In three patients, electron microscopy showed intercalated disc paleness, decreased desmosome number, and intercellular gap widening [24]. Mutations in DSG2 gene were also detected in an independent study [50]. It is interesting to note that, in this study, there was one patient with compound-heterozygous mutations in DSG2 (Fig. 1.3).

In 2005, our group identified the gene involved in ARVD1 [26]. The large critical interval for ARVD1 included 40 known genes; five of them (POMT2, KIAA0759, KIAA1036, C14orf4, and TAIL1) were unsuccessfully screened for pathogenic ARVC/D mutations [51, 52]. Among genes mapped to the ARVD1 critical region and expressed in myocardium, transforming growth factor-beta3 (TGFβ3) appeared to be

a good candidate, since it encodes a cytokine stimulating fibrosis and modulating cell adhesion. After previous analyses failed to detect any mutation in the coding region of this gene, mutation screening was extended to the promoter and untranslated regions (UTRs). A nucleotide substitution (c.-36G>A) in 5′UTR of TGFβ3 gene was detected in all affected subjects belonging to a large ARVD1 family. After the investigation was extended to 30 unrelated ARVC/D index patients, an additional mutation (c.1723C>T) was identified in the 3′ UTR of one proband. In vitro expression assays of constructs containing the mutations showed that mutated UTRs were twofold more active than wild type [26].

TGFβ3 is a member of the transforming growth factor superfamily, which includes a diverse range of proteins regulating many different physiological processes. TGFβ1, -β2, and -β3 are the prototype of the TGFβ superfamily. They inhibit proliferation in most types of cells and induce apoptosis of epithelial cells. Conversely, they stimulate mesenchymal cells to proliferate and produce extracellular matrix and they induce a fibrotic response in various tissues in vivo.

Finding TGFβ3 mutations associated with ARVC/D is very interesting, since it is well established that TGFβs stimulate mesenchymal cells to proliferate and to produce extracellular matrix components. Since mutations in UTRs of the TGFβ3 gene, detected in ARVC/D, showed enhanced gene expression in vitro, it is likely that they could promote myocardial fibrosis in vivo. Myocardial fibrosis may disrupt electrical and mechanical behavior of myocardium and extracellular matrix abnormalities may predispose to reentrant ventricular arrhythmias. In agreement with this hypothesis, endomyocardial biopsy in the two probands in which TGFβ3 UTR mutations were detected showed extensive replacement-type fibrosis. Moreover, it has been shown that TGFβs modulate expression of genes encoding desmosomal proteins in different cell types. cDNA microarray analysis, performed on RNA from cardiac fibroblasts incubated in the presence or in the absence of exogenous TGFβs, revealed increased expression of different genes, including plakoglobin [53]. Yoshida et al. [54] reported that TGFβ1 exposure of cultured airway epithelial cells increases the content of desmoplakins I and II. This suggests that regulation of cell-cell junctional complexes may be an important effect of TGFβs. Therefore, overexpression of TGFβ3, caused by UTRs mutations, might affect cell-to-cell junction stability, thus leading to disease expression similar to that observed in ARVC/D due to mutations of genes encoding desmosomal proteins.

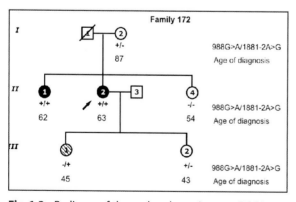

Fig. 1.3 • Pedigree of the proband carrying two DSG2 mutations (988G>A, 1881-2A>G). Hatched symbol represents an individual of unknown disease status. Presence (+) or absence (-) of the DSG2 mutation is indicated

Desmosomes are important cell-cell adhesion junctions, predominantly found in the epidermis and heart. They couple cytoskeletal elements to plasma membrane at cell-cell or cell-substrate adhesions. Whereas adherens junctions are linked with microfilaments at cell-cell interfaces, desmosomes anchor stress-bearing intermediate filaments at sites of strong intercellular adhesion. The resulting scaffold plays a key role in providing mechanical integrity to tissues such as epidermis and heart, which experience mechanical stress. Desmosomes include proteins from at least three distinct gene families: cadherins, armadillo proteins, and plakins (Fig. 1.2). Desmosomal cadherins include desmogleins and desmocollins; members of both subfamilies are single-pass transmembrane glycoproteins, mediating Ca2+-dependent cell-cell adhesion. Armadillo proteins include plakoglobin and plakophilins (PKP1-3). The plakin family proteins include desmoplakin, plectin, and the cell envelope proteins envoplakin and periplakin. Desmoplakin (involved in ARVD8), plakophilin-2 (involved in ARVD9), desmoglein-2 (involved in ARVD10), and plakoglobin (involved in Naxos syndrome, the autosomal recessive form of ARVC/D) are desmosomal proteins. Based on present evidence we may conclude that different defects in proteins of desmosomal complex lead to ARVC/D. Therefore, additional components of the desmosomal complex may be targets for pathogenic mutations leading to ARVC/D.

Molecular Pathogenesis

The reported involvement of different desmosomal proteins in ARVC/D and the discovery that some RYR2 mutations may produce ARVD2 leads us to propose a comprehensive hypothesis on the molecular pathogenesis of ARVC/D [22]. According to this hypothesis, the predililation of involvement of the right ventricle in ARVC/D might be due to greater dilatation and thinning of its wall, in comparison with the left ventricular free wall. Possibly, defective proteins in cardiac desmosomes might impair cell-to-cell contacts and, hence, might affect the response of ventricular myocardium to mechanical stretch. This alteration would occur preferably in myocardial areas subjected to high strain, like the right ventricular outflow tract, the apex, and subtricuspid areas.

According to present knowledge, mechanical forces applied to adherens junctions activate stretch-sensitive calcium channels via cadherins' mechanical intracellular signaling [55]. Data on stretch-activated channels in ventricular cardiomyocytes point to the relevance of these channels in transduction of mechanical forces into a cellular electrochemical signal, via increase of intracellular calcium concentration [56-58].

Volume overload of the right ventricle in a patient with genetically defective intercellular junctions (as in case of mutant plakoglobin, desmoplakin, plakophilin, desmoglein, or TGFβ3) would produce unusual stretching resulting in excessive calcium load. Stretching of cardiomyocytes is known to modulate the elementary calcium release process from ryanodine receptor release channels [59]. Therefore, a genetically impaired response to mechanical stress might adversely affect intracellular calcium concentration and excitation-contraction coupling, thus producing arrhythmias. On the other hand, volume overload of the right ventricle in carriers of RYR2 mutations would cause calcium overload, because of defective Ca++ homeostasis. The existence of a dominant form of ARVC/D due to RyR2 mutations supports the hypothesis of a key pathogenic role of intracellular calcium overload in the molecular pathogenesis of the disease.

Mutation Screening

We performed mutation screening in 90 unrelated probands fulfilling the International ARVC/D Task Force criteria; the screening by DHPLC and subsequent DNA sequencing involved coding sequences of known ARVC/D genes. Plakophilin-2 was involved in 21% of cases, desmoplakin-2 in 20%, desmoglein-2 in 11%, and TGFβ3 in 2% (unpublished results). In 46% of cases no mutation was detected. This is not surprising, since in 50% of reported ARVC/D loci (ARVD3, ARVD4, ARVD5, ARVD6, ARVD7) the involved gene has not been identified.

In our series of patients screened for mutations, eight compound heterozygotes were detected, suggesting that this condition may be more frequent than expected among ARVC/D patients. It is difficult to establish whether all of these cases are compound heterozygotes for pathogenic mutations, since it is almost impossible to discriminate between a rare variant with pathogenic effect and a rare DNA polymorphism.

Present knowledge on the molecular genetics of the dominant forms of ARVC/D may permit detection of asymptomatic carriers in families with ARVC/D. However, it must be noted that genotype-phenotype correlations may be established only for clearly pathogenic mutations (i.e., nonsense, frameshifts, splice-site mutations with evidence of modified RNA length, etc.) and once all genes reportedly involved in ARVC/D would have been screened.

Mutation screening is time- and effort-consuming. Routine methods (direct sequencing of coding segments or DHPLC followed by DNA sequencing) reach about 98% detection rate due to undetectable mutations in intronic sequences or in regulatory elements, or unexpected large deletions. Moreover, the presence of compound heterozygotes carrying one mutation in a known ARVD gene and one mutation in a gene still unknown might produce misleading results. Therefore, genetic assessment of asymptomatic relatives of ARVC/D patients still poses several technical, clinical, and ethical problems. However, identification of additional genes involved in dominant forms of ARVC/D and collection of data regarding pathogenic mutations in known genes will provide information to establish safe protocols for genetic investigation in families with ARVC/D, genetic counseling, and risk assessment.

Acknowledgements

The financial support of European Commission (Project QLG1-CT-2000-01091, UE) and of NIH, USA (Grant U04HL65652) is gratefully acknowledged.

P.S. Following submission of this manuscript, mutations in desmocollin-2 gene, encoding a desmosomal cadherin, have been reported to be associated with ARVC/D [60-62].

References

1. Corrado D, Basso C, Thiene G et al (1997) Spectrum of clinicopathologic manifestations of arrhythmogenic right ventricular cardiomyopathy/dysplasia: a multicenter study. J Am Coll Cardiol 30:1512-1520
2. McKenna WJ, Thiene G, Nava A et al (1994) Diagnosis of arrhythmogenic right ventricular dysplasia/cardiomyopathy. Task Force of the Working Group Myocardial and Pericardial Disease of the European Society of Cardiology and of the Scientific Council on Cardiomyopathies of the International Society and Federation of Cardiology. Br Heart J 71:215-218
3. Thiene G, Nava A, Corrado D et al (1988) Right ventricular cardiomyopathy and sudden death in young people. N Engl J Med 318:129-133
4. Basso C, Thiene G, Corrado D et al (1996) Arrhythmogenic right ventricular cardiomyopathy. Displasia, dystrophy or myocarditis? Circulation 94:983-991
5. Nava A, Rossi L, Thiene G (eds) (1997) Arrhythmogenic right ventricular cardiomyopathy/dysplasia. Elsevier, Amsterdam
6. Marcus FI, Fontaine G, Guiraudon G et al (1982) Right ventricular dysplasia. A report of 24 adult cases. Circulation 65:384-398
7. Nava A, Scognamiglio R, Thiene G et al (1988) Familial occurrence of right ventricular displasia: A study involving nine families. J Am Coll Cardiol 12:1222-1228
8. Perzanowski C, Crespo G, Yazdanfar S (2000) Images in cardiology: Familial ventricular tachycardia with mild ventricular dysfunction: A 15-year follow up of two African American brothers with arrhythmogenic right ventricular dysplasia. Heart 84:658
9. Fung WH, Sanderson JE (2001) Clinical profile of arrhythmogenic right ventricular cardiomyopathy in Chinese patients. Int J Cardiol 81:9-18
10. Obata H, Mitsuoka T, Kikuchi Y et al (2001) Twenty-seven-year follow-up of arrhythmogenic right ventricular dysplasia. Pacing Clin Electrophysiol 24:510-511
11. Rampazzo A, Nava A, Danieli GA et al (1994) The gene for arrhythmogenic right ventricular cardiomyopathy maps to chromosome 14q23-q24. Hum Mol Genet 3:959-962
12. Corrado D, Basso C, Schiavon M et al (1998) Screening for hypertrophic cardiomyopathy in young athletes. N Engl J Med 339:364-369
13. Corrado D, Fontaine G, Marcus FI et al (2000) Arrhythmogenic right ventricular dysplasia/cardiomyopathy: Need for an international registry. European Society of Cardiology and the Scientific Council on Cardiomyopathies of the World Heart Federation. J Cardiovasc Electrophysiol 11:827-832
14. Marcus F, Towbin JA, Zareba W et al (2003) Arrhythmogenic right ventricular dysplasia/cardiomyopathy (ARVD/C): A multidisciplinary study: Design and protocol. Circulation 107:2975-2978
15. Basso C, Wichter T, Danieli GA et al (2004) Arrhythmogenic right ventricular cardiomyopathy: Clinical registry and database, evaluation of therapies, pathology registry, DNA banking. Eur Heart J 25:531-534
16. Rampazzo A, Nava A, Erne P et al (1995) A new locus for arrhythmogenic right ventricular cardiomyopathy (ARVD2) maps to chromosome 1q42-q43. Hum Mol Genet 4:2151-2154
17. Severini GM, Krajinovic M, Pinamonti B et al (1996) A new locus for arrhythmogenic right ventricular dysplasia on the long arm of chromosome 14. Genomics 31:193-200
18. Rampazzo A, Nava A, Miorin M et al (1997) ARVD4, a new locus for arrhythmogenic right ventricular cardiomyopathy, maps to chromosome 2 long arm. Genomics 45:259-263
19. Ahmad F, Li D, Karibe A et al (1998) Localization of a gene responsible for arrhythmogenic right ventricular dysplasia to chromosome 3p23. Circulation 98:2791-2795

20. Li D, Ahmad F, Gardner MJ et al (2000) The locus of a novel gene responsible for arrhythmogenic right-ventricular dysplasia characterized by early onset and high penetrance maps to chromosome 10p12-p14. Am J Hum Genet 66:148-156

21. Melberg A, Oldfors A, Blomstrom-Lundqvist C et al (1999) Autosomal dominant myofibrillar myopathy with arrhythmogenic right ventricular cardiomyopathy linked to chromosome 10q. Ann Neurol 46:684-692

22. Rampazzo A, Nava A, Malacrida S et al (2002) Mutation in human desmoplakin domain binding to plakoglobin causes a dominant form of arrhythmogenic right ventricular cardiomyopathy. Am J Hum Genet 71:1200-1206

23. Gerull B, Heuser A, Wichter T et al (2004) Mutations in the desmosomal protein plakophilin-2 are common in arrhythmogenic right ventricular cardiomyopathy. Nat Genet 36:1162-1164

24. Pilichou K, Nava A, Basso C et al (2006) Mutations in desmoglein-2 gene are associated to arrhythmogenic right ventricular. Circulation 113:1171-1179

25. Tiso N, Stephan DA, Nava A et al (2001) Identification of mutations in the cardiac ryanodine receptor gene in families affected with arrhythmogenic right ventricular cardiomyopathy type 2 (ARVD2). Hum Mol Genet 10:189-194

26. Beffagna G, Occhi G, Nava A et al (2005) Regulatory mutations in transforming growth factor-beta3 gene cause arrhythmogenic right ventricular cardiomyopathy type 1. Cardiovasc Res 65:366-373

27. Stokes DL, Wagenknecht T (2000) Calcium transport across the sarcoplasmic reticulum: Structure and function of Ca2+-ATPase and the ryanodine receptor. Eur J Biochem 267:5274-5279

28. Missiaen L, Robberecht W, van den Bosch L et al (2000) Abnormal intracellular ca(2+) homeostasis and disease. Cell Calcium 28:1-21

29. Bagattin A, Veronese C, Bauce B et al (2004) Denaturing HPLC-based approach for detecting RYR2 mutations involved in malignant arrhythmias. Clin Chem 50:1148-1155

30. Priori SG, Napolitano C, Tiso N et al (2001) Mutations in the cardiac ryanodine receptor gene (hRyR2) underlie catecholaminergic polymorphic ventricular tachycardia. Circulation 103:196-200

31. Priori SG, Napolitano C, Memmi M et al (2002) Clinical and molecular characterization of patients with catecholaminergic polymorphic ventricular tachycardia. Circulation 106:69-74

32. Laitinen PJ, Brown KM, Piippo K et al (2001) Mutations of the cardiac ryanodine receptor (RyR2) gene in familial polymorphic ventricular tachycardia. Circulation 103:485-490

33. Laitinen PJ, Swan H, Kontula K (2003) Molecular genetics of exercise-induced polymorphic ventricular tachycardia: Identification of three novel cardiac ryanodine receptor mutations and two common calsequestrin 2 amino-acid polymorphisms. Eur J Hum Genet 11:888-891

34. Kopplin LJ, Tester DJ, Ackerman MJ (2004) Prevalence and spectrum of mutations in the cardiac ryanodine receptor in patients referred for long QT syndrome genetic testing. J Am Coll Cardiol 43:136A

35. Thomas NL, George CH, Lai FA (2004) Functional heterogeneity of ryanodine receptor mutations associated with sudden cardiac death. Cardiovasc Res 64:52-60

36. Leung CL, Green KJ, Liem RK (2002) Plakins: A family of versatile cytolinker proteins. Trends Cell Biol 12:37-45

37. Choi HJ, Park-Snyder S, Pascoe LT et al (2002) Structures of two intermediate filament-binding fragments of desmoplakin reveal a unique repeat motif structure. Nat Struct Biol 9:612-620

38. Virata ML, Wagner RM, Parry DA et al (1992) Molecular structure of the human desmoplakin I and II amino terminus. Proc Natl Acad Sci USA 89:544-548

39. Armstrong DK, McKenna KE, Purkis PE et al (1999) Aploinsufficiency of desmoplakin causes a striate subtype of palmoplantar keratoderma. Hum Mol Genet 8:143-148

40. Whittock NV, Ashton GH, Dopping-Hepenstal PJ et al (1999) Striate palmoplantar keratoderma resulting from desmoplakin haploinsufficiency. J Invest Dermatol 113:940-946

41. Whittock NV, Wan H, Morley SM et al (2002) Compound heterozygosity for non-sense and missense mutations in desmoplakin underlies skin fragility/woolly hair syndrome. J Invest Dermatol 118:232-238

42. Norgett EE, Hatsell SJ, Carvajal-Huerta L et al (2000) Recessive mutation in desmoplakin disrupts desmoplakin-intermediate filament interactions and causes dilated cardiomyopathy, woolly hair and keratoderma. Hum Mol Genet 9:2761-2766

43. Alcalai R, Metzger S, Rosenheck S et al (2003) A recessive mutation in desmoplakin causes arrhythmogenic right ventricular dysplasia, skin disorder, and woolly hair. J Am Coll Cardiol 42:319-327

44. Norman M, Simpson M, Mogensen J et al (2005) Novel mutation in desmoplakin causes arrhythmogenic left ventricular cardiomyopathy. Circulation 112:636-642

45. Grossmann KS, Grund C, Huelsken J et al (2004) Requirement of plakophilin 2 for heart morphogenesis and cardiac junction formation. J Cell Biol 167:149-160

46. Mertens C, Hofmann I, Wang Z et al (2001) Nuclear particles containing RNA polymerase III complexes associated with the junctional plaque protein plakophilin-2. Proc Natl Acad Sci USA 98:7795-7800

47. Syrris P, Ward D, Asimaki A et al (2006) Clinical expression of plakophilin-2 mutations in familial arrhythmogenic right ventricular cardiomyopathy. Circulation 113:356-364

48. Van Tintelen JP, Entius MM, Bhuiyan ZA et al (2006) Plakophilin-2 mutations are the major determinant of familial arrhythmogenic right ventricular dysplasia/cardiomyopathy. Circulation 113:1650-1658

49. Dalal D, Molin LH, Piccini J et al (2006) Clinical features of arrhythmogenic right ventricular dysplasia/cardiomyopathy associated with mutations in plakophilin-2. Circulation 113:1641-1649

50. Awad MM, Dalal D, Cho E et al (2006) DSG2 Mutations contribute to arrhythmogenic right ventricular dysplasia/cardiomyopathy. Am J Hum Genet 79:136-142

51. Rampazzo A, Beffagna G, Nava A et al (2003) Arrhythmogenic right ventricular cardiomyophaty type 1 (ARVD1): Confirmation of locus assignment and mutation screening of four candidate genes. Eur J Hum Gen 11:69-76

52. Rossi V, Beffagna G, Rampazzo A et al (2004) TAIL1: An isthmin-like gene, containing type 1 thrombospondin-repeat and AMOP domain, mapped to ARVD1 critical region. Gene 335:101-108

53. Kapoun AM, Liang F, O'Young G et al (2004) B-type natriuretic peptide exerts broad functional opposition to transforming growth factor-beta in primary human cardiac fibroblasts: Fibrosis, myofibroblast conversion, proliferation, and inflammation. Circ Res 94:453-61

54. Yoshida M, Romberger DJ, Illig MG et al (1992) Transforming growth factor-beta stimulates the expression of desmosomal proteins in bronchial epithelial cells. Am J Respir Cell Mol Biol 6:439-445

55. Ko K, Arora P, Lee W et al (2000) Biochemical and functional characterization of intercellular adhesion and gap junctions in fibroblasts. Am J Physiol Cell Physiol 279:C147-157

56. Gannier D, White E, Garnier F et al (1996) A possible mechanism for large stretch-induced increase in [Ca2+]i in isolated guinea-pig ventricular myocytes. Cardiovasc Res 32:158-167

57. Tatsukawa Y, Kiyosue T, Arita M (1997) Mechanical stretch increases intracellular calcium concentration in cultured ventricular cells from neonatal rats. Heart Vessels 12:128-135

58. Knoll R, Hoshijima M, Chien K (2003) Cardiac mechanotransduction and implications for heart disease. J Mol Med 81:750-756

59. Petroff MG, Kim SH, Pepe S et al (2001) Endogenous nitric oxide mechanisms mediate the stretch dependence of Ca2+ release in cardiomyocytes. Nat Cell Biol 3:867-873

60. Beffagna G, De Bortoli M, Nava A et al (2006) Mutations in desmocollin2 gene associated with arrhythmogenic right ventricular cardiomyopathy. Circulation 114:II-723-724

61. Syrris P, Ward D, Evans A et al (2006) Arrhythmogenic right ventricular dysplasia/cardiomyopathy associated with mutations in the desmosomal gene desmocollin-2. Am J Hum Genet 79:978-984

62. Henser A, Plovie E, Ellinor PT et al (2006) Mutant desmocollin-2 causes arrhythmogenic right ventricular cardiomyopathy. Am J Hum Genet 79:1081-1088

CHAPTER 2

ADVANCES IN GENETICS: RECESSIVE FORMS

Nikos Protonotarios, Adalena Tsatsopoulou

Introduction

Arrhythmogenic right ventricular cardiomyopathy/dysplasia (ARVC/D) is a genetically determined heart muscle disorder that presents clinically with ventricular arrhythmias, heart failure, and sudden death [1, 2]. The pathological process consists of progressive loss of ventricular myocardium with fibro-fatty replacement [2]. The right ventricle is mostly involved [1] but presentation of disease with predominantly left ventricular involvement has been recently reported [3].

ARVC/D usually has autosomal dominant inheritance [4]. Early gene identification efforts were hampered by low penetrance, age-related expression, and difficulty in making an accurate diagnosis [5]. The identification of ARVC/D in Greek families with an associated hair and skin phenotype facilitated recognition of the first disease-causing recessive gene, a deletion mutation in plakoglobin [6] and the subsequent finding of a C-terminal mutation in desmoplakin in Ecuadorian families [7]. The finding of disease-causing mutations in the desmosomal proteins plakoglobin and desmoplakin suggested that ARVC/D is a disease of cell adhesion and provided candidate genes for studies of autosomal dominant families.

Naxos Disease

History

In 1986, an autosomal recessive cardiocutaneous syndrome of ARVC/D associated with woolly hair and palmoplantar keratoderma was first described in families from the Greek island of Naxos [8], from which the sydrome took the name of [9]. The autosomal recessive ARVC/D in Naxos disease is similar to autosomal dominant ARVC/D with respect to age and mode of clinical presentation, distribution of right ventricular and left ventricular involvement, electrocardiographic features, natural history, and histopathology [10-12].

Following the initial presentation, families with Naxos disease phenotype were reported from other areas of the world [13-19]. In some of these families, the cardiomyopathy presented with predominantly left ventricular involvement and early morbidity overlapping clinically with dilated cardiomyopathy [13, 14]. This subtype of Naxos disease [20] was initially considered as a separate entity (Carvajal syndrome) [21].

Clinical Presentation

Woolly hair was a common finding in all affected members and it appeared at birth. Diffuse keratoderma developed later in infancy or early childhood over the pressure areas of palms and soles (Fig. 2.1). Keratoderma was characterized histologically as nonepidermolytic [22] or epidermolytic [7]. Pemphigous like vesicular lesions on palms, soles, and knees developed in some patients [16].

The cardiomyopathy usually presented with ventricular arrhythmias, electrocardiographic abnormalities, and structural alterations fulfilling the diagnostic criteria for ARVC/D [23]. The symptomatic presentation was usually with syncope and/or sustained ventricular tachycardia during adolescence and young adulthood [24]. Sudden death was the first disease manifestation in some cases. Heart disease progressed from the right to both ventricles. Left ventricular involvement ranging from regional hypokinesia, particularly of the posterior wall or apex, to global dilatation and diffuse hypokinesia was mostly related to the age of patients and to the rapidity of disease progression. Congestive heart failure developed in one fourth of patients as an end-stage feature of severe right or biventricular involvement [25]. In the Carvajal variant of Naxos disease, left ventricular involvement appeared during childhood, suggesting a rapid disease evolution.

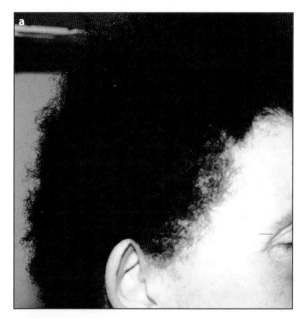

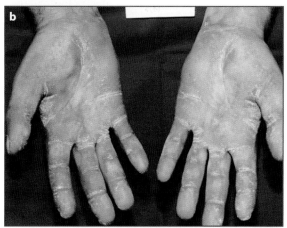

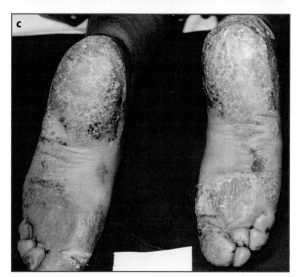

Fig. 2.1 • Cutaneous phenotype in a homozygous carrier of plakoglobin mutation. Woolly hair (**a**), striate keratoderma in the palm (**b**), diffuse keratoderma in the plantar areas (**c**)

Pathology

Cardiac pathology in patients with Naxos disease revealed typical features of ARVC/D (Fig. 2.2). The right ventricle showed extensive myocardial loss with fibrofatty replacement at subepicardial and mediomur-

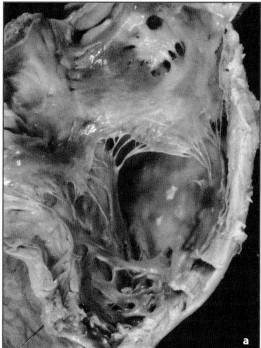

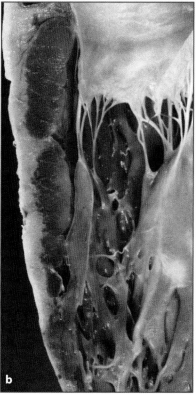

Fig. 2.2 • Gross pathology of the heart in a 33-year-old homozygous carrier of plakoglobin mutation who died in severe heart failure while waiting for heart transplantation. (**a**) The right ventricular outflow tract seen from inside. Transmural myocardial loss with fatty replacement. (**b**) Posteroapical wall of the left ventricle. Myocardial loss with fatty replacement in subepicardial layers

al layers being regionally transmural with aneurysms [26]. Strands of surviving myocytes surrounded by fibrous tissue were embedded within adipocytes. Lymphocyte infiltrates were observed particularly when the biopsy was performed at the time of clinical progression. In patients with severe biventricular involvement, the left ventricle showed extensive myocardial loss with fibrofatty replacement mainly at subepicardial layers of the postero-apical wall.

Postmortem evaluation of the heart of an adolescent with Carvajal syndrome showed biventricular involvement [21]. The right ventricle was modestly dilated with aneurysms in the outflow tract, apex, and posterior wall, known as the "triangle of dysplasia". The left ventricle was markedly dilated with aneurysms on the posterior and anteroseptal wall. Microscopic examination showed areas of extensive myocardial loss and replacement fibrosis particularly in subepicardial layers, which is identical to the pathology in ARVC/D although without the fatty component.

Molecular Genetics

The Way to Molecular Basis

The coexistence of cardiac and cutaneous abnormalities in Naxos disease suggested a common pathogenetic defect in two embryonically unrelated tissues [8]. The skin of the palms and soles as well as heart muscle are almost constantly subjected to mechanical stress or stretch demanding proper function of intercellular junctions. The identification of a mutation in the gene encoding plakoglobin, a key cell adhesion protein with a wide distribution among tissues including skin and myocardium, highlighted the pathogenesis of ARVC/D in Naxos disease [6]. Plakoglobin mutation led to consideration of ARVC/D as a disease potentially related to a cellular-adhesion defect. This finding stimulated research to find other genes encoding related proteins [27]. Since then, mutations in other desmosomal proteins including desmoplakin, plakophilin-2, and desmoglein-2 have been recognized as causative genes in families with dominant ARVC/D [28-32].

Cell-Cell Junctions

Myocardial cells are differentiated bipolar cells coupled at intercalated discs where adherence junctions, desmosomes, and gap junctions are located [33]. Adherence junctions and desmosomes provide mechanical coupling, while gap junctions serve as electrical coupling. In desmosomes, plakoglobin, plakophilin-2, and desmoplakin anchor desmin intermediate filaments to transmembrane desmosomal cadherins (desmoglein and desmocollin). Plakoglobin and plakophilin-2 are armadillo proteins located at the outer dense plaque of desmosomes and binding with the N-terminal of desmoplakin and with the C-terminal of desmosomal cadherins. Desmoplakin is a larger dumbbell-shaped molecule which makes up the inner dense plaque with its middle coiled rod domain and binds via its C-terminal with desmin intermediate filaments [34]. Plakoglobin is the only desmosomal protein also found at adherens junctions, where it is involved in linking with the actin cytoskeleton of adjacent myocardial cells [35]. Signaling to the nucleus and involvement in apoptotic mechanisms have also been attributed to plakoglobin [36]. The integrity of desmosomes is important in maintaining the normal function of gap-junction channels responsible for electrical coupling [37].

Recessive Mutations

To date, one plakoglobin mutation and three desmoplakin mutations have been implicated in recessive ARVC/D (Table 2.1).

A 2-base pair deletion mutation in plakoglobin (*2157del2TG*) was identified in 13 Greek families and one Turkish family with Naxos disease. This deletion causes a frameshift and premature termination of translation resulting in a truncated protein at the C-terminal domain [6].

A deletion mutation in desmoplakin (*7901del1G*) was identified in 3 Ecuadorian families with Carvajal syndrome [7]. This deletion causes a premature stop codon leading to a truncated desmoplakin missing the last domain of the C-terminal.

A missense mutation in desmoplakin (*G2375R*) was identified in one Arab family from Jerusalem [16]. This mutation leads to Gly2375Arg substitution in the C-terminal of the protein.

A nonsense mutation in desmoplakin (*C3799T*) in association with a polymorphism in plakoglobin (*T2089A*) was found to cause a severe form of cardiocutaneous syndrome in a Turkish family [19]. This mutation leads to loss of most of the desmoplakin isoform 1 particularly affecting the C-terminal area.

Genetic investigation in two Arab families from Israel and one family from Saudi Arabia with cardiocutaneous syndrome excluded mutations in the already-described desmosomal protein genes [15, 18].

Table 2.1 • Genotype-phenotype features in recessive ARVC/D

Mutation	PG_2157del2(TG)	DP_7901del1(G)	DP_G2375R	DP_C3799T, PG_T2089A
Country of origin (No. of families)	Greece (13), Turkey (1)	Ecuador (3)	Israel (1)	Turkey (1)
Cutaneous phenotype				
Hair abnormalities	WH	WH	WH	WH
Skin disorder	PPK	PPK	Pemphigous-like	PPK
Cardiomyopathy				
Age at earliest diagnosis (years)	13	8	16	3
Structural characteristics	Predominantly RV involvement	Predominantly LV involvement	RV involvement	Severe RV and LV involvement
Major arrhythmia	SVT	NSVT	SVT	NSVT
Major clinical events	SYNC, HF, SD	HF, SD	SD	HF

HF, heart failure; LV, left ventricular; NSVT, non-sustained ventricular tachycardia; PPK, palmoplantar keratoderma; RV, ventricular; SD, sudden death; SVT, sustained ventricular tachycardia; SYNC, syncope; WH, woolly hair.

Genotype-Phenotype

Plakoglobin Mutation

Recessive ARVC/D due to plakoglobin mutation is 100% penetrant by adolescence [23]. All homozygotes have hair and skin phenotype from infancy (Table 2.1). The right ventricle is always involved, initially with localized kinetic abnormalities at the triangle of dysplasia: the outflow tract, posterior wall, and apex. With disease progression, the right ventricle becomes dilated and hypokinetic. The left ventricle is involved later; 10% of patients have left ventricular involvement by the second decade of life, while 60% of those who survive to the fifth decade of life develop left ventricular involvement. Clinical events are usually related to episodes of sustained ventricular tachycardia of left bundle branch block morphology. Arrhythmic storms are accompanied by step-wise structural progression [24]. The involved myocardium reveals myocyte loss with fibrofatty replacement mainly at subepicardial and mediomural layers occasionally associated with inflammatory infiltrates [26]. On immunohistology the signal for plakoglobin and connexin 43 (the main gap junctional protein in ventricular myocardium) is diminished at intercellular junctions [37].

Desmoplakin Mutations

Dominant desmoplakin mutations that cause non-syndromic ARVC/D truncate either the N- or the C-terminal of the protein and result in distinctive cardiac phenotypes [28]. When the N-terminal is affected, particularly the plakoglobin binding site of desmoplakin in the outer dense plaque, the phenotype is typical for ARVC/D with respect to electrocardiographic and structural abnormalities [29]. Truncation of the molecule in the inner dense plaque results in a broader cardiac phenotype, occasionally with predominantly left ventricular involvement [3].

The identified desmoplakin mutations that cause recessive ARVC/D affect the C-terminal of the protein at the inner dense plaque of desmosomes and result in skin and hair phenotype similar to that of plakoglobin mutation and a broadened cardiac phenotype (Table 2.1) [3, 7, 16, 19]. Left ventricular involvement predominates when the mutation is predicted to disrupt the desmin-binding site at the C-terminal of desmoplakin [7, 19]. More than 90% of those affected showed left ventricular involvement by childhood or adolescence and early development of heart failure [19, 38].

Histopathologic features of a heart homozygote for *7901del1G* desmoplakin mutation were similar to those of the plakoglobin mutation, although the fatty component of the usual right ventricular replacement process was absent [21]. The immunohistochemical signal for plakoglobin, desmoplakin, and desmin at the level of intercalated disks was diminished [21].

Pathogenesis of ARVC/D

Genotype-phenotype studies in recessive ARVC/D provided insights into mechanisms of myocyte cell death and arrhythmogenesis. The observation that physical stress causes palmoplantar keratoderma provided a working hypothesis for myocyte cell death in ARVC/D. The observation that the thinnest areas of myocardium such as right ventricular free wall and left ventricular posterior wall are most often involved was considered due to these areas being more vulnerable to physical stress or stretch. The relation of a particular mutation to the clinical phenotype is of interest. The left ventricle is predominantly involved in desmoplakin mutations disrupting the cytoskeletal integrity, as are those affecting the desmin binding site at the inner dense plaque [3, 7, 19]. The mutated desmin-binding site of desmoplakin possibly affects the architecture of intermediate filaments, resulting in a DCM-like cardiac phenotype [26]. Plakoglobin mutation functioning at the outer dense plaque of desmosomes is expressed with a predominantly right ventricular phenotype that it is also observed in dominant ARVC/D caused by mutations in the N-terminal of desmoplakin, plakophilin-2, and desmoglein-2 [28-32]. Anecdotal reports suggest that fibrous rather than fatty repair occurs with rapidly progressive disease without being mutation specific [26, 29].

It has been considered that the surviving myocardial fibers, embedded within fibrous and adipose tissue, alter electrical properties and provide the substrate for slow conduction and re-entrant ventricular arrhythmias [1]. However, gap junction remodeling may be considered as an alternative pathway to intraventricular slow conduction enhancing the risk of ventricular arrhythmias [37, 39].

Conclusions

Recessive ARVC/D always presents in association with hair and skin phenotype. Woolly hair is apparent from birth and palmoplantar keratoderma or similar skin defects develop during infancy or early childhood. Mutations in genes encoding the desmosomal proteins plakoglobin and desmoplakin were identified to underlie this cardiocutaneous syndrome. The heterogeneity of cardiac phenotype may be attributed to the location of the causative mutation in the desmosomal plaque. In the plakoglobin mutation, functioning at the outer dense plaque of the desmosomes, the cardiac phenotype is that of the ordinary ARVC/D with predominantly right ventricular involvement (Naxos disease). Mutations that truncate the intermediate filament-

binding site of desmoplakin result in a cardiac phenotype with predominantly left ventricular involvement overlapping clinically with DCM (Carvajal syndrome). Thus, the phenotypic spectrum of this cell-adhesion cardiomyopathy is broader than our previous clinical view of ARVC/D as a disease of the right ventricle.

Acknowledgements

The work was supported by European Comunity research contract #QLG1-CT-2000-01091.

References

1. Marcus FI, Fontaine GH, Guiraudon G et al (1982) Right ventricular dysplasia: A report of 24 adult cases. Circulation 65:384-398
2. Thiene G, Nava A, Corrado D et al (1988) Right ventricular cardiomyopathy and sudden death in young people. N Engl J Med 318:129-133
3. Norman M, Simpson M, Mogensen J et al (2005) Novel mutation in desmoplakin causes arrhythmogenic left ventricular cardiomyopathy. Circulation 112:636-642
4. Nava A, Bauce B, Basso C et al (2000) Clinical profile and long-term follow-up of 37 families with arrhythmogenic right ventricular cardiomyopathy. J Am Coll Cardiol 36:2226-2233
5. McKenna WJ, Thiene G, Nava A et al (1994) Diagnosis of arrhythmogenic right ventricular dysplasia/cardiomyopathy. Task Force of the Working Group Myocardial and Pericardial Disease of the European Society of Cardiology and of the Scientific Council on Cardiomyopathies of the International Society and Federation of Cardiology. Br Heart J 71:215-218
6. McKoy G, Protonotarios N, Crosby A et al (2000) Identification of a deletion in plakoglobin in arrhythmogenic right ventricular cardiomyopathy with palmoplantar keratoderma and woolly hair (Naxos disease). Lancet 355:2119-2124
7. Norgett EE, Hatsell SJ, Carvajal-Huerta L et al (2000) Recessive mutation in desmoplakin disrupts desmoplakin-intermediate filament interactions and causes dilated cardiomyopathy, woolly hair and keratoderma. Hum Mol Genet 9:2761-2766
8. Protonotarios N, Tsatsopoulou A, Patsourakos P et al (1986) Cardiac abnormalities in familial palmoplantar keratosis. Br Heart J 56:321-326
9. Luderitz B (2003) Naxos disease. J Interv Card Electrophysiol 9:405-406
10. Protonotarios N, Tsatsopoulou A, Scampardonis G (1988) Right ventricular cardiomyopathy and sudden death in young people. N Engl J Med 319:175 (letter)
11. Fontaine G, Protonotarios N, Tsatsopoulou A et al (1994) Comparisons between Naxos disease and ar-

rhythmogenic right ventricular dysplasia by electrocardiography and biopsy. Circulation 90:3233

12. Fontaine G, Fontaliran F, Frank R (1998) Arrhythmogenic right ventricular cardiomyopathies: Clinical forms and main differential diagnoses. Circulation 97:1532-1535

13. Rao BH, Reddy IS, Chandra KS (1996) Familial occurrence of a rare combination of dilated cardiomyopathy with palmoplantar keratoderma and woolly hair. Indian Heart J 48:161-162

14. Carvajal-Huerta L (1998) Epidermolytic palmoplantar keratoderma with woolly hair and dilated cardiomyopathy. J Am Acad Dermatol 39:418-421

15. Djabali K, Martinez-Mir A, Horev L et al (2002) Evidence for extensive locus heterogeneity in Naxos disease. J Invest Dermatol 118:557-560

16. Alcalai R, Metzger S, Rosenheck S et al (2003) A recessive mutation in desmoplakin causes arrhythmogenic right ventricular dysplasia, skin disorder, and woolly hair. J Am Coll Cardiol 42:319-327

17. Narin N, Akcakus M, Gunes T et al (2003) Arrhythmogenic right ventricular cardiomyopathy (Naxos disease): Report of a Turkish boy. Pacing Clin Electrophysiol 26:2326-2329

18. Buhari I, Juma'a N (2004) Naxos disease in Saudi Arabia. J Eur Acad Dermatol Venereol 18:614-616

19. Uzumcu A, Norgett EE, Dindar A et al (2006) Loss of desmoplakin isoform I causes early onset cardiomyopathy and heart failure in a Naxos-like syndrome. J Med Genet 43:e5

20. Protonotarios N, Tsatsopoulou A, Fontaine G (2001) Naxos disease: Keratoderma, scalp modifications, and cardiomyopathy. J Am Acad Dermatol 44:309-310

21. Kaplan SR, Gard JJ, Carvajal-Huerta L et al (2004) Structural and molecular pathology of the heart in Carvajal syndrome. Cardiovasc Pathol 13:26-32

22. Coonar AS, Protonotarios N, Tsatsopoulou A et al (1998) Gene for arrhythmogenic right ventricular cardiomyopathy with diffuse nonepidermolytic palmoplantar keratoderma and woolly hair (Naxos disease) maps to 17q21. Circulation 97:2049-2058

23. Protonotarios N, Tsatsopoulou A, Anastasakis A et al (2001) Genotype-phenotype assessment in autosomal recessive arrhythmogenic right ventricular cardiomyopathy (Naxos disease) caused by a deletion in plakoglobin. J Am Coll Cardiol 38:1477-1484

24. Protonotarios N, Tsatsopoulou A, Gatzoulis K (2002) Arrhythmogenic right ventricular cardiomyopathy caused by a deletion in plakoglobin (Naxos disease). Card Electrophysiol Rev 6:72-80

25. Basso C, Tsatsopoulou A, Thiene G et al (2001) "Petrified" right ventricle in long-standing Naxos arrhythmogenic right ventricular cardiomyopathy. Circulation 104:e132-e133

26. Protonotarios N, Tsatsopoulou A (2004) Naxos disease and Carvajal syndrome: Cardiocutaneous disorders that highlight the pathogenesis and broaden the spectrum of arrhythmogenic right ventricular cardiomyopathy. Cardiovasc Path 13:185-194

27. Schonberger J, Seidman CE (2001) Many roads lead to a broken heart: The genetics of dilated cardiomyopathy. Am J Hum Genet 69:249-260

28. Rampazzo A, Nava A, Malacrida S et al (2002) Mutation in human desmoplakin domain binding to plakoglobin causes a dominant form of arrhythmogenic right ventricular cardiomyopathy. Am J Hum Genet 71:1200-1206

29. Bauce B, Basso C, Rampazzo A et al (2005) Clinical profile of four families with arrhythmogenic right ventricular cardiomyopathy caused by dominant desmoplakin mutations. Eur Heart J 16:1666-1675

30. Gerull B, Heuser A, Wichter T et al (2004) Mutations in the desmosomal protein plakophilin-2 are common in arrhythmogenic right ventricular cardiomyopathy. Nat Genet 36:1162-1164

31. Syrris P, Ward D, Asimaki A et al (2006) Clinical expression of Plakophilin-2 mutations in familial arrhythmogenic right ventricular cardiomyopathy. Circulation 113:356-364

32. Pilichou K, Nava A, Basso C et al (2006) Mutations in desmoglein-2 gene are associated with arrhythmogenic right ventricular cardiomyopathy. Circulation 113:1171-1179

33. Perriard JC, Hirschy A, Ehler E (2003) Dilated cardiomyopathy: A disease of the intercalated disc? Trends Cardiovasc Med 13:30-38

34. Green KJ, Gaudry CA (2000) Are desmosomes more than tethers for intermediate filaments? Nat Rev Mol Cell Biol 1:208-216

35. Zhurinsky J, Shtutman M, Ben-Ze'ev A (2000) Plakoglobin and β-catenin: Protein interactions, regulation and biological role. J Cell Sci 113:3127-3139

36. Brancolini C, Sgorbissa A, Schneider C (1998) Proteolytic processing of the adherens junctions components β-catenin and γ-catenin/plakoglobin during apoptosis. Cell Death Differ 5:1042-1050

37. Kaplan SR, Gard JJ, Protonotarios N et al (2004) Remodeling of myocyte gap junctions in arrhythmogenic right ventricular cardiomyopathy due to a deletion in plakoglobin (Naxos disease). Heart Rhythm 1:3-11

38. Duran M, Avellan F, Carvajal L (2000) Dilated cardiomyopathy in the ectodermal dysplasia. Electroechocardiographic observations in palmo-plantar keratoderma with woolly hair. Rev Esp Cardiol 53:1296-1300

39. Wichter T, Schulze-Bar E, Eckardt L et al (2002) Molecular mechanisms of inherited ventricular arrhythmias. Hertz 27:712-739

CHAPTER 3
GENOTYPE-PHENOTYPE CORRELATIONS

Barbara Bauce, Andrea Nava

Introduction

The recent genetic discoveries in arrhythmogenic right ventricular cardiomyopathy/dysplasia (ARVC/D) permit genotype-phenotype correlation in an increasing number of subjects, providing better knowledge of the diagnostic criteria, natural history, and ethiopathogenesis of the disease. Three different groups of genes have been found to be linked to ARVC/D: the ryanodine receptor-2 gene (RyR2), the gene encoding for the growth factor TGFbeta 3 and five genes encoding for intercellular junction proteins (plakoglobin, desmoplakin, plakophilin-2, desmoglein-2, and desmocollin-2) [1-8]. Mutations of all these genes lead to the pathogenetic process that is the basis of the disease, consisting of myocyte death followed by myocardial atrophy and fibrofatty replacement [9, 10] (Fig. 3.1). These discoveries have confirmed the genetic heterogeneity of ARVC/D [11].

In our series of patients with ARVC/D, a mutation of a known gene can be identified in about 50% of cases, indicating that additional disease genes have still to be detected. Genetic analysis of affected families found the presence of RyR2 mutations in 28%, of TGFbeta 3 in 4%, and a gene encoding for desmosomal proteins (desmoplakin, plakophilin-2 and desmoglein-2) in 68%.

ARVC/D Linked to Mutations of RyR2 Gene

Mutations of the RyR2 gene cause effort-induced polymorphic ventricular arrhythmias (PVA) associated with mild alterations of the right ventricle or with normal hearts [12-16]. The RyR2 receptor is involved in the calcium release from the sarcoplasmic reticulum. Mutations of this gene cause malfunction of the receptor resulting in intracellular calcium overload [17, 18]. The calcium overload may induce both cellular injury that triggers apoptosis and electrical instability due to after-depolarization potentials.

Ventricular arrhythmias are usually induced during exercise testing and the heart rate threshold at which they appear is different in each subject. This heart rate can be quite low, even below 100 bpm, and these subjects are particularly at risk of sudden death, since it is common to reach this rate in normal life. Beta-blockers have a role in raising the heart rate threshold, thus they have a preventive effect on the onset of arrhythmias. Bauce et al. studied eight families with RyR2 mutations [14] (Fig. 3.2). A total of 43 subjects were found to carry a RyR2 mutation; among these, 28 (65%, 13 males and 15 females; mean age 28±12 years) presented with effort-induced arrhythmic symptoms or signs (PVA in 26 cases and isolated syncopal episodes in 2) (Fig. 3.3). Among the 26 subjects with PVA during exercise, 15 presented with polymorphic ventricular complexes, either isolated or in couplets, whereas in ten subjects, PVA progressed to nonsustained ventricular tachycardia (VT). In one patient a sustained VT was induced. PVA were re-

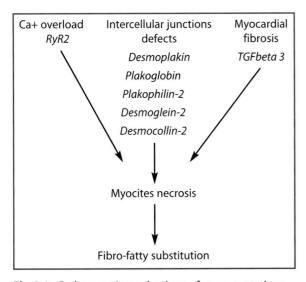

Fig. 3.1 • Pathogenetic mechanisms of genes mutations

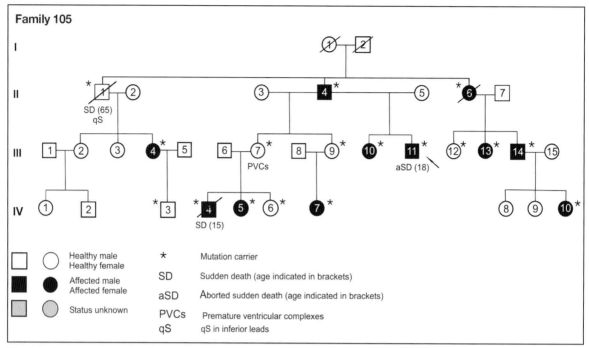

Fig. 3.4 • Pedigree of one family carrying a mutation of the desmoplakin gene. Subjects II-1, and III-7, who carried the DSP mutation, did not fulfil the diagnostic criteria. However, the former died suddenly while the latter showed PVCs at 24-h ambulatory ECG. Reproduced from [20] with permission from Oxford University Press

gression. Moreover, ARVC/D caused by DSP mutations was found to be characterized by a high occurrence of SD as the first clinical manifestation and that left ventricular involvement is not a rare feature of the disease.

Syrris et al. published a genotype-phenotype correlation study of nine families carrying PKP2 mutations [22]. Among the 34 subjects with a PKP2 mutation, 32 had clinical evaluation and 17 (53%) were found to fulfil the ARVC/D diagnostic criteria. An additional nine presented some cardiac signs of the disease. Right ventricular structural abnormalities were present in 20 (62%), mutations carriers and abnormal ECG/SAECG features in 21 (66%).

Antoniades et al. studied 22 PKP2 carriers and 26 homozygous JUP carriers and found a similar cardiac phenotype [23]. Moreover, T-wave inversion in leads V1-V3, right ventricular wall motion abnormalities and frequent ventricular complexes were the most sensitive and specific markers for identification of mutation carriers.

The desmoglein-2 gene mutation was recently identified by Pilichou et al., who found this gene in 8 probands (5 males and 3 females). The mean age at diagnosis/symptom onset was 38±20 years with a range of 11 to 63 years [7]. The clinical data showed that the first symptom consisted of sustained VT in three patients, palpitations in three, and chest pain with increased serum markers of myocardial necrosis in presence of angiographically normal coronary arteries in one; the remaining patient was asymptomatic. In addition, skin and hair were normal in all. There was a significant difference in the mean age at symptom onset/diagnosis between males and females (26±13 years vs. 58±4 years, respectively, p=0.001). All patients showed ECG abnormalities, and late potentials were detected in seven subjects. Ventricular arrhythmias were recorded in all probands and ranged from isolated monomorphic PVCs, nonsustained VT, and sustained VT with left bundle-branch block morphology. Abnormal echocardiographic findings were present in all probands, with right ventricular kinetic abnormalities involving only one region in one patient and ≥2 regions in the remaining seven. Left ventricular involvement was present in half of the patients. Family members of the two index cases were studied and five additional subjects were found to carry a DSG2 mutation; of these, two were classified as affected.

ARVC/D Linked to Mutations of TGFbeta 3 Gene

Mutations of TGFbeta 3 has been found in a small percentage of ARVC/D patients (4%). Beffagna et al. [6] found a proband in one family with mutations of this gene. Clinical analysis of 12 TGFbeta 3 mutation carriers lead to a diagnosis of ARVC/D in nine subjects (75%). The 12-lead ECG, SAECG, and 2D-echo findings were similar to those reported in DSP and DSG2 carriers. TGFbeta 3 is a member of the transforming growth factor family, a large group of regulatory cytokines that has a pivotal role in tissue development and homeostasis [24]. TGFbeta 3 induces a fibrotic response in various tissues in vivo [25] by promoting expression of extracellular matrix genes and by suppressing the activity of genes such as matrix metalloproteinases, which are involved in extracellular matrix degradation [26, 27]. On the basis of this information, we hypothesized that mutations in the TGFbeta 3 gene, which increases expression in vitro, could promote myocardial fibrosis in vivo.

Impact of Genetic Results on Clinical Evaluation of Patients with ARVC/D

Increasing knowledge of the disease from studies of genotype-phenotype correlation should facilitate assessment of the incidence of the disease, modality of disease expression and clinical presentation, the rate of disease progression, the incidence of sudden death and heart failure, as well as evaluation of electrical instability. In addition, it should clarify the role of important diagnostic features as the ECG, echocardiogram, signal-averaged ECG, and cardiac magnetic resonance.

The prevalence of ARVC/D has been estimated to be about 1:5000; however, the detection of several subjects carrying a gene mutation but without clinical signs of ARVC/D (healthy carriers) or with a mild form of the disease suggests that this prevalence is greatly underestimated, at least by 50%.

The above-cited genotype-phenotype correlation studies confirmed that ARVC/D is characterized by a wide clinical spectrum. Some genetically affected patients can have no symptoms, nor ventricular arrhythmias, syncopal episodes, sudden death, or chest pain. Moreover, analysis of the age of patients at disease onset showed that the disease rarely appeared before the age of 10, whereas the majority of patients showed clinical signs of the disease between 10 and 20 years of age. Sudden death or aborted sudden

death almost always occurred in subjects without a previous diagnosis and rarely in already diagnosed patients; congestive heart failure was quite rare. The degree of arrhythmic risk is difficult to quantify; however, our data confirmed previous observations regarding its relation to the extent of the disease, presence of complex ventricular arrhythmias and episodes of the "acute phase" of the disease, that in many cases were not predictable. Moreover, evaluation of families carrying DSP and PKP2 mutations showed that ECG/SAECG and 2D-echo finding were normal in a significant percentage of mutation carriers [7, 22]. Thus these diagnostic tools may not be helpful in disease diagnosis.

The presence of healthy carriers or of mutation carriers that show some clinical signs of the disease without fulfilling the diagnostic criteria, led us to reconsider the Task Force criteria published in 1994. It is important to stress that these criteria were established when no genetic data on ARVC/D were known. It is clear that additional studies on genotype-phenotype correlation will facilitate new diagnostic protocols. At this time there are no new clinical diagnostic tools available.

These new protocols should consider a scale that, on the basis of presence of one or more criteria, could define different degrees of severity of the disease (mild, moderate, severe). The presence of genetic mutations should be considered a major criterion of the disease; consequently even a healthy genetic carrier should have a major criterion of the disease.

In clinically affected patients, genetic information does not modify the clinical management; that is always related to the disease extent and the degree of electrical instability. However, the detection of a genetic mutation in a subject with no clinical signs of the disease (so-called healthy carrier) can lead to a difficult management decision for the physician and the patient. The aim of management should be the avoidance of those factors that may worsen the extent of the disease and prevent the onset of ventricular arrhythmias. At present we do not have impressive data on pejorative factors, but the hypothesis that myocardial cells stretching due to strenuous physical activity can play a role in favoring the onset or progression of the pathologic process has been advanced. It seems reasonable to advise these subjects to limit their physical activity. It is also advisable to suggest frequent noninvasive clinical evaluation (ECG, SAECG, Holter, stress test, 2D-Ecocardiogram) in the follow-up.

Results of genotype-phenotype studies in ARVC/D families should help to establish appropriate clinical management in mutations carriers.

In our experience the detection of a genetic mutation in a proband or family member may pose different management problems depending on circumstances as described below:

1. *Presence of an ARVC/D genetic mutation in an affected proband.* The proband usually has an overt form of the disease. In this subject, genetic result leads only to a confirmation of the disease diagnosis but it does not modify the clinical management that is related to the extent of the disease and degree of electrical instability. The degree of electrical instability is assessed on the basis of disease extent as well as presence of sustained ventricular tachycardia or previous ventricular fibrillation. If an ICD is indicated, we always prescribe antiarrhythmic drug therapy because we are aware that each ICD shock can create a new scar in a myocardium that already has a pathologic process.

2. *Detection of a genetic mutation in a subject, usually a family member, with no clinical signs of the disease.* This situation can be due to the young age of the subject who has not yet developed the disease or to the fact that the mutation is characterized by a low expression. There are no guidelines for management of these healthy carriers of the disease. Since a myocardial stretching may facilitate the onset and progression of the disease, as also confirmed by recent studies on animal models carrying a mutation [28], in these kind of subjects we allow only a limited physical activity without isotonic efforts, whereas a competitive physical activity is always prohibited.

3. *Identification of a genetic mutation in a subject with minor signs of the disease.* In this case we can assume that a mild anatomic abnormality is present. This patient may be asymptomatic and we strongly suggest only mild physical activity and a systematic clinical evaluation. The detection of ventricular arrhythmias has to lead the physician to start an antiarrhythmic therapy and to suggest the avoidance of physical activity. On the basis of the degree of electrical instability, we consider the choice of drugs as a pyramid, which presents at the apex the association between amiodarone+beta-blockers, then Class I antiarrhythmic drugs associated with beta-blockers, then sotalol, and finally Class I antiarrhythmic drugs alone.

4. *Identification of a genetic mutation in family members with an overt form of the disease* (previously unknown). In these cases there is a strong correlation between the presence of a gene mutation and disease expression; thus, the clinical management will be the same as that of the proband.

In a family member who does not carry a genetic mutation, genetic analysis provides a definitive and rewarding answer. As a consequence, subjects do not need to be followed. Moreover, they may lead a normal life and family planning, being assured that they will not transmit ARVC/D to their children.

In subjects classified as affected, physical activity must be prohibited, both in competitive as well as noncompetitive sports. A major management problem is the detection of a genetic mutation in professional athletes, since avoidance of sports activity in these individuals has important economic and legal consequences. Finally, a clinical comparison among subjects carrying different mutations has been attempted, with the aim of ascertaining if these mutations can be characterized by different degrees of risk for sudden death; RyR2 mutations are always potentially dangerous both in the presence or absence of effort-induced PVA. Subjects carrying this mutation must be treated with beta blockers, which have been shown to be effective in the majority of cases, and to avoid physical activity.

For subjects carrying DSP, PKP2, DSG2, and TGf-beta3 mutations, our preliminary data has not shown significant clinical differences among the different gene mutations; nonetheless, analysis of larger series of patients with long follow-up may provide genetic-phenotype correlations.

In conclusion, advances in the genetics of ARVC/D has not helped the clinical management of affected patients, since therapeutic decisions relate to clinical features and degree of electrical instability. At this time, we are not able to modify the disease progression with certainty. Nonetheless, genetic analysis of family members allows the early detection of subjects at risk of life-threatening ventricular arrhythmias and sudden death. In these subjects it is important to eliminate those factors that theoretically favor the onset of the clinical disease. We do not have a clear knowledge on pejorative factors, even if we hypothesize that myocardial cell stretching due to strenuous physical activity can favor the onset of the pathologic process. In these subjects physical activity has to be limited or prohibited; moreover, they must be followed systematically with frequent noninvasive clinical evaluations with the aim of promptly identifying the onset of electrical instability and in order to prevent serious life threatening ventricular arrhythmia by antiarrhythmic therapy.

Genotype-phenotype correlation studies are providing important new information that will be completed when all affected subjects are genetically characterized. Moreover, long follow-up studies will provide important information that will help in deciding the best therapeutic strategies for ARVC/D patients.

References

1. McKoy G, Protonotarios N, Crosby A et al (2000) Identification of a deletion in plakoglobin in arrhythmogenic right ventricular cardiomyopathy with palmoplantar keratoderma and woolly hair (Naxos disease). Lancet 355:2119-2124

2. Tiso N, Stephan DA, Nava A et al (2001) Identification of mutations in the cardiac ryanodine receptor gene in families affected with arrhythmogenic right ventricular cardiomyopathy type 2 (ARVD2). Hum Mol Genet 10:189-194

3. Rampazzo A, Nava A, Malacrida S et al (2002) Mutation in human desmoplakin domain binding to plakoglobin causes a dominant form of arrhythmogenic right ventricular cardiomyopathy. Am J Hum Genet 71:1200-1206

4. Alcalai R, Metzger S, Rosenheck S et al (2003) A recessive mutation in desmoplakin causes arrhythmogenic right ventricular dysplasia, skin disorder, and woolly hair. J Am Coll Cardiol 42:319-327

5. Gerull B, Heuser A, Wichter T et al (2004) Mutations in the desmosomal protein plakophilin-2 are common in arrhythmogenic right ventricular cardiomyopathy. Nat Genet 36:1162-1164

6. Beffagna G, Occhi G, Nava A et al (2005) Regulatory mutations in transforming growth factor-β3 gene cause arrhythmogenic right ventricular cardiomyopathy type 1. Cardiovasc Res 65:366-373

7. Pilichou K, Nava A, Basso C et al (2006) Mutations in desmoglein-2 gene are associated with arrhythmogenic right ventricular cardiomyopathy. Circulation 113:1171-1179

8. Syrris P, Ward D, Evans A et al (2006) Arrhythmogenic right ventricular dysplasia/cardiomyopathy associated with mutations in the desmosomal gene desmocollin-2. Am J Hum Genet 79:978-984

9. Thiene G, Nava D, Corrado D et al (1988) Right ventricular cardiomyopathy and sudden death in young people. N Engl J Med 318:129-133

10. Basso C, Thiene G, Corrado D et al (1996) Arrhythmogenic right ventricular cardiomyopathy. Dysplasia, dystrophy, or myocarditis? Circulation 94:983-991

11. Nava A, Bauce B, Basso C et al (2000) Clinical profile and long-term follow-up of 37 families with arrhythmogenic right ventricular cardiomyopathy. J Am Coll Cardiol 36:2226-2233

12. Nava A, Canciani B, Daliento L et al (1988) Juvenile sudden death and effort ventricular tachycardias in a family with right ventricular cardiomyopathy. Int J Cardiol 21:111-126

13. Bauce B, Nava A, Rampazzo A et al (2000) Familial effort polymorphic ventricular arrhythmias in apparently normal heart map to chromosome 1q42-q43. Am J Cardiol 85:573-579

14. Bauce B, Rampazzo A, Basso C et al (2002) Screening for RyR2 mutations in families with effort-induced polymorphic ventricular arrhythmias and sudden death: Early diagnosis of asymptomatic carrier. J Am Coll Cardiol 40:341-349

15. Priori S, Napolitano C, Tiso N et al (2001) Mutations in the cardiac ryanodine receptor gene (hRyR2) underlie catecholaminergic polymorphic ventricular tachycardia. Circulation 103:196-200

16. Laitinen P, Brown K, Piippo K et al (2001) Mutations of the cardiac ryanodine receptor (RyR2) gene in familial polymorphic ventricular tachycardia. Circulation 103:485-490

17. Tunwell RE, Wickenden C, Bertrand BM et al (1996) The human cardiac muscle ryanodine receptor-calcium release channel: Identification, primary structure and topological analysis. Biochem J 18:477-487

18. Marks AR, Priori S, Memmi M et al (2002) Involvement of the cardiac ryanodine receptor/calcium release channel in catecholaminergic polymorphic ventricular tachycardia. J Cell Physiol 190:1-6

19. Protonotarios N, Tsatsopoulou A, Anastasakis A et al (2001) Genotype-phenotype assessment in autosomal recessive arrhythmogenic right ventricular cardiomyopathy (Naxos disease) caused by a deletion in plakoglobin. J Am Coll Cardiol 38:1477-1484

20. Bauce B, Basso C, Rampazzo A et al (2005) Clinical profile of four families with arrhythmogenic right ventricular cardiomyopathy caused by dominant desmoplakin mutations. Eur Heart J 26:1666-1675

21. McKenna WJ, Thiene G, Nava A et al (1994) Diagnosis of arrhythmogenic right ventricular dysplasia/cardiomyopathy. Br Heart J 71:215-218

22. Syrris P, Ward D, Asimaki A et al (2006) Clinical expression of plakophilin-2 mutations in familial arrhythmogenic right ventricular cardiomyopathy. Circulation 113:356-364

23. Antoniades L, Tsatsopoulou A, Anastasakis A et al (2006) Arrhythmogenic right ventricular cardiomyopathy caused by deletions in plakophilin-2 and plakoglobin (Naxos disease) in families from Greece and Cyprus: Genotype-phenotype relations, diagnostic features and prognosis. Eur Heart J 27:2208-2216

24. Sporn A, Roberts AB (1992) Transforming growth factor-beta: Recent progress and new challenges. J Cell Biol 119:1017-1021

25. Leask A, Abraham DJ (2004) TGF-beta signaling and the fibrotic response. FASEB J 18:816-827

26. Varga J, Jimenez SA (1986) Stimulation of normal human fibroblast collagen production and processing by transforming growth factor-beta. Biochem Biophys Res Commun 138:974-980

27. Overall CM, Wrana JL, Sodek J (1989) Independent regulation of collagenase, 72-kDa progelatinase, and metalloendoproteinase inhibitor expression in human fibroblasts by transforming growth factor-beta. J Biol Chem 264:1860-1869

28. Kirchhof P, Fabritz L, Zwiener M et al (2006) Age- and training-dependent development of arrhythmogenic right ventricular cardiomyopathy in heterozygous plakoglobin-deficient mice. Circulation 114:1799-1806

CHAPTER 4

AUTOPSY AND ENDOMYOCARDIAL BIOPSY FINDINGS

Cristina Basso, Gaetano Thiene

Introduction

According to the 1995 WHO classification, arrhythmogenic right ventricular cardiomyopathy/dysplasia (ARVC/D) is defined as a heart muscle disorder characterized by progressive fibrofatty replacement of right ventricular myocardium, initially with typical regional and later global right and some left ventricular involvement, with relative sparing of the septum [1]. The residual myocytes interspersed among adipocytes and fibrous tissue provides the ideal substrate for re-entrant life-threatening ventricular arrhythmias [2-8]. In 1982, Marcus et al. [2] reported the first clinical series in adults, pointing out the peculiar fatty "dysplasia" of the right ventricular free wall in the absence of an ischemic milieu. In their original series, morphologic findings were obtained from 13 adult patients, 12 who had surgery and one who died because of pulmonary embolism and had postmortem investigation. Aneurysms were described in the so-called triangle of dysplasia, i.e., the right ventricular outflow tract, the apex, and the inferior wall. Furthermore, a marked decrease in myocardial fibers with myocardium usually replaced by fibrosis and fat was evident. In the areas of "dysplasia," there was thickened whitish sclerotic endocardium. At higher magnification, hypertrophy or degeneration of the few remaining myocytes with dysmorphic and picnotic nuclei was detected, as well as a variable amount of histiocytic and lymphocytic inflammatory infiltrates.

The morphologic features of the disease have been systematically assessed only in the late 1980s. Thiene and collaborators [3] investigated a series of juvenile sudden deaths that occurred in the Veneto region in Italy and recognized that the disease is a major cause of sudden death in the young, ranking second only to atherosclerotic coronary artery disease. They described two distinct patterns of ARVC/D, based upon the nature of myocardial tissue replacement, i.e., mostly fatty tissue (fatty or lipo-matous pattern) or fibrous and fatty tissue (fibro-fatty or fibrolipomatous pattern).

In this chapter we will focus the attention on what has been learned about the pathology of ARVC/D, from postmortem or from endomyocardial biopsy (EMB) investigation. In particular we will deal with the gross and histologic diagnostic criteria, to clarify the significance of fatty infiltration and to assess whether the involvement of the right ventricle must be considered the *conditio sine qua non* for diagnosing ARVC/D. The discovery of disease-causing genes and the feasibility of genetic analysis even at postmortem and/or in family members of deceased patients is helpful to clarify this issue.

The need to adopt strict criteria for diagnosis is important for the forensic and the general pathologist. These criteria are also vital both for epidemiologic purposes and for clinical implications, since the identification of a genetic disease as a cause of death represents the starting point for familial screening and sudden death prevention. International Registries and tissue banks have been established [9, 10], with the aim of providing not only clinical but also morphologic diagnostic criteria for ARVC/D.

Gross and Histologic Diagnosis

The pathologic diagnosis of ARVC/D in autopsy hearts or those explanted at the time of cardiac transplantation has been traditionally based upon gross and histologic evidence of transmural fatty or fibrofatty myocardial replacement of the right ventricular free wall. This could be considered a myocardial dystrophy, extending from the epicardium towards the endocardium, sparing only the trabecular myocardium [3-8].

Table 4.1 summarizes the main pathologic features as observed in the original Padua series. At

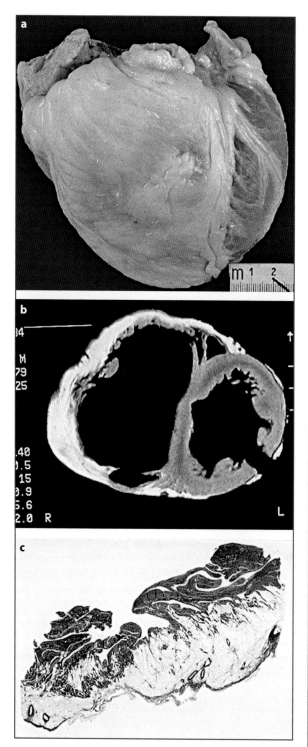

gross examination, the right side of the heart appears yellowish or whitish suggesting fatty or fibro-fatty replacement (Fig. 4.1). Right ventricular aneurysms, whether single or multiple (Figs. 4.2, 4.3) are considered a pathognomonic feature of ARVC/D. The heart weight is almost normal according to sex and age, but right ventricular enlargement, whether mild, moderate or severe, is a constant finding. The right ventricular dystrophic process can be diffuse or segmental, whereas left ventricular involvement may not be seen on gross examination, thus explaining its underestimated prevalence (see below). The ventricular septum may be involved in about 20% of cases

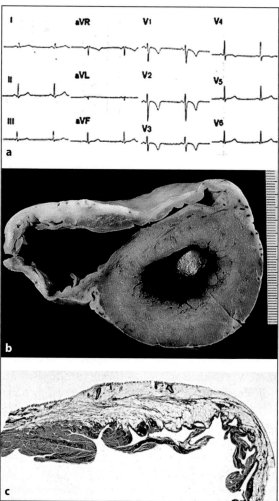

Fig. 4.1 • A 49-year-old woman who was transplanted due to heart failure and refractory ventricular arrhythmias. (**a**) External view of the native heart specimen obtained at cardiac transplantation: note the yellow appearance of the *right side* of heart. (**b**) In vitro spin-echo cardiac magnetic resonance, short axis, shows massive right ventricular dilatation and full-thickness myocardial atrophy with fatty tissue replacement. (**c**) Panoramic histologic section of the right ventricular free wall shows transmural fibro-fatty replacement (Heidenhain trichrome)

Fig. 4.2 • A 17-year-old boy who died suddenly while playing soccer. (**a**) Basal 12 lead ECG shows inverted T waves in the right precordial leads up to V4. (**b**) Transverse section of the heart specimen showing extreme thinning of the right ventricular free wall accounting for anterior and posterior (subtricuspid) aneurysms. (**c**) Panoramic histologic section of the anterior right ventricular free wall shows transmural fibro-fatty replacement (fibro-fatty variant) (Heidenhain trichrome)

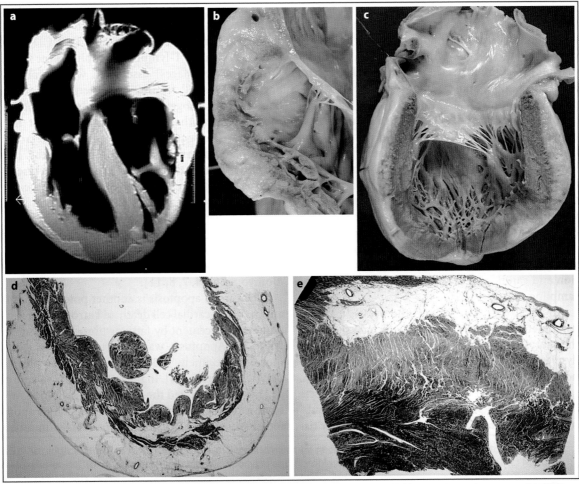

Fig. 4.3 • A 40-year-old man, previously asymptomatic, who died suddenly at rest. (**a**) In vitro spin-echo cardiac magnetic resonance, four-chamber cut, shows increased high intensity signal in both ventricles, either transmural (*right*) or subepicardial (*left*). (**b**) View of the right ventricular inflow with fatty appearance of the lateral wall, subtricuspid aneurysm and endocardial fibrous thickening. (**c**) View of the postero-lateral left ventricular free wall: note the wave front extension of fat from the epicardium towards the endocardium. (**d**) Panoramic histologic section of the right ventricular free wall shows transmural fibro-fatty replacement (Heidenhain trichrome). (**e**) Panoramic histologic section of the left ventricular free wall with fibro-fatty replacement in the outer layer (Heidenhain trichrome)

and the left ventricle in nearly half of cases [4, 5] (Table 4.1).

Hearts with end-stage disease and congestive heart failure, obtained either at autopsy or at cardiac transplantation [4, 11], consistently show biventricular involvement. There are usually multiple right ventricular aneurysms and a parchment-like appearance of the free wall. Intracavitary mural thrombi may be present and may be a source of pulmonary embolism. Thickening of the endocardium is a frequent finding, most probably as a result of fine thrombus deposition and organization, usually in conjunction with aneurysms and/or severe dilatation. As a consequence, the trabeculae are shrunk and the intertrabecular spaces appear enlarged, thus explaining the feature of deep fissures at angiography. The

Table 4.1 • Main clinical-pathologic features in 30 ARVC/D cases

M/F	2/1
Age range (mean)	15-65 (28)
Mode of death or failure	
Sudden death	24(80%)
Congestive heart failure	6 (20%)
Heart weight range (gr, mean)	270-660 (400)
RV aneurysms (triangle of dysplasia)	15 (50%)*
Inferior	12
Infundibular	8
Apical	6
LV involvement	14 (47%)**
Septal involvement	6 (20%)
Patchy inflammation***	20 (67%)

Note: when considering only the fibro-fatty variant, values are * 78%; ** 78%; and *** 100%; *LV* left ventricle; *RV* right ventricle

Pure Fatty Infiltration of the Right Ventricle vs. ARVC/D

At present, considerable importance is given to the finding of fatty infiltration of the myocardium, since cardiac magnetic resonance imaging has the ability to identify adipose tissue in vivo with consequent diagnostic and therapeutic implications. It is still a matter of debate whether fatty infiltration of the right ventricle per se should be considered a morphologic hallmark of ARVC/D [19]. We must recognize that the original distinction in two histologic variants, i.e., fatty and fibro-fatty, has been a source of confusion, since it has not been sufficiently appreciated that even in the fatty variant a certain amount of replacement-type fibrosis and myocyte abnormalities should be found to label it as ARVC/D [3].

Several authors reported that fat is a normal finding in the heart in a large series of patients, particularly at older age, and since they were not convinced of the clinical or pathological significance of isolated fat infiltration, they concluded that this entity is different from ARVC/D [20-24]. In particular, Burke et al. [23] found that, in autopsy hearts of people dying suddenly with pure fatty infiltration, the right ventricular myocardium was of normal or increased thickness, the left ventricle was mostly normal and there was no inflammation or myocyte atrophy. Moreover, the authors pointed out that while up to 15% fatty replacement is distinctly abnormal in the right ventricular outflow tract or posterior wall, it is probably normal in the anterior wall near the apex. Tansey et al. [24] found that 85% of hearts from people who died of noncardiac causes contained at least some intramyocardial fatty tissue, in the absence of fibrosis or inflammation, with significantly more fat replacement noted in the right ventricle of older subjects and in females than in males.

Massive fatty infiltration of the right ventricle, without any evidence of fibrosis and myocyte degeneration, represents a questionable cause of sudden death and does not have a familial tendency [21] (Fig. 4.6). In this condition, the myocytes seem to be pushed apart rather than replaced and they appear structurally normal. In contrast to fatty infiltration of the right ventricle, both the so-called fatty and the fibro-fatty ARVC/D variants consistently show degenerative changes of the myocytes and nuclei, often resembling those observed in dilated cardiomyopathy [25].

Thus, in addition to fat, two additional histologic features are essential in order to provide an unequivocal diagnosis of ARVC/D: (a) replacement-type fibrosis; and/or (b) degenerative changes of the

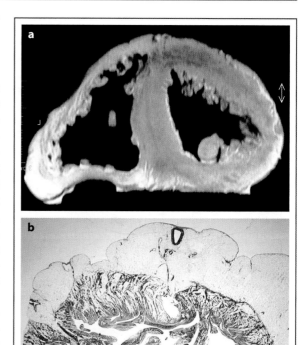

Fig. 4.6 • Adipositas cordis in a 46-year-old obese woman (**a**) In vitro spin-echo cardiac magnetic resonance, short axis cut, shows transmural high intensity signal in the right ventricle, with preserved wall thickness. (**b**) Panoramic histologic section of the right ventricular free wall shows increased epicardial fat and finger-like fat infiltration of the underlying myocardium, in the absence of fibrous tissue (Heidenhain trichrome)

myocytes. On this basis, it is clear that newly available cardiac imaging techniques, which are able to detect not only fatty tissue deposition but also fibrous tissue, such as cardiac magnetic resonance with gadolinium enhancement, could play a key role in differential diagnosis [19]. A corollary is that the finding of fatty infiltration of the right ventricular myocardium in the absence of wall motion abnormalities should be interpreted with caution.

In a patient with sudden death, where extensive right ventricular fatty infiltration is observed in the heart, it would be preferable to state this finding without implying a cause and effect relationship. In other words, this would not necessarily indicate that death was due to ARVC/D [19]. If pathologists would ascribe sudden death as due to ARVC/D based on simple observation of adipose infiltration, there will be a huge increase in its frequency as a cause of sudden death which in most instances will be totally spurious, as forecast by Davies [26]. Noteworthy, a recent forensic autopsy investigation reported an extremely high incidence (more than 10%) of ARVC/D in people aged 1-65 years who died suddenly in France: in the majority of cases there was not any evidence of fibrous tissue replacement [27].

Nowadays, disease-causing genes are potentially available for mutational analysis [28-33], even at postmortem or in family members of sudden death cases. In the reported genotyped ARVC/D forms, due to desmosomal protein encoding genes, in which the heart was available for morphological investigation, the specimens were characterized by biventricular involvement, typical fibro-fatty replacement, myocyte death and nuclear abnormali-

ties [34-36]. Noteworthy, if cardiac arrest occurs in the early phase of the disease, we have observed massive myocyte injury, with early fibrous tissue replacement and very few adipocytes [36] (Fig. 4.7). These data are consistent with those by Fletcher et al. [37], who found that the pathology of ARVC/D varies with age in both ventricles, fibrosis being the earliest hallmark of ARVC/D in younger patients, and fatty infiltration being more prominent in older patients. Similar findings were reported in an earlier histomorphometric EMB study from our group, demonstrating a higher amount of fat in older patients [38]. Thus, the changing face of the disease

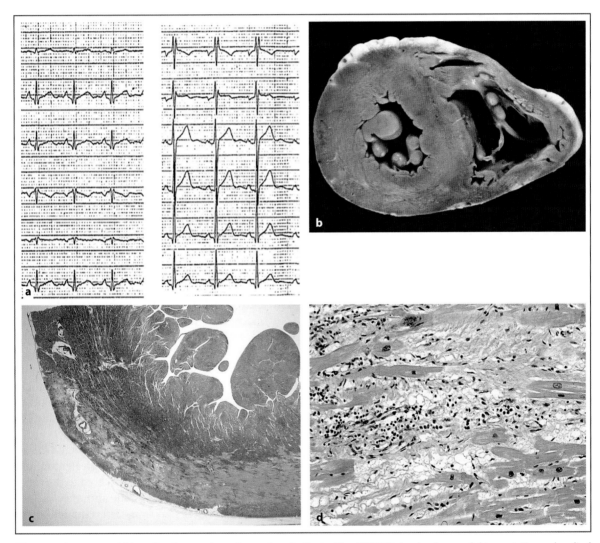

Fig. 4.7 • A 15-year-old boy, family member of a proband affected by ARVC/D due to desmoplakin mutation, who died suddenly at rest despite negative cardiological screening. (**a**) 12 lead ECG with incomplete right bundle branch block. (**b**) Cross section of the heart: there is no macroscopic evidence of fatty tissue infiltration or aneurysm, whereas a gray band is evident in the subepicardial postero-lateral region. (**c**) Panoramic histologic view of the postero-lateral left ventricular wall showing a subepicardial band of acute-subacute myocyte necrosis with loose fibrous tissue and granulation tissue (trichrome Heidenhain). (**d**) Myocyte necrosis, myocytolysis, and polymorphous inflammatory infiltrates together with fibrous and fatty tissue repair are visible at higher magnification (haematoxylin-eosin)

morphology, depending on its stage, should be taken into consideration, when evaluating a case of sudden death due to ARVC/D.

Recently, Garcia Gras et al. [39], reported their findings with heterozygous desmoplakin-deficient mice. They showed excess adipocytes and fibrosis in the myocardium, increased myocyte apoptosis, cardiac dysfunction, and ventricular arrhythmias, mimicking the phenotype of human fibro-fatty ARVC/D. The authors provided evidence that expression and nuclear localization of PPAR-γ, a major regulator of adipogenesis, was restricted to fibrotic areas in desmoplakin-deficient mouse hearts, suggesting a possible origin of adipocytes from fibrocytes or pre-fibroblasts, which are considered adipocyte progenitor cells, rather than cardiac myoblasts or resident and circulating mesenchymal stem cells. This possibility is strengthened by the colocalization of adipocytes and fibrosis both in the hearts of desmoplakin-deficient mice and in the myocardium of human patients affected by ARVC/D.

ARVD2 [40] is an exception to the unifying hypothesis that desmosomal protein abnormalities cause ARVC/D. This is due to a defective ryanodine cardiac receptor 2 (RYR2) gene, which regulates the release of Ca++ from sarcoplasmic reticulum to cytosol for excitation-contraction coupling. This variant is clinically characterized by effort-induced polymorphic ventricular arrhythmias, whereas the resting 12 lead ECG is normal. In a minority of cases, there is mild right ventricular involvement. Pathologically, the heart is usually normal or shows segmental right ventricular fatty infiltration at the apex. Thus, the question is whether this disease is truly an ARVC/D variant [40, 41]. In an index case with effort-induced polymorphic ventricular arrhythmias, d'Amati et al. [42], in addition to segmental fibro-fatty replacement, reported a specific morphological substrate consisting of calcium phosphate deposits within cardiac myocytes. Thus ARVD2 variant should be viewed as an ion channel disease, with some secondary myocyte injury related to the underlying molecular defect.

Left Ventricular Involvement

ARVC/D has been classically defined as a selective disorder predominantly affecting the right ventricle [1]. Since the early description in the 1980s, left ventricular involvement has been recognized clinically with greater and greater frequency [2, 43-45].

From the pathological point of view, several case reports of ARVC/D with histologic abnormalities of

the left ventricle have been published [46-53], even in the absence of heart failure.

In the Padua series, Basso et al. [4] indicated that left ventricular free wall involvement is present in nearly half of cases, all with a fibro-fatty pattern (Table 4.1) (Figs. 6.2, 6.3, 6.8). Hearts with left ventricular involvement were from older individuals, were slightly heavier and more likely associated with a clinical picture of congestive heart failure. Corrado et al. [7] found a 76% incidence (32 cases) of left ventricular involvement in a study of 42 hearts from six European centers, all with fibro-fatty or mainly fibrous pattern. Fifteen showed only histologic changes, whereas 17 had both gross and histologic evidence of left ventricular involvement.

A study from Canada by Lobo et al. [54] found that 45% of hearts of ARVC/D showed left ventricular fibrous scars, although coronary atherosclerosis coexisted in some. In another North American series by Burke et al. [23], microscopic subepicardial left ventricular involvement was present in 64% of fibro-fatty ARVC/D. In a French series of sudden death due to ARVC/D, Fornes and colleagues [55] reported a 40% incidence of left ventricular disease. However, in all series a severe diffuse biventricular involvement, mimicking dilated cardiomyopathy requiring heart transplantation, appears to be rare. Recently, d'Amati et al. [25], in a series of transplanted hearts, found grossly biventricular involvement in 87% of cases with the so-called cardiomyopathic pattern vs. 9% of those with the "infiltrative" (fatty) pattern.

To characterize the pathological features of left ventricular involvement in this disease, Lobo et al. [56] reviewed 17 hearts with ARVC/D, all with involvement of the left ventricle, seven of whom had evidence of left ventricular disease only at histology. In the involved areas, the left ventricle or ventricular septum were of nearly normal thickness. Full thickness transmural fatty replacement of the left ventricular myocardium was never observed nor were left ventricular aneurysms. At histology, the myocardial changes of the left ventricular free wall were typically subepicardial or midmural, with a greater amount of fibrous tissue deposition as compared to the right. On the basis of these findings, the authors concluded that pathologists may miss left ventricular involvement on gross examination, thus suggesting that multiple histological sections from the septum and left ventricular free walls should always be taken and observed.

There is a question of whether we should recognize within the spectrum of ARVC/D a condition of "pure" left ventricular involvement, without any ev-

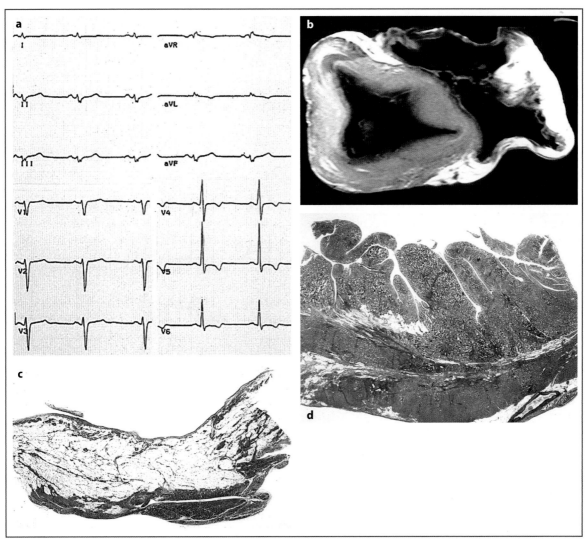

Fig. 4.8 • A 35-year-old man who died suddenly with an in vivo diagnosis of ARVC/D with biventricular involvement belonging to a family found positive at genetic screening for desmoplakin mutation. (**a**) 12 lead ECG shows low voltage QRS complexes and inverted T waves in the lateral leads. (**b**) In vitro spin-echo cardiac magnetic resonance, short axis cut, shows biventricular dilatation, transmural fatty infiltration of the right ventricular free wall and spots of fatty tissue in the postero-lateral left ventricular free wall. (**c**) Panoramic histologic section of the right ventricular free wall transmural fibro-fatty replacement of the myocardium (Heidenhain trichrome). (**d**) Panoramic histologic section of the left ventricular lateral wall: fibro-fatty with prevalent fibrous tissue replacement is evident in the subepicardial and midmural layers (Heidenhain trichrome)

idence of right ventricular abnormalities, and whether we should update the disease nomenclature [57, 58]. The diagnosis of ARVC/D has been always a challenge both clinically and at autopsy. For this reason, standardized diagnostic criteria have been proposed and, as far as pathology is concerned, the presence of "transmural fatty or fibro-fatty myocardial replacement of the right ventricular free wall" has been usually considered the *conditio sine qua non* for diagnosis. This could explain why several cases with isolated left ventricular disease escaped the diagnosis of ARVC/D and were labeled as chronic myocarditis. Interestingly, in a study of ARVC/D as a

cause of sudden death in Spain, Aguilera et al. [59] widened the inclusion criterion, by considering subepicardial or transmural fibro-fatty replacement of the ventricular, either left or right, myocardium. Based upon this definition, they found that ARVC/D accounted for 21 out of 264 (6.8%) sudden deaths in people less than 35 years of age. Noteworthy, it was mostly consistent with biventricular disease (62%), whereas isolated left ventricular or right ventricular involvement were each present in 19% of cases.

Collett et al. [60] reported two cases of sudden cardiac death with histopathological analysis, one showing extensive left ventricular fibrolipomatous infiltration in the setting of a completely normal right ventricle. In 1995 Okabe et al. [61] first proposed the possibility of isolated "arrhythmogenic left ventricular dysplasia," by reporting an unusual case of a patient who presented with ventricular tachycardia originating from the left ventricle who had severe left ventricular dysfunction and who eventually developed intractable heart failure. At autopsy, there was fibro-fatty replacement confined to the left ventricle, with normal coronary arteries. Since then there have been other articles, mostly single case reports with isolated or prevalent left ventricular involvement [62-65]. Recently our group reported the autopsy findings of a proband who died suddenly and belonged to a family with desmoplakin mutation, that showed massive left ventricular myocardial injury and only mild right ventricular involvement [36]. Soon after, Norman et al. [57] reported a family with a desmoplakin mutation, in which the proband presented with sudden death and there was fibro-fatty replacement of the left ventricular myocardium, thus introducing the term of arrhythmogenic left ventricular cardiomyopathy.

We must acknowledge that the left ventricle is more commonly involved in ARVC/D than initially thought and it should be carefully studied with pathologic investigation, both in patients dying suddenly and in those who die or are transplanted due to congestive heart failure. As emphasized previously, in the few publications in which the hearts came from genotyped patients, there was evidence of biventricular disease, either prevalent right or left. More often left ventricular involvement consists of either isolated or prevalent fibrous tissue deposition in the subepicardial or midmural layers, as compared to the usual pathology from the right side. These data suggest that the various locations and amounts of the fibro-fatty tissue are different expressions of the same disease entity. Therefore, consideration should be given to the use of terms like arrhythmogenic cardiomyopathy [66] or desmosomal cardiomyopathy [67].

In Vivo Tissue Characterization by EMB

A definitive diagnosis of ARVC/D relies on histological demonstration of fibro-fatty replacement of ventricular myocardium and it is listed among the major Task Force diagnostic criteria [68].

In vivo, the pathological specimens are obtained through EMB. Right ventricular EMB is a well-established procedure in the diagnosis of heart muscle disease and seems to be particularly helpful in sus-

pected ARVC/D because of the peculiar topographic and histologic features of the disease. The fibro-fatty replacement is almost transmural exclusively in the right ventricular free wall, whereas the septum is usually spared and the left ventricular free wall, when affected, shows involvement of the subepicardial-mid layers. To avoid false negative results, biopsies should not be taken from the septum, but the bioptome should be directed to the free wall, with the potential risk of perforation and hemopericardium. However, clinically relevant complications from EMB sampling are rare and are estimated at 1%-2%, with death as an exceptionally rare event (less than 0.2%) [69].

In the 1994 Task Force diagnostic criteria only a qualitative analysis of EMB samples was mentioned in terms of fibro-fatty replacement [68]. However, we should recognize that the histopathologic findings of fatty or fibrous tissue in the myocardium is far from specific, since fatty infiltration frequently occurs in the right ventricle in the elderly and obese population [70], and fibrosis can be observed in many cardiomyopathic and noncardiomyopathic conditions [71-75].

The key to diagnosis pertains to the site and quantity rather than to quality of myocardial tissue replacement [76]. Quantitative diagnostic parameters have been established by histomorphometric analysis of EMBs from patients with suspected ARVC/D, dilated cardiomyopathy and controls. Angelini et al. [76, 77] obtained the following diagnostic parameters in ARVC/D: myocardial atrophy with residual myocytes less than 45% of the EMB cross sectional area, fibrous tissue >40% and fatty tissue>3%, with a 67% sensitivity and a 92% specificity for at least one parameter. It should be emphasized that the morphometric analysis was a mean of the evaluation of all the specimens drawn from the different sites of the right ventricle. It is known that there is a difference in the percentage of tissue parameters among the different specimens, since the disease is frequently segmental and, at times, only one specimen can be informative (Figs. 6.9, 6.10).

In 1992, Pinamonti et al. [78] reported moderate-severe fatty infiltration in 50% of EMBs taken from 25 ARVC/D patients, and it was associated with fibrosis in about half of the cases. No fat was detected in six left ventricular EMBs, but fibrosis associated with hypertrophy and myocyte attenuation was evident. Similar features were found in the Mayo Clinic experience, who reported right ventricular EMB findings with adequate tissue sampling in 13 affected patients [79]. Since the authors considered the presence of abnormal amounts of adipose tissue as diagnostic in either EMB specimens or explanted hearts, only 54% of patients had characteristic histo-

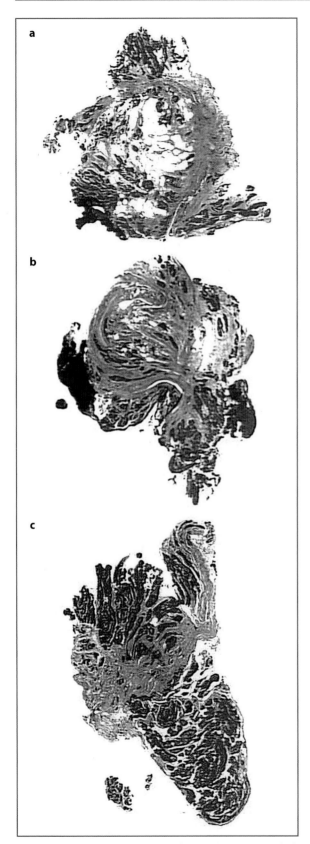

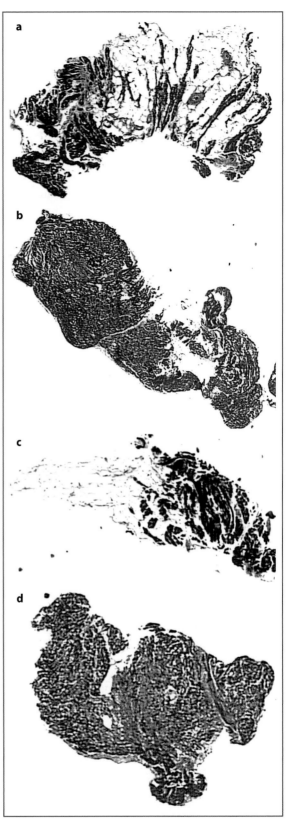

Fig. 4.9 • Endomyocardial biopsy findings in a proband affected by a diffuse form of ARVC/D: all the three bioptic samples (**a**, **b**, **c**) present extensive fibro-fatty tissue replacement

Fig. 4.10 • Endomyocardial biopsy findings in a proband affected by a localized form of ARVC/D: only two (**a**, **c**) out of four bioptic samples have either extensive or focal fibro-fatty tissue replacement, whereas the remaining two are normal (**b**, **d**)

logic features of ARVC/D, while in the remaining 46% only myocyte hypertrophy and interstitial fibrosis were detected. In four patients who had left ventricular EMB, no fatty infiltration was evident, and only myopathic changes were present.

In the series by Wichter et al. [80], abnormal fibro-fatty or fatty tissue infiltration exceeding an area of 25% in one or more biopsy samples, taken from different regions of the right ventricle, was considered a diagnostic feature of ARVC/D. Based upon this definition, EMB resulted diagnostic in 66% of patients, whereas it was normal in 28% and nonspecific in 6%.

Daliento et al. [38] compared EMB findings in 12 young vs. 17 adult patients with ARVC/D. By strictly applying the histomorphometric criteria [76], only 25% of the young and 35% of the adult patients would have had a histopathologic diagnosis at EMB. No difference was found as far as the amount of myocardium was concerned, whereas in the younger group a greater amount of fibrous tissue and a lower amount of fatty tissue were found. In ten young patients there were no adipocytes. The low prevalence of diagnostic EMBs on the basis of histomorphometric data may be the result of either sampling error in segmental forms of ARVC/D or of the fact that, in the early stages of the disease, histological abnormalities may be restricted to subepicardial regions which are not accessible through EMB.

In a clinical-pathologic study correlating EMB findings with cardiac imaging and electrocardiographic data, fibrous substitution (>30%) was a significant univariate predictor of late potentials in the signal-averaged electrocardiogram and of reduced right ventricular ejection fraction, whereas fatty tissue, traditionally considered a more specific histomorphometric parameter, did not correlate with any clinical feature [81]. This is in contrast with the findings by Chimenti et al. [82], who demonstrated more evident fatty replacement in the EMB samples taken from the areas with more prominent morphofunctional abnormalities.

To clarify the issue, we recently carried out an in vitro EMB study by simulating endocardial sampling in archival heart specimens in different sites of the right ventricle as well as in the left ventricle [83]. According to our data, a ≤64% of residual myocardium in right ventricular samples should be considered as a diagnostic cut-off for ARVC/D, with a sensitivity of 80% and a specificity of 90%. Mean fatty tissue is a less reliable diagnostic histologic parameter, since there are no statistically significant differences when comparing ARVC/D vs. the adipositas cordis and the elderly, whereas fibrous tissue is in-

creased both in ARVC/D and in dilated cardiomyopathy. When considering the sampling site from the right ventricular apex, the amount of fatty tissue in ARVC/D is higher than in dilated cardiomyopathy, but no significant differences are found vs. controls, adipositas cordis and the elderly, thus indicating that fatty tissue is mostly nonspecific, particularly at the apex, whereas the residual myocardium and fibrous tissue appear the most relevant diagnostic parameters. Finally, no significant differences were found among the groups when considering the septum and the left ventricle, clearly confirming that septal and left ventricular EMB are not useful for diagnostic purposes in ARVC/D. Although histomorphometric evaluation is mandatory, a careful qualitative assessment of residual myocytes as well as of characteristics of fibrosis and adipocytes may be also of help and sometimes crucial to the final correct diagnosis (Fig. 4.4).

EMB for Differential Diagnosis Between ARVC/D and Other Arrhythmias with Right Ventricular Origin

EMB can aid in the differential diagnosis between ARVC/D and other diseases that can mimic ARVC/D, such as dilated cardiomyopathy, myocarditis, and idiopathic right ventricular outflow tract tachycardia.

Nava et al. [84] first demonstrated the role of EMB in revealing concealed forms of ARVC/D as a cause of apparently idiopathic ventricular arrhythmias, since they observed myocardial atrophy with fibrous-fatty substitution by right ventricular EMB. Recently, by correlating abnormal voltage mapping with myocardial atrophy and fibrofatty replacement at EMB, we also confirmed an underlying segmental form of ARVC/D at risk of life-threatening events in a subgroup of patients with apparently idiopathic right ventricular outflow tract tachycardia [85].

Chimenti et al. [82] found that only 30% of patients with sporadic ARVC/D had diagnostic histologic features of ARVC/D at EMB, while the majority had myocarditis according to Dallas criteria. That myocarditis can mimic the clinical picture of ARVC/D was also reported recently by our group in a study comparing CARTO electroanatomic mapping with EMB features [86]. The differential diagnosis is important, since prognosis and treatment are different.

Sarcoidosis deserves special mention because affected patients may present with clinical and morphological features of ARVC/D, including typical ECG features like epsilon wave and left bundle branch block ventricular tachycardia [87-89]. Recently, Koplan et al. [89] reported a series of eight patients with recurrent monomorphic ventricular tachycardia due to cardiac sarcoid, two of whom had a previous presumptive diagnosis of ARVC/D. A differential diagnosis by EMB is important, since treatment with corticosteroids may benefit patients with sarcoidosis, although results of this therapy remain controversial.

Idiopathic giant cell myocarditis may be confused with sarcoidosis, although the former is a much more fulminant disease. Okura et al. [90] recently compared the two entities and found that both conditions frequently had ventricular tachycardia, although a longer duration of symptoms and the presence of heart block should suggest sarcoidosis.

EMB to Validate Cardiac Imaging Techniques for Tissue Characterization

EMB is the only tool available for in vivo tissue characterization of the right ventricular free wall. However, it is an invasive procedure which carries a certain risk of complications, thus raising ethical concerns. For these reasons, efforts have been made to identify an alternative diagnostic tool able to provide an in vivo tissue characterization and EMB has been used as the reference standard to validate the sensitivity and specificity.

Among imaging techniques, cardiac magnetic resonance has been first employed for differentiating fatty tissue from normal myocardium, through spin echo T1-weighted pulse sequences, but its diagnostic accuracy remains uncertain [91]. Our group first compared the diagnostic accuracy of EMB vs. spin echo cardiac magnetic resonance in patients with the clinical diagnosis of ARVC/D and we found that EMB sensitivity was higher than that of spin echo magnetic resonance (89% vs. 56%) in diagnosing ARVC/D [92]. More recently, the additional diagnostic value of cardiac magnetic resonance has been shown using delayed-enhancement after contrast medium gadolinium administration in order to evaluate the presence of fibrous tissue replacement. To this regard, Tandri et al. [93] reported an excellent correlation between delayed-enhancement magnetic resonance and histopathologic findings on EMB. This resulted in the superiority of the former technique in diagnosing ARVC/D, since it can reveal segmental forms, which could be not be detected by EMB due to sampling error, as well as left ventricular involvement. The latter finding is important, since left ventricular involvement may not be detected by EMB due to subepicardial-midwall location of fibro-fatty replacement.

Finally, we demonstrated the value of three-dimensional electro-anatomic voltage mapping for the diagnosis of ARVC/D, by showing that right ventricular fibro-fatty myocardial replacement at EMB corresponds to positive CARTO mapping with low voltage areas [85].

In conclusion, EMB is a relatively safe interventional procedure, which is useful to assess and diagnose ARVC/D. However, since it is an invasive procedure, we must consider ethical and legal issues when advising the procedure. EMB can be useful in patients presenting with ventricular arrhythmias when a diagnosis of ARVC/D is suspected but not established with other noninvasive techniques. Both the clinician and the pathologist should appreciate that the interpretation of EMB specimens requires knowledge of the patient's clinical history as well as the location of the biopsy. The recognition of ARVC/D and the differential diagnosis with other diseases, such as myocarditis and sarcoidosis, influences the type of therapy, risk stratification, and prognosis.

Acknowledgements

This study was supported by Ministry of Health and Telethon, Rome, and ARVC/D Project, QLG1-CT-2000-01091 5th Framework Programme European Commission, Bruxelles

References

1. Richardson P, McKenna WJ, Bristow M et al (1996) Report of the 1995 WHO/ISFC task force on the definition of cardiomyopathies. Circulation 93:841-842
2. Marcus FI, Fontaine G, Guiraudon G et al (1982) Right ventricular dysplasia. A report of 24 adult cases. Circulation 65:384-398
3. Thiene G, Nava A, Corrado D et al (1988) Right ventricular cardiomyopathy and sudden death in young people. N Engl J Med 318:129-133
4. Basso C, Thiene G, Corrado D et al (1996) Arrhythmogenic right ventricular cardiomyopathy. Dysplasia, dystrophy or myocarditis? Circulation 94:983-991
5. Thiene G, Basso C (2001) Arrhythmogenic right ventricular cardiomyopathy. An update. Cardiovasc Pathol 10:109-111
6. Nava A, Rossi L, Thiene G (eds) (1997) Arrhythmogenic right ventricular cardiomyopathy/dysplasia. Elsevier, Amsterdam
7. Corrado D, Basso C, Thiene G et al (1997) Spectrum of clinicopathologic manifestations of arrhythmogenic right ventricular cardiomyopathy/dysplasia: A multicenter study. J Am Coll Cardiol 30:1512-1520

70. Kitzman DW, Scholz DG, Hagen PT et al (1988) Age-related changes in normal human hearts during the first 10 decades of life. Part II (Maturity): A quantitative anatomic study of 765 specimens from subjects 20 to 99 years old. Mayo Clin Proc 63:137-146

71. Unverferth DV, Baker PB, Swift SE et al (1986) Extent of myocardial fibrosis and cellular hypertrophy in dilated cardiomyopathy. Am J Cardiol 57:816-820

72. Olsen EG (1979) The pathology of cardiomyopathies. A critical analysis. Am Heart J 98:385-392

73. Roberts WC, Ferrans UJ, Buja LM (1974) Pathologic aspects of the idiopathic cardiomyopathies. Adv Cardiol 13:349-367

74. Edwards WD (1987) Cardiomyopathies. Hum Pathol 18:625-635

75. Gravanis MB, Ansari AA (1987) Idiopathic cardiomyopathies. A review of pathologic studies and mechanisms of pathogenesis. Arch Pathol Lab Med 111:915-929

76. Angelini A, Basso C, Nava A, Thiene G (1996) Endomyocardial biopsy in arrhythmogenic right ventricular cardiomyopathy. Am Heart J 132:203-206

77. Angelini A, Thiene G, Boffa GM et al (1993) Endomyocardial biopsy in right ventricular cardiomyopathy. Int J Cardiol 40:273-282

78. Pinamonti B, Sinagra G, Salvi A et al (1992) Left ventricular involvement in right ventricular dysplasia. Am Heart J 123:711-724

79. Kullo IJ, Edwards WD, Seward JB (1995) Right ventricular dysplasia: The Mayo Clinic Experience. Mayo Clin Proc 70:541-548

80. Wichter T, Hindricks G, Lerch H et al (1994) Regional myocardial sympathetic dysinnervation in arrhythmogenic right ventricular cardiomyopathy. An analysis using 123I-meta-iodobenzylguanidine scintigraphy. Circulation 89:667-683

81. Turrini P, Angelini A, Thiene G et al (1999) Late potentials and ventricular arrhythmias in arrhythmogenic right ventricular cardiomyopathy. Am J Cardiol 83:1214-1219

82. Chimenti C, Pieroni M, Maseri A et al (2004) Histologic findings in patients with clinical and instrumental diagnosis of sporadic arrhythmogenic right ventricular dysplasia. J Am Coll Cardiol 43:2305-2313

83. Basso C, Ronco F, Abudureheman A, Thiene G (2006) In vitro validation of endomyocardial biopsy for the in vivo diagnosis of arrhythmogenic right ventricular cardiomyopathy. Eur Heart J 27:960

84. Nava A, Thiene G, Canciani B et al (1992) Clinical profile of concealed form of arrhythmogenic right ventricular cardiomyopathy presenting with apparently idiopathic ventricular arrhythmias. Int J Cardiol 35:195-206

85. Corrado D, Tokajuk B, Leoni L et al (2005) Differential diagnosis between idiopathic right ventricular outflow tract tachycardia and ARVC/D by 3-d electroanatomic voltage mapping. Eur Heart J 26:373 (Abstract)

86. Corrado D, Basso C, Leoni L et al (2005) Three-dimensional electroanatomic voltage mapping increases accuracy of diagnosing arrhythmogenic right ventricular cardiomyopathy/dysplasia. Circulation 111:3042-3050

87. Ott P, Marcus FI, Sobonya RE et al (2003) Cardiac sarcoidosis masquerading as right ventricular dysplasia. Pacing Clin Electrophysiol 26:1498-1503

88. Santucci P, Morton JB, Picken MM et al (2004) Electroanatomic mapping of the right ventricle in a patient with giant epsilon wave, ventricular tachycardia and cardiac sarcoidosis. J Cardiovasc Electrophysiol 15:1091-1094

89. Koplan BA, Soejima K, Baughman K et al (2006) Refractory ventricular tachycardia secondary to cardiac sarcoid: Electrophysiologic characteristics, mapping, and ablation. Heart Rhythm 3:924-929

90. Okura Y, Dec GW, Hare JM et al (2003) A clinical and histopathologic comparison of cardiac sarcoidosis and idiopathic giant cell myocarditis. J Am Coll Cardiol 41:322-329

91. Bluemke DA, Krupinski EA, Ovitt T et al (2003) MR Imaging of arrhythmogenic right ventricular cardiomyopathy: Morphologic findings and interobserver reliability. Cardiology 99:153-162

92. Menghetti L, Basso C, Nava A et al (1996) Spin-echo nuclear magnetic resonance for tissue characterisation in arrhythmogenic right ventricular cardiomyopathy. Heart 76:467-470

93. Tandri H, Saranathan M, Rodriguez ER et al (2005) Noninvasive detection of myocardial fibrosis in arrhythmogenic right ventricular cardiomyopathy using delayed-enhancement magnetic resonance imaging. J Am Coll Cardiol 45:98-103

CHAPTER 5

CELL ADHESION PATHOLOGY

Jeffrey E. Saffitz

Introduction

Significant progress has been made in identifying single gene mutations responsible for causing human cardiomyopathies. Although many of these monogenic cardiomyopathies are rare, insights into pathogenesis by identification of the responsible mutations can provide clues about mechanisms in more common forms of heart disease. We have studied a group of human cardiomyopathies caused by mutations in genes encoding proteins that function as linkers in cell-cell adhesion junctions. These heart diseases, which we have termed *cell-cell junction cardiomyopathies*, are caused by mutations in intracellular proteins that link adhesion molecules at adherens junctions and desmosomes to the myocyte cytoskeleton. Among the genes implicated in these diseases are those encoding desmoplakin, plakoglobin, and plakophilin-2. These mutations have both dominant and recessive patterns of inheritance and are associated with clinical phenotypes of arrhythmogenic right ventricular cardiomyopathy/dysplasia (ARVC/D) or dilat cardiomyopathy (DCM), with or without hair and skin abnormalities [1]. Common features of the cell-cell junction cardiomyopathies are a high incidence of syncope, ventricular arrhythmias, and sudden cardiac death. This observation suggests that alterations in intercellular adhesion caused by defects in cell-cell mechanical junctions may create anatomic substrates that are particularly conducive to the development of lethal ventricular arrhythmias. Our work in this area has focused on the hypothesis that defective mechanical linkage in the cell-cell junction cardiomyopathies causes remodeling of gap junctions, which, in turn, can give rise to conduction abnormalities that may contribute to the high incidence of sudden death in these patients.

Electrical Coupling at Gap Junctions in the Heart

Cardiac muscle is not a true electrical syncytium. Rather, it is composed of individual cells, each invested with a continuous lipid bilayer which provides a considerable degree of electrical insulation. Electrical activation of the heart requires intercellular transfer of current, a process that can only occur at gap junctions [2]. Thus, the number, size, and distribution of gap junctions are important determinants of impulse propagation in cardiac muscle. Furthermore, alterations in the structure or function of gap junctions can give rise to conduction disturbances that may contribute to arrhythmogenesis.

There is an intimate structural, functional, and spatial relationship between gap junctions and mechanical junctions in cardiac myocytes. Cardiac myocytes are connected by extremely large intercellular junctions, which, presumably, have evolved to subserve the specialized electrical and contractile function of these cells. For example, because cardiac myocytes contract, they require more extensive and robust adhesion junctions than noncontractile cells in other solid organs. It is no surprise, therefore, that adherens junctions and desmosomes, organelles responsible for physically connecting one cardiac myocyte to another, are highly concentrated at the ends of individual cells where they form elaborate complexes that can be readily identified at the light microscopic level of resolution and which have been given a specific name – the *intercalated disk*. Intercalated disks are composed mainly of arrays of adherens junctions, each located at the end of a row of sarcomeres. These junctions act as bridges which link actin filaments within sarcomeres of neighboring cells. Interspersed among the adherens junctions are desmosomes, which also provide mechanical coupling and link cell-cell adhesion junctions to desmin filaments of the cytoskeleton. Because electrical activation of the heart requires intercellular transfer of current, cardiac myocytes also have a special requirement for extensive electrical coupling. Indeed, gap junctions interconnecting ventricular myocytes are among the largest in living systems, presumably reflecting a need for many low-resistance electrical communicating channels between cells to ensure safe conduction.

However, membrane regions containing gap junctions are rigid and nonfluid because of the high concentration of protein within the lipid bilayer, and as a result, these regions are vulnerable to shear stress. It is no surprise, therefore, that gap junctions in cardiac myocytes are located at intercalated disks where they are virtually surrounded by mechanical junctions. Presumably, these mechanical junctions act like "spot welds" to create membrane domains that are protected from shear stress caused by contractile activities of neighboring cells and which facilitate assembly and maintenance of large arrays of intercellular electrical channels. On the basis of these and related observations, we have proposed that the extent to which cardiac myocytes can become electrically coupled depends on their degree of mechanical coupling [3]. As shown in Fig. 5.1, this hypothesis provides a mechanistic link between contractile dysfunction and electrical dysfunction in the cell-cell junction cardiomyopathies. A genetic defect in a protein in cell-cell adhesion junctions may lead to unstable mechanical linkage between cells and/or discontinuities between cell-cell junctions and the cardiac myocyte cytoskeleton. Such defective mechanical linkage may lead to diminished force transmission which, in turn, can lead to myocyte injury, tissue remodeling, and a clinical picture characterized by contractile dysfunction and cardiomyopathy. In addition, abnormal mechanical linkage can destabilize the sarcolemmas of adjacent cells. This may lead to gap junction remodeling which could contribute to slow conduction, arrhythmias, and sudden death in patients with cell-cell junction cardiomyopathies. As briefly presented below, we have tested this hypothesis through multiple approaches. First, we have characterized the distribution of intercalated disk proteins in cardiac tissues from patients and have shown that, as a general rule, the cell-cell junction cardiomyopathies are associated with remodeling of gap junctions. Second, we have identified electrophysiological phenotypes in genetically engineered mouse models of the human cardiomyopathies. Third, we have elucidated signaling pathways that coordinately regulate expression of mechanical and electrical junction proteins in cardiac myocytes in response to mechanical stress.

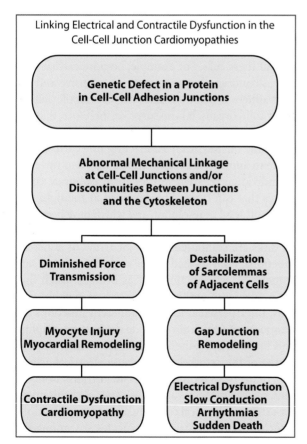

Fig. 5.1 • A flow chart illustrating a proposed mechanism linking electrical and contractile dysfunction in the cell-cell junction cardiomyopathies

Altered Expression and Distribution of Cell-Cell Junction Proteins in Human Cardiomyopathies

To test the hypothesis that defects in the adhesion junction-cytoskeleton network disrupt gap junctions, we analyzed ventricular tissues from patients with Naxos disease, a cardiocutaneous syndrome consisting of the clinical triad of woolly hair, palmoplantar keratoderma, and ARVC/D [4]. Patients with Naxos disease are readily identified early in life because of the distinctive cutaneous features (the disease is 100% penetrant) [5, 6]. Naxos disease is associated with a particularly high incidence of sudden cardiac death. Approximately 60% of affected children present with syncope and/or aborted sudden death, and the annual risk of arrhythmic death is 2.3% [6]. Naxos disease is caused by a recessive mutation in the gene encoding plakoglobin [7]. The mutation is a deletion of nucleotides 2157 and 2158 which causes a frame-shift resulting in premature termination and expression of a truncated protein lacking 56 residues at the C-terminus [7]. We characterized the distribution of cell-cell junction proteins in fixed ventricular tissues from autopsy of Naxos disease patients using confocal immunofluorescence microscopy, and also performed immunoblotting analysis on frozen, unfixed cardiac tissue from an affected child who died of acute leukemia before overt clinical or pathological evidence of ARVC/D had developed. Im-

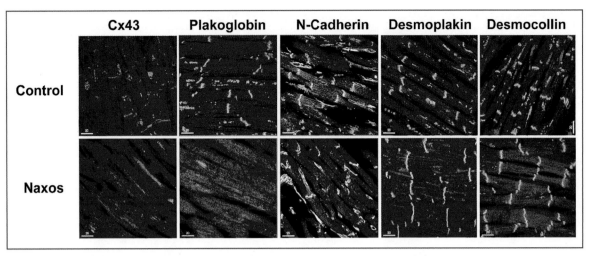

Fig. 5.2 • Representative confocal microscopy images of left ventricle from control and Naxos disease stained with specific antibodies against selected intercellular junction proteins

munoreactive signal for plakoglobin, the mutant protein in Naxos disease, was dramatically reduced at intercalated disks in both ventricles from all Naxos disease patients whereas signals for N-cadherin, desmoplakin and desmocollin-2 appeared to be normal (Fig. 5.2) [4]. There was also a striking reduction in the amount of junctional signal for connexin43 (Cx43), the major ventricular gap junction protein, in both the right and left ventricles in Naxos disease, including the individual who died before ARVC/D had become manifest clinically or pathologically (Fig. 5.2) [4]. Electron microscopy revealed smaller and fewer gap junctions interconnecting ventricular myocytes, providing independent evidence of gap junction remodeling. Immunoblotting revealed that truncated plakoglobin was expressed abundantly in the myocardium even though it failed to localize normally at intercellular junctions. Similarly, although Cx43 signal at gap junctions was dramatically reduced, total Cx43 protein content assessed by immunoblotting showed little or no reduction. However, the highly phosphorylated P2-isoform of Cx43, which is selectively located in the junctional pool, was missing [4]. These observations suggest that remodeling of gap junctions in Naxos disease is not related to changes in Cx43 expression *per se*, but rather to an inability to assemble and/or maintain large gap junction channel arrays. The degree of gap junction remodeling observed in Naxos disease patients is sufficient to cause conduction slowing, which could contribute to the characteristic widening of the QRS complex in the right precordial leads. Although uncoupling at gap junctions may not, by itself, cause arrhythmias, it could produce a substrate that promotes arrhythmias when combined with a "second

insult" such as the pathological changes in the right ventricle in ARVC/D.

We have also characterized the distribution of cell-cell junction proteins in Carvajal syndrome, a cardiocutaneous syndrome characterized by woolly hair, palmoplantar keratoderma, and a diffuse cardiomyopathy that is distinct from ARVC/D [8]. Complex ventricular arrhythmias and conduction disturbances are prominent in Carvajal syndrome. Affected children usually die before the age of 20, apparently due to both pump dysfunction and lethal arrhythmias [8]. Carvajal syndrome is caused by a recessive single nucleotide deletion mutation in desmoplakin leading to a premature stop-codon and truncation of the C-terminal desmin-binding domain [9]. We described the pathology of Carvajal syndrome and analyzed the distribution of cell-cell junction proteins in the heart of an 11-year-old girl from Ecuador [10]. The heart was markedly enlarged. The left ventricle was widely dilated and showed shallow posterior and antero-septal aneurysms with mural thrombosis (Fig. 5.3). The right ventricle also showed discrete aneurysms involving inferior, atypical, and infundibular regions (Fig. 5.3). Interestingly, these same right ventricular areas also show the greatest abnormalities in ARVC/D (the so-called triangle of dysplasia), but there was no gross or microscopic evidence of fatty replacement of right or left ventricular muscle in Carvajal Syndrome. Confocal microscopy revealed that immunoreactive signals for both desmoplakin (the mutant protein) and plakoglobin were markedly diminished at intercalated disks, presumably reflecting altered interactions between these two binding partners [10]. The intermediate filament protein desmin was distributed in a normal sarcomeric pattern but it failed to local-

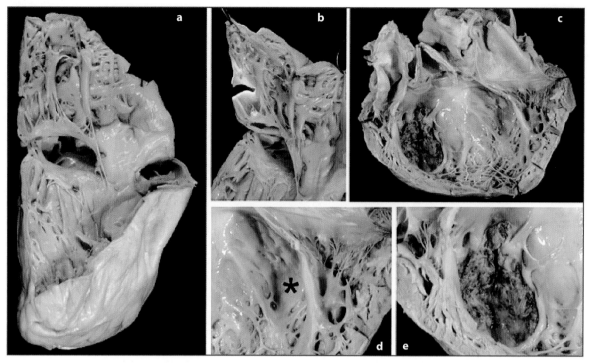

Fig. 5.3 • Gross photographs of the right (**a**, **b**) and left (**c-e**) sides of the heart in Carvajal syndrome. Both ventricles contained discrete regions of aneurysmal wall thinning. Affected areas included the subtricuspid posterior right ventricle (transilluminated area in **b**), the posterior basal portion of the left ventricle (area marked by *asterisk* in **d**), and the antero-septal portion of the left ventricle which was lined by a mural thrombus (**e**)

ize properly at intercalated disks. This indicates that interactions between desmin and desmoplakin are disrupted in Carvajal Syndrome, which, according to our hypothesis, would cause remodeling of gap junctions. As predicted, Cx43 signal at junctions was markedly diminished. These results provide further evidence that abnormal protein-protein interactions at intercellular junctions cause both contractile and electrical dysfunction in Carvajal Syndrome.

Taken together, our studies of human cell-cell junction cardiomyopathies have led to two major conclusions: (1) remodeling of gap junctions is a consistent and prominent feature of the cell-cell junction cardiomyopathies, and (2) specific patterns of abnormal localization of mechanical junction proteins at intercalated disks correlate with cardiomyopathy disease phenotypes.

Mouse Models of Human Cardiomyopathies

Delineation of structural and molecular pathology in human tissues is essential to understanding the cell-cell junction cardiomyopathies; yet to elucidate mechanisms of disease, we have turned to analysis of mouse models.

The first mouse line we characterized was a model of human desmin-related cardiomyopathy created by X.J. Wang in the laboratory of Jeffrey Robbins [11]. We were attracted to this model because we anticipated that it might exhibit altered desmin-desmosome interactions and, therefore, recapitulate Carvajal syndrome. Human desmin-related skeletal and cardiomyopathies have been attributed to a 7-amino acid deletion mutation (R173-E179) and several missense mutations in desmin. To determine whether the R173-E179 deletion was sufficient to cause desmin-related cardiomyopathy, Wang et al. [11] produced transgenic mice with cardiac-specific expression of the 7-amino acid deletion mutation in desmin (D7-des) implicated in the human disease. In their initial description of this model, they showed that D7-des mice exhibit features of human desmin-related cardiomyopathy including intracellular accumulation of desmin, disruption of the desmin filament network, misalignment of myofibrils, and diminished responsiveness to α-adrenergic agonist stimulation [11].

To test the hypothesis that expression of D7-des disrupts the linkage between desmosomes and the cytoskeleton and leads to remodeling of gap junctions, we characterized the expression and localization of intercellular junction proteins and searched for an elec-

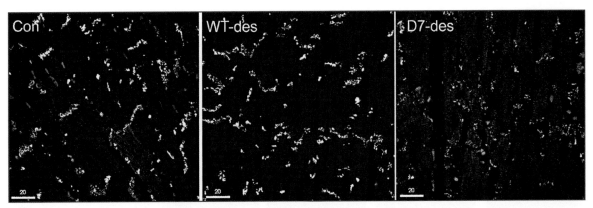

Fig. 5.4 • Representative confocal immunofluorescence images showing the amount of Cx43 immunoreactive signal at cell-cell junctions in left ventricular myocardium from a nontransgenic control mouse (Con), a transgenic mouse expressing wild-ype desmin (WT-des), and a transgenic mouse expressing D7-des

trophysiological phenotype [12]. As predicted by studies of the human cell-cell junction cardiomyopathies, Cx43 signal at intercalated disks was decreased by approximately threefold in D7-des hearts due to significant reductions in both the number and mean size of individual gap junctions (Fig. 5.4). The amount of immunoreactive signal at intercalated disks was also reduced significantly for selected adhesion molecules and linker proteins of both desmosomes and adherens junctions, and desmin-desmosomal interactions were completely disrupted [12]. Quantitative electron microscopy showed decreased gap junction density in D7-des mice, providing independent evidence of gap junction remodeling, but immunoblotting showed no reduction in the total tissue content of Cx43 and mechanical junction proteins. These observations are consistent with findings in Naxos disease, suggesting that diminished localization of cell-cell junction proteins at intercalated disks is not due to insufficient protein expression but, rather, to failure of these proteins to assemble properly within electrical and mechanical junctions. We also showed, using optical mapping, that remodeling of gap junctions in D7-des mice slows ventricular conduction [12]. These results indicate, therefore, that a defect in a protein conventionally thought to fulfill a strictly mechanical function in the heart can also lead to electrophysiological alterations that may contribute to arrhythmogenesis.

Mechanisms Regulating Expression of Cell-Cell Junction Proteins in Response to Mechanical Load

To elucidate mechanisms regulating expression of intercellular junction proteins, we developed an in vitro system in which monolayers of neonatal rat ventricular myocytes are grown on silicone membranes and subjected to uniaxial pulsatile stretch [13]. Imposition of this mechanical load rapidly induces a hypertrophic response which can be rigorously quantified and characterized. An important feature of this response is a marked increase in Cx43 expression and enhanced intercellular coupling. After only 1h of stretch (110% of resting length at 3 Hz), expression of Cx43 is increased by approximately twofold, resulting in a significant increase in both the number of gap junctions and the velocity of impulse propagation [13]. We have shown previously that upregulation of Cx43 expression is mediated by stretch-induced secretion of vascular endothelial growth factor (VEGF) which acts in an autocrine fashion [14]. Incubation of cells with exogenous VEGF for 1h increases Cx43 expression by an amount roughly equal to that seen after 1h of pulsatile stretch. Moreover, stretch-induced upregulation of Cx43 expression can be blocked by stretching cells in the presence of anti-VEGF or anti-VEGF receptor antibodies.

To determine whether stretch-induced formation of new gap junctions requires concomitant assembly of new mechanical junctions, we measured changes in mechanical junction protein expression in cells subjected to stretch [15]. The amounts of plakoglobin, desmoplakin, and N-cadherin at cell-cell junctions all increased by at least twofold in myocytes subjected to 1h of pulsatile stretch (Fig. 5.5). However, VEGF secretion plays no role in this process. For example, addition of exogenous VEGF does not affect plakoglobin, desmoplakin, or N-cadherin expression, nor is stretch-induced upregulation of these proteins blocked by anti-VEGF antibodies. To further define the responsible mechanisms, we studied the role of focal adhesion kinase (FAK), which is phosphorylated in response to integrin engagement and activates

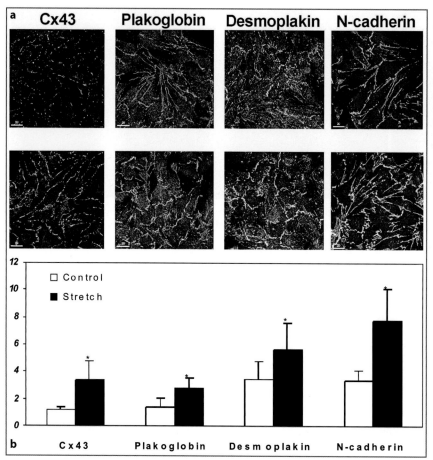

Fig. 5.5 • Representative confocal immunofluorescence images (**a**) (top = control, bottom = stretch and quantitative confocal microscopy data (**b**) showing the effects of stretch on expression of Cx43 and the mechanical junction proteins, plakoglobin, desmoplakin, and N-cadherin. *p<0.05 compared with control

multiple intracellular signaling molecules including src kinase. We infected cardiac myocytes with an adenovirus containing GFP-FRNK, a GFP-tagged dominant-negative inhibitor of FAK-dependant signaling, and then subjected cells to pulsatile stretch [15]. FRNK blocked stretch-induced upregulation of both electrical (Cx43) and mechanical (N-cadherin, desmoplakin, and plakoglobin) junction proteins. Infection of cells with virus expressing GFP alone had no effect. Addition of exogenous VEGF to FRNK-infected cells upregulated expression of Cx43 but not mechanical junction proteins. Conditioned medium removed from uninfected cells after 1h of stretch increased Cx43 expression when added to nonstretched cells, and this effect was blocked by anti-VEGF antibodies, but stretch-conditioned medium from FRNK-infected cells had no effect on Cx43 expression. Thus, secretion of VEGF in response to stretch requires activation of FAK. Finally, the src kinase inhibitor PP2 blocked stretch-induced upregulation of mechanical junction proteins but not Cx43 [15]. These results indicate that mechanical load regulates expression of both electrical and mechanical junctions proteins, but by disparate mechanisms. Cx43 expression is regulated by autocrine actions of chemical mediators secreted during stretch, whereas adhesion junction proteins are regulated by intracellular mechanotransduction pathways initiated via FAK and dependent on downstream activation of src kinase.

Conclusions

We have proposed a unified hypothesis that links contractile and electrical dysfunction in the cell-cell junction cardiomyopathies. It is based on the premise that the extent to which cardiac myocytes are coupled mechanically at cell-cell adhesion junctions is a key determinant of the extent to which they can be coupled electrically at gap junctions. Our observations in several human cardiomyopathies indicate that genetic defects in linker proteins such as desmoplakin and plakoglobin can create anatomic substrates of sudden death by remodeling gap junctions. Molecular mechanisms responsible for gap junction remodeling in the cell-cell junction cardiomyopathies are unknown. One possibility is that rates of C×43 synthesis and degradation are unaffected but connexin molecules are unable to assemble properly in gap junctions. It must also be considered, however, that C×43 gene expression may be altered in the cell-cell junction cardiomyopathies. Plakoglobin and other members of the catenin family fulfill both structural and nuclear signaling roles [16]. Disease-related mutations may shift the relative proportions of these proteins within junctional and cytosolic pools, which, in turn, could affect nuclear signaling mediated by plakoglobin, or β-catenin or other related proteins. If, for example, β-catenin substitutes for mutant plakoglobin within cell-cell junctions, then the resultant decrease in the cytosolic pool of β-catenin could lead to diminished expression of C×43 and other proteins under the control of β-catenin signaling. Thus, it is possible and perhaps even likely that both altered mechanical integrity and altered nuclear signaling underlie the pathogenesis of contractile and electrical dysfunction in heart muscle diseases caused by mutations in cell-cell junction proteins.

Acknowledgements

Work in the author's laboratory was supported by grants from the National Institutes of Health, March of Dimes, American Heart Association, and the Sarnoff Endowment.

References

1. Protonotarios N, Tsatsopoulou A (2004) Naxos disease and Carvajal syndrome: cardiocutaneous disorders that highlight the pathogenesis and broaden the spectrum of arrhythmogenic right ventricular cardiomyopathy. Cardiovasc Pathol 13:185-194
2. Saffitz JE, Lerner DL, Yamada KA (2004) Gap junction distribution and regulation in the heart. In: Zipes DP, Jalife J, (eds) Cardiac electrophysiology: From cell to bedside, 4th edn. Saunders, Philadelphia pp 181-191
3. Saffitz JE (2005) Dependence of electrical coupling on mechanical coupling in cardiac myocytes: insights gained from cardiomyopathies caused by defects in cell-cell connections. Ann N Y Acad Sci 1047:336-344
4. Kaplan SR, Gard JJ, Protonotarios N et al (2004) Remodeling of myocyte gap junctions in arrhythmogenic right ventricular cardiomyopathy due to a deletion in plakoglobin (Naxos disease). Heart Rhythm 1:3-11
5. Protonotarios N, Tsatsopoulou AA, Gatzoulis KA (2002) Arrhythmogenic right ventricular cardiomyopathy caused by a deletion in plakoglobin (Naxos disease). Card Electrophysiol Rev 6:72-80
6. Protonotarios N, Tsatsopoulou A, Anastasakis A et al (2001) Genotype-phenotype assessment in autosomal recessive arrhythmogenic right ventricular cardiomyopathy (Naxos disease) caused by a deletion in plakoglobin. J Am Coll Cardiol 38:1477-1484
7. McKoy G, Protonotarios N, Crosby A et al (2000) Identification of a deletion in plakoglobin in arrhythmogenic right ventricular cardiomyopathy with palmoplantar keratoderma and woolly hair (Naxos disease). Lancet 355:2119-2124
8. Carvajal-Huerta L (1998) Epidermolytic palmoplantar keratoderma with woolly hair and dilated cardiomyopathy. J Am Acad Dermatol 39:418-421
9. Norgett EE, Hatsell SJ, Carvajal-Huerta L et al (2000) Recessive mutation in desmoplakin disrupts desmoplakin-intermediate filament interactions and causes dilated cardiomyopathy, woolly hair and keratoderma. Hum Mol Genet 9:2671-2766
10. Kaplan SR, Gard JJ, Carvajal-Huerta L et al (2004) Structural and molecular pathology of the heart in Carvajal syndrome. Cardiovasc Pathol 13:26-32
11. Wang X, Osinska H, Dorn GW 2nd et al (2001) Mouse model of desmin-related cardiomyopathy. Circulation 103:2402-2407
12. Gard JJ, Yamada K, Green KG et al (2005) Remodeling of gap junctions and slow conduction in a mouse model of desmin-related cardiomyopathy. Cardiovasc Res 67:539-547
13. Zhuang J, Yamada KA, Saffitz JE et al (2000) Pulsatile stretch remodels cell-to-cell communication in cultured myocytes. Circ Res 87:316-322
14. Pimentel RC, Yamada KA, Kléber AG et al (2002) Autocrine regulation of C×43 expression by VEGF. Circ Res 90:671-677
15. Yamada K, Green KG, Samarel AM et al (2005) Distinct pathways regulate expression of cardiac electrical and mechanical junctions proteins in response to stretch. Circ Res 97:346-353
16. Conacci-Sorrell M, Zhurinsky J, Ben-Ze'ev A (2002) The cadherin-catenin adhesion system in signaling and cancer. J Clin Invest 109:987-991

CHAPTER 6

ULTRASTRUCTURAL SUBSTRATES

Elzbieta Czarnowska, Mila Della Barbera, Gaetano Thiene, Marialuisa Valente, Cristina Basso

Introduction

There have been extensive studies on the morphological findings and pathogenesis of ARVC/D [1-3]. However, little attention has been directed toward the ultrastructural features of the disease.

The histopathological features of the cardiomyocytes in ARVC/D include loss of myofibrils, cellular hypertrophy or degeneration with dystrophic or pyknotic nuclei, and histochemically proven apoptosis [4-6]. Attention is currently focused on the structure of intercalated discs (IDs) and sarcoplasmic reticulum (SR) due to the gene mutations that have been discovered both in the autosomal recessive (Naxos Disease) and dominant forms of ARVC/D. These mutations affect plakoglobin in Naxos disease [7], desmoplakin [8-11], plakophilin-2 [12], desmoglein-2 [13], and the cardiac ryanodine receptor (RyR2) [14]. Moreover, mutations have been found at the regulatory site of the TGFβ3 [15]. Overexpression of TGFβ3 might explain increased fibrosis and affect cell-cell junction stability in ARVC/D.

ARVC/D has been rarely investigated at the ultrastructural level [16-18]. Therefore, analysis of cardiomyocyte ultrastructure, particularly in endomyocardial biopsy (EMB) tissue and in sections where cardiomyocytes exhibit normal structure under light microscopy, might identify primary cellular defects. This paper reviews cardiomyocyte structure as analyzed by electron microscopy in EMB samples obtained from adolescents and adult patients with a clinical diagnosis of ARVC/D [19].

General Characteristics

To identify specific features of cardiomyocytes in right ventricular tissue obtained from hearts of children and adults with ARVC/D, EMB samples were compared with those from patients with dilated cardiomyopathy (DCM). Donor hearts at cardiac transplantation served as normal control [19].

Adult cardiomyocytes in a normal heart are covered by a ~50-nm thick surface coat, also termed glycocalyx, which forms a continuous layer on the cell membrane. The cardiomyocyte membrane shows specialized regions including the transverse tubular system, termed T-tubules, and the ID. Cells are characterized by a well-developed regular sarcomeric apparatus, oval mitochondria distributed between contractile fibrils, single glycogen particles, and a regular sarcoplasmic reticulum network. Oval nuclei are located in the cell center. Single Golgi apparatus, consisting of flattened cisterns, rough endoplasmic reticulum and single lipofuscin granules are localized in the perinuclear space.

In ARVC/D, there was no impairment of cell membrane continuity or dilatation of sarcoplasmic reticulum cisterns. The T-tubules were normal and there was a variable amount of lipofuscin granules. The nuclei were often highly convoluted and contained dense aggregates of chromatin below the nuclear membrane. In single cardiomyocytes not exhibiting myolytic features, dilated T-tubules and numerous profiles of Golgi apparatus and vacuoles were present (Fig. 6.1a) Abundant glycogen and variously sized lipid droplets were seen in many myocytes. Irregular organization of contractile filaments and widening of Z bands were observed in ARVC/D hearts, similar to that seen in DCM hearts. A characteristic feature of ARVC/D was thickening of the glycocalyx covering the cell membrane in some normal cardiomyocytes (Fig. 6.1b) and a pale structure of ID junctions. Giant lipid droplets were present in some cardiomyocytes (Fig. 6.1c). Such features were not found in DCM. The general characteristics of ARVC/D cardiomyocytes in comparison with DCM and donor transplanted hearts (controls) are presented in Table 6.1.

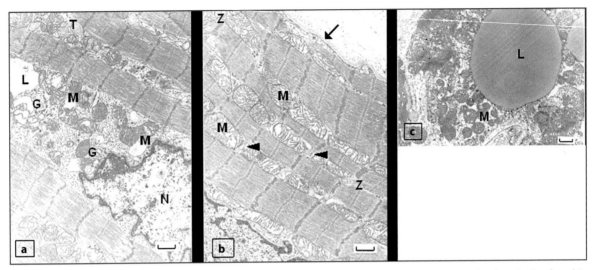

Fig. 6.1 • Electron microscopic images of human ARVC/D cardiomyocytes. **a** Perinuclear region with injured mitochondria (*M*), numerous Golgi (*G*), lipid droplets (*L*), dilated T-tubules (*T*) and highly convoluted nuclear (*N*) membrane. Bar = 600 nm. **b** Widened Z-bands (*Z*), normal mitochondria (*M*) and T-tubules (*arrowhead*), thick glycocalyx (*arrow*) that covers cell membrane. Bar = 600 nm. **c** Cardiomyocyte from ARVC/D heart with giant lipid droplets (*L*) and numerous mitochondria (*M*) and disarrangement of contractile fibrils. Bar = 2 μm

Table 6.1 • General ultrastructural findings

Cell structure	Characteristic	ARVC/D; (21 pts); (%)	DCM; (10 pts); (%)	Controls; (10 pts); (%)
Cell membrane	Continuous	100	100	100
Glycocalyx	Thickening	57	0	0
Nucleus	Highly convoluted	100	35%	5
	Oval in single cells	28,5	0	Numerous
T- tubules	Dilated	76,2	80	0
Sarcoplasmic reticulum	Normal	100	100	100
Mitochondria	Polymorphic	28,5	33,3	10
	Irregular cristae	23,8	13,3	0
	Increased number	80,8	100	37,4
Sarcomers	Normal	90	33,3	100
	Contraction bands	100	30	6,5
Lipofuscin	Various number	100	80	30
Glycogen	Abundant in some cells	100	60	30
Lipid droplets	Various size in single cells	85,7	60	20
	Giant	14	0	0
Vacuoles	Various size	76,2	30	0
Golgi	Numerous	33,3	Single	Single
ID junctions	Pale	80,8	0	0

ARVC/D, arrhythmogenic right ventricular cardiomyopathy; *DCM*, dilated cardiomyopathy; *Pts*=patients

Intercalated Disc Junctions

The ID is the area of end-to-end connections between cardiomyocytes, and consists of three junctional complexes: desmosomes, fascia adherens, and gap junction (also called the nexus). The desmosome is composed of a cytoplasmic electron-dense plaque of intracellular filaments containing desmoplakin, plakoglobin, plakophilin, and transmembrane calcium-sensitive proteins, i.e., desmoglein and desmocollin. In addition to cell-to-cell adhesion, this type of junction provides a structural connection to the intermediate filaments system (i.e., desmin) [20, 21] responsible for mechanical cell-cell stability. The fascia adherens junction consists of complex proteins that link a transmembrane protein, N-cadherin, to catenin and further to sarcomeric actin. This structure transmits contractile force across the sarcolemma [20]. The gap junction consists of transmembrane channels called connexons, which do not connect to the cytoskeleton system, but allow intercellular metabolic communication by transmitting small molecules and electrical stimuli [22].

The growing interest in the intercellular junction is due, in part, to the identification of desmosomal protein-encoding gene mutations in ARVC/D. Also there is evidence that plakoglobin null-mutant mouse embryos show decreased myofiber compliance and reduced cell-cell adhesion as a consequence of defects in desmosome number and structure [23]. Impairment of myocyte cell-to-cell adhesion has been advocated as a possible common pathway in ARVC/D, since failure of desmosome to couple cells will invariably lead to tissue and organ fragility.

The major ultrastructural findings reported in ARVC/D were "pale" junctional structures and flattened ID convolutions [16, 17]. "Paleness" of desmosomes and fascia adherens at the cytoplasmic plaque was confirmed in our study (Fig. 6.2a); however, morphometric analysis of samples from 21 ARVC/D hearts showed normal convoluted ID in comparison with normal hearts (Table 6.2). These findings suggest an abnormal composition of proteins located in the plaque area, i.e., cadherins and cytoplasmic tails of β-catenin, respectively.

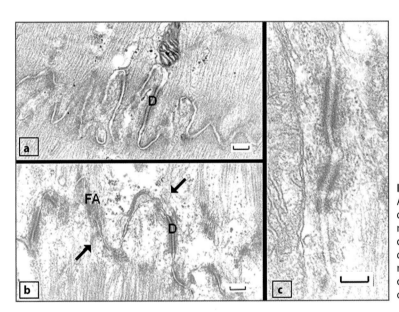

Fig. 6.2 • ID region of cardiomyocytes from ARVC/D hearts. **a** Pale ID with visible long desmosome (*D*) Bar = 200 nm. **b** Abnormal junctional structures of the ID: the fascia adherens junction (*FA*) and long desmosome (*D*) and intersected actin filaments (*arrows*) Bar = 200 nm. **c** Fragment of the ID exhibiting desmosomes of various length. Bar = 200 nm

Table 6.2 • Ultrastructural morphometry of ID junctions

ID	ARVC/D (21)	DCM (10)	Controls (10)	*p* ARVC/D vs. Controls	*p* ARVC/D vs. DCM	*p* DCM vs. Controls
Convolution index	3,0 ± 0,9	2,8 ± 0,5	2,8 ± 0,6	0.34	0.18	0.76
D mean length (μm)	0,31 ± 0,08	0,23 ± 0,1	0,16 ± 0,08	<0.001	0.04	0.11
n. D/10 μm unity length	3,34 ± 0,9	4,2 ± 0,8	5,54 ± 2,3	0.01	0.02	0.10
D percent length of ID (%)	9,8 ± 3,2	8,4 ± 2,2	5,7 ±1,4	<0.001	0.16	0.008
Nexus mean length (μm)	0,34 ± 0,15	0,31 ± 0,07	0,32 ± 0,16	0.78	0.47	0.69
n. Nexus/10 μm unity length	0,29 ± 0,86	0,23 ± 0,32	0,78 ± 0,54	0.03	0.64	0.02
Nexus percent length of ID (%)	1,2 ± 1,8	1,14 ± 1,5	3,0 ± 2,5	0.07	0.93	0.08
D mean gap (nm)	29,33 ± 8,95	24,21±2,1	21,78 ± 3,42	0.004	0.03	0.19
FA mean gap (nm)	41,49 ± 20,36	28,39 ± 5,1	27,18 ± 10,72	0.03	0.02	0.67

After Bonferroni correction, only *p* ≤0.016 are significant.
D, desmosome; *DCM*, dilated cardiomyopathy; *FA*, fascia adherens; *n*, number; *ID*, intercalated disc

Other characteristic features of ID in ARVC/D hearts are abnormally elongated desmosomes (Figs. 6.2a, b) and a series of short desmosomes (Fig. 6.2c), similar to those observed in Carvajal syndrome, which is related to desmoplakin mutation [8, 24]. The biological significance of these abnormalities is unknown. Desmosomes were often abnormally displaced from the cell membrane to the cell contractile apparatus area and, simultaneously, desmin filaments in the proximity of these desmosomes were intersected. Morphometric analysis confirmed an increase of mean desmosome length and revealed a decreased number of desmosomes and widened gaps between membranes of adjoining cells (Table 6.2). These features probably influence the mechanical coupling of adjoining cells. Additionally, impaired desmin organization in the proximity of desmosomes may affect the mechanical strength that can be provided by normal junctions [21].

At the level of the fascia adherens, widening of the ID gap (Table 6.2) and abnormal organization of actin filaments have been observed in ARVC/D (Fig. 6.2b) These might be due to a specific impairment of fascia adherens protein, but might also be the result of a "symbiotic" relationship with a defect of desmosome structure.

The length and ultrastructure of nexuses seem to be normal, while their number is decreased in ARVC/D, as shown by morphometric analysis. In Naxos disease, a decrease of both average profile length and number of nexuses was observed by Kaplan et al. [25] in a patient who died before ARVC/D became clinically manifest. They suggested that abnormal linkage between mechanical junctions and the cytoskeleton due to mutant plakoglobin was responsible for this remodeling. The decreased number of nexuses probably led to increased tissue anisotropy, which may potentially account for lack of homogeneity in the propagation of action potentials.

In summary, remodeling of cellular junctions seen at the ultrastructural level probably affects the response of myocardial tissue to mechanical stretching and electrical conduction. This might explain why structural abnormalities occur mainly in areas subjected to high strain, i.e., in the triangle of dysplasia (the right ventricular outflow, the apex and subtricuspid area).

Noteworthy, in nearly half of the cases, we found evidence of desmosomal gene mutations, i.e., desmoplakin, plakophilin-2, and desmoglein-2. Desmosome remodeling was present at the ultrastructural level in both gene-positive and gene-negative ARVC/D patients. This supports the view that other ARVC/D genes are as yet undiscovered.

Cytoskeleton

In addition to ID proteins, the cytoskeleton of cardiomyocytes consists of a sarcomeric skeleton (e.g., titin, α-actinin), true cytoskeletal proteins (i.e., intermediate filaments, microtubules, and actin), and membrane-associated proteins (e.g., dystrophin, spectrin, talin, vinculin) [26]. This complex network stabilizes cellular organelles, maintains cell size and shape, and plays an active role during contraction/relaxation and intracellular signaling [27, 28]. The perisarcomer cytoskeleton anchors to the lateral cell membrane in areas called costameres, which are composed of focal adhesion proteins. Therefore, the cytoskeleton responds to the physical and biochemical properties of the extracellular matrix.

Ultrastructural analysis of ARVC/D revealed an irregular or decreased cytoskeleton in the region of the Z band and cell membrane invaginations that form T-tubules (Fig. 6.3), as well as in the perinuclear area in many cardiomyocytes. The lateral costameres in some cells were numerous while in others, with decreased invagination of cell-membrane-forming T-tubules, were single or aggregated in the area of the cell membrane outside of the Z-band region (Fig. 6.3). These were not related to the presence of collagen in the extracellular space. Cytoskeletal alterations have been reported to be responsible for cellular contractile dysfunction [27, 29]. It is also known that costameres are responsible for cell structural and functional integrity since they are involved in fixation of sarcomeres to the lateral sarcolemma and stabilization of T-tubules [27, 30]. It is not clear if the varied number of

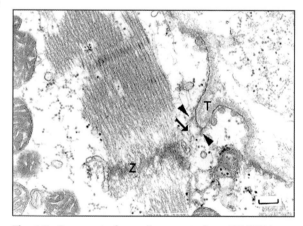

Fig. 6.3 • Fragment of a cardiomyocyte from ARVC/D heart in the region of cell membrane invagination forming T-tubule (*T*) with impaired intermediate filaments (*arrow*) connecting a Z-band region across the enlargement of interfibrillary space to cell membrane costameres (*arrowheads*) and impaired Z-band (*Z*) and actin arrangement. Bar = 150 nm

costamere junctions in cardiomyocytes of ARVC/D is related to the loss of intermediate filaments or abnormal strength linkage with extracellular matrix due to increasing fibrosis as the disease progresses. From experimental cell biology, it is known that an increased stiffness on the extracellular matrix induces a stronger integrin cytoskeleton link [31]. The number and quality of extracellular matrix binding components via membrane integrins with cell cytoskeleton affects a variety of intracellular signaling events. Both diminished cytoskeleton and increased or diminished number of costamere junctions could be related to cell death.

Cell Death

The mechanism of cell death by apoptosis is generally accepted as a cause of cardiomyocyte loss in ARVC/D, which has been confirmed by the histochemical TUNEL method [4-6]. Nonetheless, typical ultrastructural features of apoptosis are rarely seen in ultrathin sections. This is probably due to the fact that only a small tissue area is analyzed under an electron microscope. Results obtained by TUNEL method on endomyocardial biopsy suggest that apoptotic cardiomyocyte nuclei are present in 35% of ARVC/D cases with a mean apoptotic index of 25% [5]. Mallat et al. [4] found apoptotic cells in 75% of autopsy samples, in areas of myocardium not containing adipocytes and fibrosis and which exhibited little or no dysplasia. The factors triggering apoptosis have not been systematically investigated.

The most common ultrastructural feature of cardiomyocyte nuclei in ARVC/D is their highly convoluted membrane and abnormal condensation of chromatin with a granular or cord-like appearance (Fig. 6.1a). Yamamoto et al. [32] described two types of these abnormal nuclei: one dislocated to the cell periphery, extruded and comet-like in shape, and the second with typical preapoptotic features. Our findings are in agreement with these observations (Figs. 6.4a, b) [19]. The significance of nuclear morphological abnormalities remains unknown. The influence of an impaired cytoskeleton on nuclei morphology and fate cannot be excluded.

Cardiomyocyte Dedifferentiation

Some cardiomyocytes in ARVC/D are characterized by cellular hypertrophy, disruption of sarcomeres, depletion of myofibrils, and T-tubular membrane invaginations of the sarcolemma and sarcoplasmic reticulum. There are also oval nuclei with homogenously dispersed chromatin resembling nuclei of fetal cardiomyocytes. These nuclei contain mitochondria of various size and shape with normal cristae (Fig. 6.5a), and often abundant glycogen. The above-

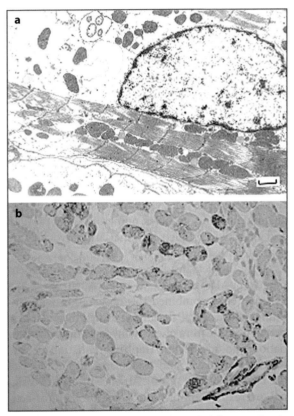

Fig. 6.5 • Features of cardiomyocytes dedifferentiation in ARVC/D heart. **a** Fragment of cardiomyocyte from ARVC/D heart characterized by oval nuclei exhibiting widespread chromatin, various size mitochondria, vacuoles, no T-tubules and myocytolysis of contractile fibrils. Bar = 2 μm. **b** Expression of smooth muscle α-actin in cardiomyocytes in ARVC/D heart at immunostain

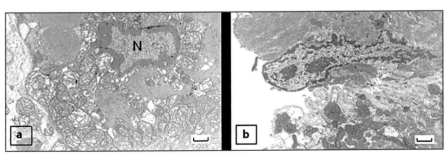

Fig. 6.4 • Electron microscopic images of nuclei of dying cardiomyocytes in ARVC/D hearts. **a** Apoptotic nuclei (*N*) with condensed chromatin beneath nuclear membrane. Bar = 2 μm. **b** A nucleus protruded from cardiomyocyte with irregular outline of tail segment directed to cell body. Bar = 2 μm

not a perfect recreation of the human condition, it serves as a proof of concept. Another model described by Bierkamp et al. better correlated with the Naxos phenotype, including the heart and skin defects [41].

Desmoplakin Mutant Murine Model

Desmoplakin (DSP), localized to chromosome 6p24, was initially identified as the mutant gene causing autosomal recessive Carvajal syndrome [20, 21] and later shown to cause autosomal dominant ARVD8 [14]. Desmoplakin is a major component of desmosomes, complex intercellular junctions assembled through cooperative interactions between multiple proteins [22, 23]. The majority of patients with DSP have the classic form of ARVC/D, although a substantial number of affected individuals have associated LV disease [42].

Using the Cre-LoxP system [43], a cardiac-restricted exon 2 deletion in DSP was created in mice by Garcia-Gras et al. [44]. These animals were engineered by crossing mice in which the second exon of the murine DSP gene is flanked by loxP sequence (floxed DP mice; 129/SvJ strain) with mice expressing Cre recombinase under the control of the a-MHC promoter (a-MHC-Cre mice; FVB/N strain). Homozygous ($DP^{-/-}$) mutant mice had a high rate of embryonic lethality, consistent with that previously reported by Gallicano et al. [45, 46] in germline DP-null mice. These homozygous mutant mouse embryos exhibited growth arrest at embryonic stage E10-E12, appeared pale, had no circulating red blood cells in organs, and were growth retarded. Histopathologic evaluation revealed poorly formed hearts with no chamber specification and unorganized cardiac myocytes. In addition, red blood cells were localized to the pericardial sac instead of within the cardiac chambers. Furthermore, an excess number of cells resembling adipocytes, dispersed between myocytes and localized to adjacent areas, were also detected. In comparison, cardiac phenotype was normal in $DP^{+/+}$ and $DP^{+/-}$ embryos, with and without the a-MHC-Cre transgene. Those $DP^{-/-}$ mice surviving the embryonic period (approximately 5% of the litter) died typically within the first 2 weeks from birth. On the other hand, $DP^{+/-}$ mice were born with normal development but had age-dependent penetrance of heart involvement, including a 20% incidence of SCD by 6 months of life. Gross pathologic analysis of both $DP^{+/-}$ and $DP^{-/-}$ animals demonstrated grossly enlarged cardiac chambers and increased heart weight with increased heart weight-to-body ratio, being highest in the homozygous mutants and lowest in the WT animals. Both RV and LV were enlarged equally and this enlargement occurred at approximately the same age. The gross anatomic findings were further supported by echocardiographic measurements, which revealed thin ventricular walls, increased LV end-diastolic and end-systolic dimensions, and depressed systolic function with reduced ejection fraction. Furthermore, baseline resting electrocardiographic evaluation identified spontaneous ventricular ectopy, including premature ventricular contractions, ventricular couplets and short runs of VT in heterozygous mutants but no ventricular arrythmias in WT mice. Histologic examination revealed poorly organized myocytes with large areas of patchy fibrosis; in the $DP^{-/-}$ animals, fibrosis was seen in up to 30%-40% of the myocardium. Excess accumulation of fat droplets was notable in both $DP^{-/-}$ and $DP^{+/-}$ mutant mice using Oil Red O staining, and was seen predominantly at the site of fibrosis.

In addition to these pathologic abnormalities, the authors showed that JUP, a member of the armadillo repeat protein family that plays a role in regulation of gene expression, interacts and competes with β-catenin, the effector of the canonical Wnt signaling [47], having a negative effect on this pathway. They were able to show that plakoglobin was translocated to the nucleus in cardiac-restricted DP-deficient mice and that expression levels of gene targets of the canonical Wnt/β-catenin pathway (c-myc and cyclin D1) were reduced (Fig. 7.1). Expression of adipogenic genes were increased, as was TUNEL-positive cells, but in the absence of DNA laddering consistent with low levels of apoptosis.

Another animal model of mutant desmoplakin was recently described by our group [48]. This model, a transgenic mouse with cardiac-restricted overexpression of a C-terminal DSP mutant (R2834H), demonstrated histological evidence of increased cardiomyocyte apoptosis, cardiac fibrosis, and lipid accumulation (Fig. 7.2). Echocardiography and cardiac magnetic resonance imaging revealed ventricular enlargement and cardiac dysfunction of both ventricles, which was confirmed on necropsy (Fig. 7.2). RV wall thickness was also reduced. The mutant mice also displayed interruption of the DSP-desmin interaction at intercalated disks and marked ultrastructural abnormalities of the intercalated disks. The intercalated disks were irregularly shaped with markedly widened gaps

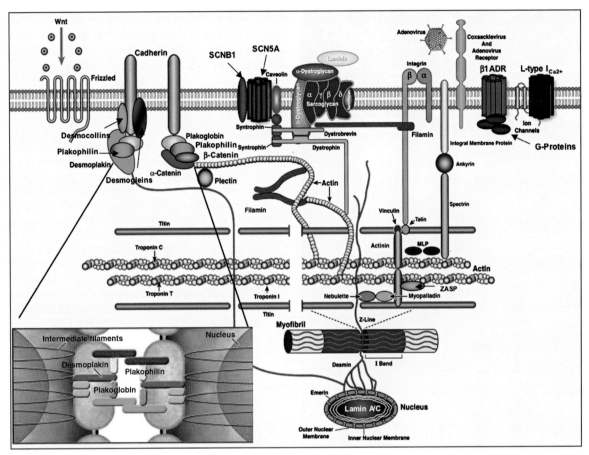

Fig. 7.1 • Cardiomyocyte architecture. This illustration shows the various proteins that contribute to the function of the cardiomyocyte. In the extracellular matrix, α2-laminin interacts with the intrasarcolemmal dystrophin-associated protein complex via partnering with α-dystroglycan. The α-dystroglycan interfaces with the β-dystroglycan and sarcoglycan complex, which binds dystrophin and binds with the sarcomere via the actin cytoskeleton. Interactions with the nucleus also occur. At the periphery, the desmosomal proteins are seen (*left*) and include cadherin, desmocollin, desmoglein, plakoglobin, plakophilin, and desmoplakin, the latter interacting with the *Wnt* pathway. The interactions between these desmosomal proteins is shown in the expanded view at the *bottom left* of the figure

between adjacent anchoring sarcomeres, affecting both the adherens junctions and desmosomes (Fig. 7.2). In addition, changes in other desmosomal and junctional components were notable, including increased expression and redistribution of JUP, PKP2, and β-catenin, as well as changes in gap junction components including redistribution of connexin 43.

Conclusions

The animal models described in this chapter support the notion that ARVC/D is a disease of the desmosome. Although the only model to date that appears to recapitulate ARVC/D in part is that of desmoplakin, the cumulative message of these desmosome-mutant mice is that disruption of desmosome func-

tion leads to cardiomyopathy. The fact that fibrous infiltration is common in all, that there is myocardial thinning in all, and that the desmoplakin model has abnormalities of lipid accumulation in the myocardium, is sufficient to state that these models provide the necessary proof of concept that the "final common pathway" of ARVC/D is desmosomal dysfunction; in other words, ARVC/D is a disease of the desmosome. Future human and animal models will continue to focus on desmosomal and other adherens junction proteins and other genes responsible for this disorder is likely to be identified. The next series of important steps in better understanding the paradigm of this disorder include defining the mechanisms responsible for the fatty infiltrative process, the mechanisms responsible for the disruption of the junctions and intercalated disks, and the mechanisms responsible for the development of arrhythmias [49,

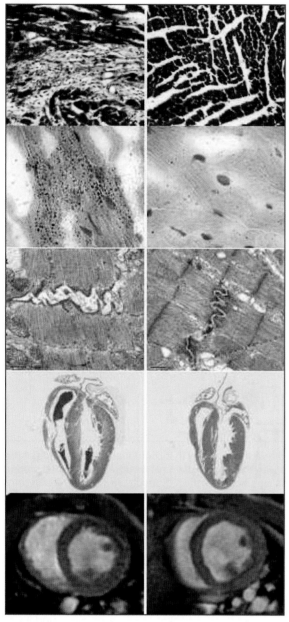

Fig. 7.2 • Desmoplakin (DSP) transgenic mouse model. In this model by Yang et al., comparison between the normal (*right*) and mutant (*left*) mice demonstrates fibrosis (*top left*), lipid infiltration (*second panel, left*), intercalated disk disruption (*third panel, left*), and right ventricular dilation and thinning by cardiac pathology with H&E stain (*fourth panel, left*) and cardiac MRI (*bottom left*) in the mutant animal, recapitulating the human condition

that probably bind to these important channels [11]. Once determined, these models will enable targeted therapies to be developed, leading to more predictable and better survival of affected individuals.

References

1. Marcus FI, Fontaine GH, Guiraudon G et al (1982) Right ventricular dysplasia: A report of 24 adult cases. Circulation 65:3884-3898
2. Thiene G, Nava A, Corrado D et al (1988) Right ventricular cardiomyopathy and sudden death in young people. New Engl J Med 318:129-133
3. Peters S, Trummel M, Meyners W (2004) Prevalence of right ventricular dysplasia-cardiomyopathy in a non-referral hospital. Int J Cardiol 97:499-501
4. Corrado D, Basso C, Thiene G et al (1997) Spectrum of clinicopathologic manifestations of arrhythmogenic right ventricular cardiomyopathy/dysplasia: A multi-center study. J Am Coll Cardiol 30:1312-1520
5. Corrado D, Basso C, Schiavon M et al (1998) Screening for hypertrophic cardiomyopathy in young athletes. N Engl J Med 339:364-369
6. Tabib A, Loire R, Chalabreysse L et al (2004) Circumstances of death and gross and microscopic observations in a series of 200 cases of sudden death associated with arrhythmogenic right ventricular cardiomyopathy and/or dysplasia. Circulation 108:3000-3005
7. Corrado D, Leoni L, Link MS et al (2003) Implantable cardioverter-defibrillator therapy for prevention of sudden death in patients with arrhythmogenic right ventricular cardiomyopathy/dysplasia. Circulation 108:3084-3091
8. Suzuki H, Sumiyoshi M, Kawai S et al (2000) Arrhythmogenic right ventricular cardiomyopathy with an initial manifestation of severe left ventricular impairment and normal contraction of the right ventricle. Jpn Circ J 64:209-213
9. Basso C, Thiene G, Corrado D et al (1996) Arrhythmogenic right ventricular cardiomyopathy. Dysplasia, dystrophy, or myocarditis? Circulation 94:983-991
10. Bowles NE, Ni J, Marcus F, Towbin JA (2002) The detection of cardiotropic viruses in the myocardium of patients with arrhythmogenic right ventricular dysplasia/cardiomyopathy. J Am Coll Cardiol 39:892-895
11. Bowles NE, Bowles KR, Towbin JA. (2000) The "final common pathway" hypothesis and inherited cardiovascular disease. The role of cytoskeletal proteins in dilated cardiomyopathy. Herz 25:168-175
12. Towbin JA, Bowles NE (2001) Arrhythmogenic inherited heart muscle diseases in children. J Electrocardiol 34:151-165
13. Bowles NE, Bowles K, Towbin JA (2000) Prospects for gene therapy for inherited cardiomyopathies. Prog Pediatr Cardiol 12:133-145
14. Rampazzo A, Nava A, Malacrida S et al (2002) Mutation in human desmoplakin domain binding to plakoglobin

50]. Our "final common pathway" hypothesis would suggest that these rhythm disturbances are likely to occur from secondary disruption of ion channel function (cascade events) and we predict that one or more ion channels will be found to be dysfunctional based on abnormal interactions with the desmosome, intercalated disks, or specific cadherin proteins causes a dominant form of arrhythmogenic right ventricular cardiomyopathy. Am J Hum Genet 7:1200-1206

15. Gerull B, Heuser A, Wichter T et al (2004) Mutations in the desmosomal protein plakophilin-2 are common in arrhythmogenic right ventricular cardiomyopathy. Nat Genet 36:1162-1164

16. Dalal D, Molin LH, Piccini J et al (2006) Clinical features of arrhythmogenic right ventricular dysplasia /cardiomyopathy associated with mutations in plakophilin-2. Circulation 113:1641-1649

17. Pilichou K, Nava A, Basso C et al (2006) Mutations in desmoglein-2 gene are associated with arrhythmogenic right ventricular cardiomyopathy. Circulation 113:1171-1179

18. McKoy G, Protonotarios N, Crosby A et al (2000) Identification of a deletion in plakoglobin in right ventricular cardiomyopathy with palmoplantar keratoderma and woolly hair (Naxos disease). Lancet 355:2119-2124

19. Protonotarios N, Tsatsopoulou A, Patsourakos P et al (1986) Cardiac abnormalities in familial palmoplantar keratosis. Br Heart J 56:321-326

20. Carvajal-Huerta L (1998) Epidermolytic palmoplantar keratoderma with woolly hair and dilated cardiomyopathy. J Am Acad Dermatol 44:309-311

21. Norgett EE, Hatsell SJ, Carvajal-Guerta L et al (2000) Recessive mutation in desmoplakin disrupts desmoplakin-intermediate filament interactions and causes dilated cardiomyopathy, woolly hair and keratoderma. Hum Mol Genet 9:2761-2766

22. McMillan JR, Shimizu H (2001) Desmosomes: Structure and function in normal and diseased epidermis. J Dermatol 28:291-298

23. Green KJ, Gaudry CA (2000) Are desmosomes more than tethers for intermediate filaments? Nat Rev Mol Cell Biol 1:208-216

24. Beffagna G, Occhi G, Nava A et al (2005) Regulatory mutations in transforming growth factor-beta3 gene cause arrhythogenic right ventricular cardiomyopathy type 1. Cardiovasc Res 65:366-373

25. Tiso N, Stephan DA, Nava A et al (2001) Identification of mutations in the cardiac ryanodine receptor gene in families affected with arrhythmogenic right ventricular cardiomyopathy type 2 (ARVD2). Hum Mol Genet 10:189-194

26. Laitinen PJ, Swan H, Piippo K et al (2004) Genes, exercise and sudden death: Molecular basis of familial catecholaminergic polymorphic ventricular tachycardia. Ann Med 36:81-86

27. Priori SG, Napolitano C, Memmi M et al (2002) Clinical and molecular characterization of patients with catecholaminergic polymorphic ventricular tachycardia. Circulation 106:8-10

28. Dalloz F, Osinska H, Robbins J (2001) Manipulating the contractile apparatus: Gentically defined animal models of cardiovascular disease. J Mol Cell Cardiol 33:9-25

29. Maass A, Leinwand LA (2000) Animal models of hypertrophic cardiomyopathy. Curr Opin Cardiol 15:189-196

30. Thierfelder L, Watkins H, MacRae C et al (1994) Alpha-tropomyosin and cardiac troponin T mutations cause familial hypertrophic cardiomyopathy: A disease of the sarcomere. Cell 77:701-712

31. Roopnarine O, Leinwand LA (1998) Functional analysis of myosin mutations that cause familial hypertrophic cardiomyopathy. Biophys J 75:3023-3030

32. Asano Y, Takashima S, Asakura M et al (2004) *Lamr1* functional retroposon causes right ventricular dysplasia in mice. Nat Genet 36:123-130

33. Kannankeril PJ, Mitchell BM, Goonasekera SA et al (2006) Mice with the R176Q cardiac ryanodine receptor mutation catecholamine-induced ventricular tachycardia and cardiomyopathy. Proc Natl Acad Sci USA 103:12179-12184

34. Appleton GO, Li Y, Taffet GE, Hartley CJ et al (2004) Determinants of cardiac electrophysiological properties in mice. J Intervent Card Electrophysiol 11:5-14

35. Hatzfeld M (2007) Plakophilins: Multifunctional proteins or just regulators of desmosomal adhesion? Biochim Biophys Acta 1773:69-77

36. Hatzfeld M (1999) The armadillo family of structural proteins. Int Rev Cytol 186:179-224

37. Grossmann KS, Grund C, Huelsken J et al (2004) Requirement of plakophillin 2 for heart morphogenesis and cardiac junction formation. J Cell Biol 167:149-160

38. Cowin P, Kapprell HP, Franke WW et al (1986) Plakoglobin: A protein common to different kinds of intercellular adhering junctions. Cell 46:1063-1073

39. Zhurinsky J, Shtutman M, Ben-Ze'ev A (2000) Plakoglobin and beta-catenin: Protein interactions, regulation and biological roles. J Cell Sci 113:3127-3139

40. Ruiz P, Brinkmann V, Ledermann B et al (1996) Targeted mutation of plakoglobin in mice reveals essential functions of desmosomes in the embryonic heart. J Cell Biol 135:215-225

41. Bierkamp C, McLaughlin KJ, Schwarz H et al (1996) Embryonic heart and skin defects in mice lacking plakoglobin. Dev Biol 180:780-785

42. Norman M, Simpson M, Mogensen J et al (2005) Novel mutation in desmoplakin causes arrhythmogenic left ventricular cardiomyopathy. Circulation 112:636-642

43. Agah R, Frenkel PA, French BA et al (1997) Gene recombination in postmitotic cells. Targeted expression of Cre recombinase provokes cardiac-restricted, site-specific rearrangement in adultventricular muscle in vivo. J Clin Invest 100:169-179

44. Garcia-Gras E, Lombardi R, Giocondo MJ et al (2006) Suppression of canonical Wnt/b-catenin signaling by nuclear plakoglobin recapitulates phenotype of arrhythmogenic right ventricular cardiomyopathy. J Clin Invest 116:2012-2021

45. Gallicano GI, Kouklis P, Bauer C et al (1998) Desmoplakin is required early in development for assembly of desmosomes and cytoskeletal linkage. J Cell Biol 143:2009-2022

46. Gallicano GI, Bauer C, Fuchs E (2001) Rescuing desmoplakin function in extra-embryonic ectoderm

reveals the importance of this protein in embryonic heart, neuroepithelium, skin, and vasculature. Development 128:929-941

47. Klymkowsky MW, Williams BO, Barish GD et al (1999) Membrane-anchored plakoglobins have multiple mechanisms of action in Wnt signaling. Mol Biol Cell 10:3151-3169

48. Yang Z, Bowles NE, Scherer SE et al (2006) Desmosomal dysfunction due to mutations in desmoplakin cause arrhythmogenic right ventricular dysplasia/cardiomyopathy. Circ Res 99:646-655

49. MacRae CA, Birchmeier W, Thierfelder L (2006) Arrhythmogenic right ventricular cardiomyopathy: Moving toward mechanism. J Clin Invest 116:1825-1828

50. Nerbonne JM (2004) Studying cardiac arrhythmias in the mouse – a reasonable model for probing mechanisms? Trends Cardiovasc Med 14:83-93

CHAPTER 8

SPONTANEOUS ANIMAL MODELS

Philip R. Fox, Cristina Basso, Gaetano Thiene, Barry J. Maron

Spontaneous Cardiovascular Disease in Animals

Cardiovascular disease occurs commonly in companion animals, particularly in domestic cats and dogs [1]. Myocardial disease represents a substantial portion of these disorders, many of which closely resemble cardiomyopathies in human patients [2]. Such disorders in cat, include hypertrophic [3, 4], dilated [5], restrictive [6, 7], and arrhythmogenic right ventricular cardiomyopathies (ARVC/D) [8]. A heritable form of hypertrophic cardiomyopathy associated with a cardiac myosin binding protein C mutation has been recently reported in the Maine Coon cat breed [4]. In dogs, chronic myxomatous valve disease is the most prevalent cardiac disorder [9, 10], but cardiomyopathies occur frequently, particularly within certain medium and large-sized breeds [10]. Familial forms of dilated cardiomyopathy have been described in the Doberman Pinscher [11], Irish wolfhound [12], and Great Dane [13], and a familial form of ARVC/D has been reported in the boxer breed [14, 15]. Dysplastic conditions of the right ventricle (RV) have been described in other mammals including minks [16] and rodents. In mice, ARVC/D has been associated with mutation of the gene laminin receptor [17]. One of the authors (PF) has observed a case of ARVC/D in a primate.

Recently, the canine genome has been mapped using a boxer dog [18], and the US National Human Genome Research Institute has recognized the canine to be an unrivaled model for the study of human disease. Detailed investigations of the genetic basis of ARVC/D in the boxer dog should now be possible. Spontaneous ARVC/D in cats [8] – and particularly dogs [15], have strikingly similar clinical and pathologic features to this condition in humans [19]. Because the pathology of ARVC/D in both the canine and feline models is characterized by myocyte injury and repair, these models provide the opportunity to investigate the ultrastructural features as well as the underlying molecular basis of these changes. Moreover, the high familial incidence of ventricular arrhythmias and sudden death in boxer dogs with ARVC/D makes this model particularly suited for studying the electrophysiologic mechanisms of arrhythmias, the efficacy of antiarrhythmic drugs and therapies, and strategies directed to modify the progression of disease or clinical outcome. Thus, the study of cardiomyopathies in these animals should serve to increase the understanding of the genetic basis of human disease, including development of improved diagnostic assays and assessment of clinical therapies.

Etiology and Pathogenesis of ARVC/D

In humans ARVC/D is familial in approximately 30%-50% of patients, suggesting that genetic factors may play an important role in this condition [20, 21]. To date, six candidate genes have already been identified including ryanodine receptor (*RyR2* on 1q42), plakoglobin (*JUP* on 17q21), desmoplakin (*DSM* on 6p24), plakophilin-2 (*PKP2* on 12p11), transforming growth factor β3 gene (*TGFβ3* on 14q24.3), and desmoglein-2 (DSG2 on 18) [22-27]. In dogs, cardiac RyR2 message and protein expression are differentially expressed across the cardiac walls in normal hearts, with the RV containing significantly lower concentration. In the canine model of ARVC/D, the message and protein expression of the RyR were reduced in all chambers. Thus, the increased susceptibility of the RV to ARVC/D may be associated with the lower baseline protein concentration of RyR2 in the normal RV compared to the left ventricle (LV) and interventricular septum [28]. Recently, boxer dogs with ARVC/D were found to have substantially reduced quantities of calstabin-2, a regulatory molecule of RYR2, in cardiac myocytes [29].

Pathophysiology

Progressive atrophy of the RV myocardium with fibrous and/or fatty replacement are common sequelae of ARVC/D in cats [8], dogs [15], and humans

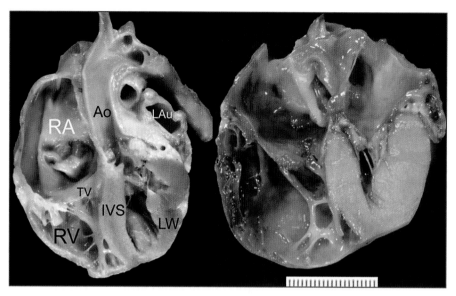

Fig. 8.1 • Hearts from two cats with ARVC/D and congestive heart failure. There is severe right atrial and right ventricular dilatation, and thinned, translucent right ventricular walls associated with marked trabecular flattening; the septo-parietal bands appear prominent. ECG showed ventricular tachycardia (left bundle branch block morphology)

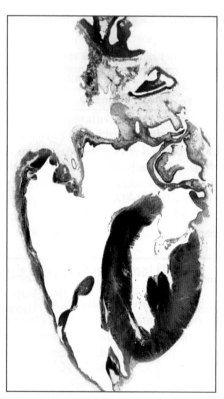

Fig. 8.2 • Whole heart histological section from a cat with ARVC/D and ventricular ectopy. There is anterior and apical RV free wall thinning and aneurysm. Heidenhain trichrome stain. From [8] with permission

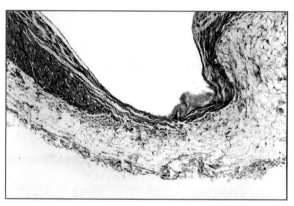

Fig. 8.3 • Higher magnification (×45) of the apical aneurysm from Fig. 8.2. There is severe transmural fibrofatty replacement with organized mural thrombosis and thickened epicardium. Heidenhain trichrome stain. From [8] with permission

ment-type fibrosis (Figs. 8.2, 8.3). The fatty pattern within the RV wall and trabeculae is characterized by multifocal or diffuse areas of adipose cell infiltration with only mild patchy fibrosis. Islands of myocytes are often surrounded by fat or fibrofatty tissue. In both forms, residual surviving myocytes are usually scattered within the areas of fibrosis or fat, and fibro-fatty replacement usually extends from the epicardium toward the endocardium. Focal or multifocal RV myocarditis is most prevalent in ARVC/D cats with the fibro-fatty pattern. It consists mostly of T lymphocytes associated with myocyte cell death and mild-to-severe fibrous tissue deposition. Similar findings may be also present in left and right atrial walls, as well as LV free wall and ventricular septum. Fatty infiltration is occasionally present in the LV free wall but not in the ventricular septum. Abnormal intramural small vessels, with thickened walls (due primarily to medial hypertrophy), are uncommon. Apoptotic myocytes have been identified by TUNEL histochemical investigation in 75% of affected cats.

ARVC/D in Dogs

It has been noted for many years that some dogs, in particular the boxer breed, were predisposed to ventricular arrhythmias with syncope, sudden death, or heart failure [38-44]. Initially described as "boxer cardiomyopathy" [38], the clinicopathologic features were recently clarified as ARVC/D (Table 8.1) [15]. In addition to the boxer breed, where ARVC/D is recognized most commonly, canine ARVC/D has also been observed in the English bulldog and Labrador retriever.

Clinical Manifestations

Affected boxer dogs may die suddenly and unexpectedly during vigorous exercise, leisurely walking, or while sleeping. Persistently high sympathetic tone was not found to be a consistent feature of boxer dogs with ARVC/D [45]. Syncope is common and has been recorded in approximately half of severely affected dogs, including up to two-thirds of those that subsequently died suddenly, but there was no significant difference in the mode of death, sudden vs. nonsudden, in dogs with this symptom. Although less common, congestive heart failure may occur when systolic dysfunction is present.

Physical Examination

Commonly, the physical examination is unremarkable. Tachycardia may be detected and abnormal jugular venous pulse may accompany arrhythmias. In some dogs, auscultation may reveal an S3 gallop or soft, systolic, regurgitant heart murmur heard loudest over the tricuspid valve. Signs that may be associated with heart failure include tachypnea, ascites, hepatosplenomegaly, jugular venous distension, and respiratory crackles.

Electrocardiography

Ventricular premature complexes (PVCs) with left bundle branch block morphology are commonly detected during 24-h Holter ECG recording [43] and may occur in up to three-quarters of affected boxer dogs. This arrhythmia is consistent with RV origin [44]. Ventricular tachycardia with left bundle branch block occurs in almost half of ARVC/D dogs (Fig. 8.4). One of the authors (PF) considers such arrhythmias in the boxer breed as surrogate markers of ARVC/D, particularly in combination with familial history of this disease, or with other clinical signs such as syncope or heart failure. Other arrhythmias including PVCs of right bundle branch block morphology as well as supraventricular arrhythmias may also be observed, particularly if myocardial failure and severe atrial dilation are present. The role of the ECG in screening and assessing animal models of ARVC/D, however, has not been clarified. QT interval duration and dispersion have not been found to correlate with disease severity [46], although the use of signal-averaged ECG may identify some individual dogs at risk for sudden death [47].

Radiography

Thoracic radiographs are often unremarkable. Some affected dogs may have right-sided heart enlargement. Animals with myocardial failure have generalized cardiac enlargement and pulmonary edema may be detected. With right-sided congestive heart failure, pericardial, pleural, or abdominal effusion is present.

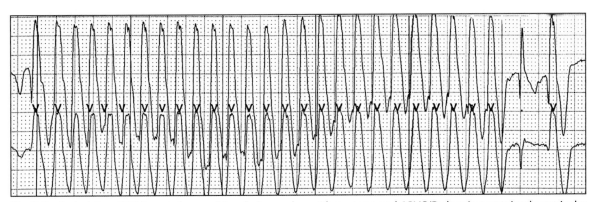

Fig. 8.4 • Ambulatory ECG from a 5-year-old male boxer dog with syncope and ARVC/D showing sustained ventricular tachycardia (up to 300bpm) with left bundle branch block pattern

Echocardiography

Transthoracic echocardiographic examination is frequently unremarkable. RV dilation or thinning of apical RV myocardium is evident in some dogs, and animals with myocardial failure display reduced systolic function and cardiac chamber dilation.

Magnetic Resonance Imaging

ARVC/D hearts display high transmural signal intensity in the anterolateral and/or infundibular regions of RV. This is particularly evident in hearts with fatty replacement, and corresponds anatomically to those areas of RV fat identified with histopathology (Fig. 8.5) [15].

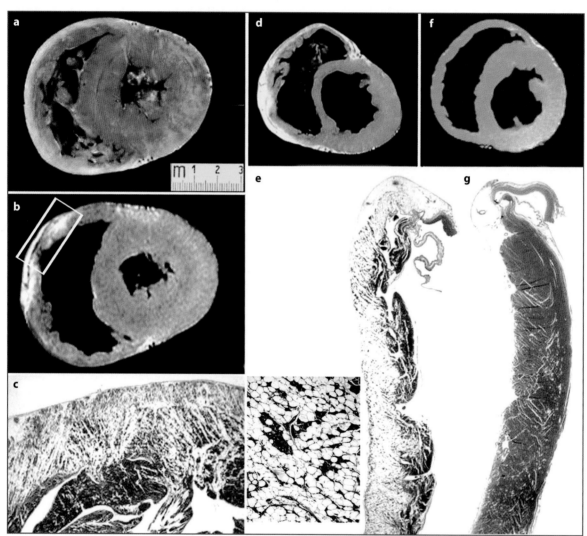

Fig. 8.5 • Pathologic findings in two boxer dogs with the fatty pattern of ARVC/D, and a control dog. **a, b,** and **c** are from a 9-year-old female boxer dog with ventricular tachycardia and sudden death during physical activity. **a,** Gross heart specimen cut in cross section. **b,** T1-weighted postmortem MRI corresponding to the same cross-sectional plane shown in **a.** RV cavity is dilated but wall thickness is normal. **c,** Low-power histopathologic section of RV wall from the region of bright MRI signals (delineated by the *box* shown in **b**); marked transmural fatty replacement is evident (original magnification ×3). **d** and **e** are from a 12-year-old female boxer dog with ventricular tachycardia and congestive heart failure. **d,** Cross-sectional MRI image showing bright, high-intensity signal in the RV infundibulum. **e,** Panoramic histopathologic section from region of bright MRI signals demonstrating massive, diffuse fatty replacement of atrophic myocardium (magnification ×3). Insert shows small islands of a few surviving myocytes surrounded by fat (magnification ×10). **f** and **g** are from a normal control dog. **f.** Cross-sectional MRI showing absence of bright MRI signals in RV wall. **g,** Panoramic histopathologic section demonstrating normal RV myocardial architecture (magnification ×3). Staining for **c, e,** and **g** is with trichrome Heidenhain. From [15] with permission

Therapy

Heart failure can occur in dogs with ARVC/D, particularly when left ventricular dysfunction is present. Standard therapy includes diuretics, angiotensin-converting enzyme inhibitors, and digitalis. The calcium channel agent diltiazem is added to control ventricular heart rate when atrial fibrillation occurs.

There is substantial spontaneous variability in the frequency of ventricular arrhythmias in boxer dogs with ARVC/D, and changes of up to 80% in PVC frequency have been recorded by Holter monitor [48]. Several antiarrhythmic drugs have been studied in boxer dogs with ARVC/D with regard to their effects on heart rate, the frequency of PVCs, the severity of arrhythmia, and the influence on syncope. Treatment with mexiletine combined with atenolol, or with sotalol alone, significantly reduced the frequency of PVCs, arrhythmia severity, and heart rate. In contrast, treatment with either atenolol or procainamide did not significantly affect these parameters. Neither of these treatment groups significantly affected the occurrence of syncope [49].

Gross Pathology

RV chamber dilatation is evident in approximately one-third of affected dogs. Infundibular aneurysms may be present but are uncommon. In a study that compared hearts from ARVC/D boxer dogs and controls, there was no significant difference with regard to heart weight (252±35 vs. 245±63 g), RV wall thickness (4.3±1.2 vs. 3.7±0.9 mm), or LV thickness (11.4±1.9 mm vs. 11.7±1.2 mm) [15].

Histopathology

Histopathologic lesions closely resemble those characteristic of human patients with ARVC/D [30-32]. Most distinguishing is substantial replacement of RV cardiac myocytes by adipose or fibrous tissue which occur in two patterns: a fatty form in approximately two-thirds and a fibro-fatty form in approximately one-third of cases [15].

The fatty form is characterized by diffusely distributed, multifocal regions of adipose cell replacement within the RV wall and trabeculae, extending from epicardium toward endocardium, in association with tiny patchy fibrosis (Fig. 8.5). The fibro-fatty form consists of focal or diffuse regions of adipose cell replacement associated with extensive areas of replacement fibrosis (Fig. 8.6). Both

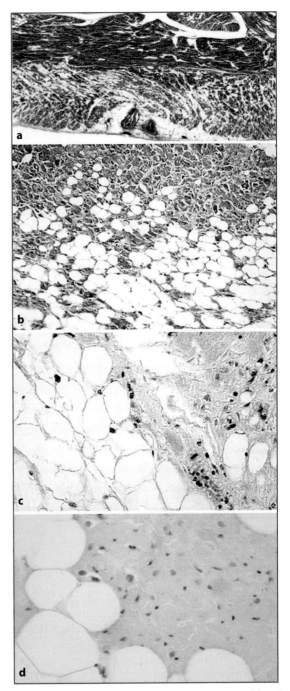

Fig. 8.6 • Histopathology of RV wall from an 8-year-old male boxer dog with sustained ventricular tachycardia (180bpm), syncope, and sudden death. **a**, Low power photomicrograph. Diffuse myocardial loss associated with adipose tissue and replacement-type fibrosis representative of the fibro-fatty form of ARVC/D was present in the subepicardium and mid-mural wall, (trichrome Heidenhain stain, magnification ×3) **b**, Surviving, atrophic myocytes surrounded by, and interspersed within, fat and patchy fibrous replacement tissue (trichrome Heidenhain stain, magnification ×25); **c**, Myocarditis characterized by patchy, mononuclear cellular inflammatory infiltrate (CD45RO) (magnification ×40). **d**, Brown-staining TUNEL-positive apoptotic myocyte nuclei (magnification ×40). From [15] with permission

the fatty and fibro-fatty forms are characterized by surviving myocytes embedded within regions of fibrous tissue. In ARVC/D dogs, mean percentage of area of RV fat did not differ significantly between anterolateral (46.7±19.7%) and infundibular (45.2±12.2%) sites, but was lower in the posterior wall (29.2±18.9%) ($p \leq 0.008$). Replacement of RV myocardium by fat was diffuse (involving ≥2 regions) in 70% of affected dogs, and segmental in the remaining 30% [15].

LV lesions may be present in up to half of ARVC/D hearts and consisted largely of focal, fibrous tissue replacement with some mild fatty tissue replacement. In left or right atrial walls, approximately one-third of ARVC/D boxer dogs display myocyte loss with fatty or fibro-fatty replacement [15]. Myxomatous degeneration of the mitral valve leaflets can occur as a normal aging change in older dogs.

Myocarditis characterized by focal or multifocal T-lymphocytic infiltrates (CD45, CD45RO, and CD43 positive) and associated with myocyte death, has been identified in the RV of almost two-thirds of ARVC/D boxer dogs. Myocarditis is often present in the LV free wall and in the atria. Myocyte apoptosis has been identified in 39% of ARVC/D hearts. In boxer dogs with ARVC/D that died suddenly there was a significantly greater percent of dogs with myocarditis (9/9; 100%) vs. those who did not die suddenly (7/14; 50%; $p=0.04$). The fibrofatty form was also more prominent in dogs with (6/9; 67%) than in those without sudden cardiac death (2/14; 14%) ($p=0.02$).

Conclusions

We reported novel, spontaneous animal models of ARVC/D, sudden death, and heart failure in both cats and boxer dogs. These spontaneous models closely resemble the clinical and pathological features of the human disease. In particular, they are characterized by ventricular tachycardia of suspected RV origin and structural abnormalities distinguished by RV enlargement and aneurysms, myocyte loss with fatty or fibrofatty replacement, myocarditis, and apoptosis. In the boxer dog series, several of these animals were related, suggesting that canine ARVC/D is inherited. These animal models of human ARVC/D constitute a new and potentially useful investigative tool to understand the complex clinical and pathogenic mechanisms responsible for sudden death and disease progression.

References

1. Fox PR, Sisson D, Moise N, eds (1999) Textbook of canine and feline cardiology, 2nd edn. WB Saunders, Philadelphia
2. Maron BJ, Towbin JA, Thiene G et al (2006) Contemporary definitions and classification of the cardiomyopathies. An American Heart Association Scientific Statement from the Council on Clinical Cardiology, Heart Failure and Transplantation Committee; Quality of care and outcomes research and functional genomics and translational biology interdisciplinary working groups, and council on epidemiology and prevention. Circulation 113:1807-1816
3. Fox PR, Liu SK, Maron BJ (1995) Echocardiographic assessment of spontaneously occurring feline hypertrophic cardiomyopathy: An animal model of human disease. Circulation 92:2645-2651
4. Meurs KM, Sanchez X, David RM et al (2005) A cardiac myosin binding protein C mutation in the Maine Coon cat with familial hypertrophic cardiomyopathy. Hum Mol Genet 14:3587-3593
5. Pion PD, Kittleson MD, Rogers QR et al (1987) Myocardial failure in cats associated with low plasma taurine: A reversible cardiomyopathy Science 237:764-768
6. Fox PR (2000) Feline cardiomyopathies. In: Ettinger SJ, Feldman EC (eds) Textbook of veterinary internal medicine, 5th edn, WB Saunders, Philadelphia, pp 896-923
7. Fox PR (2004) Endomyocardial fibrosis and restrictive cardiomyopathy: Pathologic and clinical features. J Vet Cardiol 6:25-31
8. Fox PR, Maron BJ, Basso C et al (2000) Spontaneous occurrence of arrhythmogenic right ventricular cardiomyopathy in the domestic cat: A new animal model of human disease. Circulation 102:1863-1870
9. Detweiler DK, Patterson DF (1965) The prevalence and types of cardiovascular disease in dogs. Ann NY Acad Sci 127:481-516
10. Buchanan JW (1999) Prevalence of cardiovascular disorders. In: Fox PR, Sisson D, Moise NS (eds) Textbook of canine and feline cardiology principles and practice, 2nd edn, WB Saunders, Philadelphia, pp 457-470
11. Meurs KM, Magnon AL, Spier AW et al (2001) Evaluation of the cardiac actin gene in Doberman Pinschers with dilated cardiomyopathy Am J Vet Res 62:33-36
12. Vollmar AC (2000) The prevalence of cardiomyopathy in the Irish wolfhound: A clinical study of 500 dogs. J Am Anim Hosp Assoc 36:125-132
13. Meurs KM, Miller MW, Wright NA (2001) Clinical features of dilated cardiomyopathy in Great Danes and results of a pedigree analysis: 17 cases (1990-2000). J Am Vet Med Assoc 218:729-732
14. Meurs KM, Spier AW, Miller MW et al (1999) Familial ventricular arrhythmias in boxers. J Vet Intern Med 13:437-439

15. Basso C, Fox PR, Meurs KM et al (2004) Arrhythmogenic right ventricular cardiomyopathy causing sudden cardiac death in boxer dogs: A new animal model of human disease. Circulation 109:1180-1185

16. Ishikawa S, Zu Rhein GM, Gilbert EF (1977) Uhl's anomaly in the mink. Partial absence of the right atrial and ventricular myocardium. Arch Pathol Lab Med 101:388-390

17. Asano Y, Takashima S, Asakura M et al (2004) Lamr1 functional retroposon causes right ventricular dysplasia in mice. Nat Genet 36:123-130

18. Lindblad-Toh K, Wade CM, Mikkelsen TS et al (2005) Genome sequence, comparative analysis and haplotype structure of the domestic dog. Nature 438:745-746

19. Nava A, Rossi L, Thiene G (eds) (1997) Arrhythmogenic right ventricular cardiomyopathy/dysplasia. Elsevier, Amsterdam

20. Nava A, Bauce B, Basso C et al (2000) Clinical profile and long term follow-up of 37 families with arrhythmogenic right ventricular cardiomyopathy. J Am Coll Cardiol 36:2226-2233

21. Hamid MS, Norman M, Quraishi A et al (2002) Prospective evaluation of relatives for familial arrhythmogenic right ventricular cardiomyopathy/dysplasia reveals a need to broaden diagnostic criteria. J Am Coll Cardiol 40:1445-1450

22. McKoy G, Protonotarios N, Crosby A et al (2000) Identification of a deletion in plakoglobin in arrhythmogenic right ventricular cardiomyopathy with palmoplantar keratoderma and woolly hair (Naxos disease). Lancet 355:2119-2124

23. Tiso N, Stephan DA, Nava A et al (2001) Identification of mutations in the cardiac ryanodine receptor gene in families affected with arrhythmogenic right ventricular cardiomyopathy type 2 (ARVD2). Hum Mol Gen 10:189-194

24. Rampazzo A, Nava A, Malacrida S et al (2002) Mutation in human desmoplakin domain binding to plakoglobin causes a dominant form of arrhythmogenic right ventricular cardiomyopathy. Am J Hum Genet 71:1200-1206

25. Beffagna G, Occhi G, Nava A et al (2005) Regulatory mutations in transforming growth factor-[beta]3 gene cause arrhythmogenic right ventricular cardiomyopathy type 1. Cardiovasc Res 65:366-373

26. Gerull B, Heuser A, Wichter T et al (2004) Mutations in the desmosomal protein plakophilin-2 are common in arrhythmogenic right ventricular cardiomyopathy. Nat Genet 36:1162-1164

27. Pilichou K, Nava A, Basso C et al (2006) Mutations in Desmoglein-2 gene are associated to arrhythmogenic right ventricular cardiomyopathy. Circulation 113:1171-1179

28. Meurs KM, Lacombe VA, Dryburgh K et al (2006) Differential expression of the cardiac ryanodine receptor in normal and arrhythmogenic right ventricular cardiomyopathy canine hearts. Hum Genet 120:111-118

29. Oyama MA, Reiken S, Meurs KM et al (2006) Arrhythmogenic right ventricular cardiomyopathy in boxer dogs is associated with calstabin2 (FKBP12.6) deficiency. J Vet Int Med 20:747 (Abstr)

30. Thiene G, Nava A, Corrado D et al (1988). Right ventricular cardiomyopathy and sudden death in young people. N Engl J Med 318:129-133

31. Basso C, Thiene G, Corrado D et al (1996) Arrhythmogenic right ventricular cardiomyopathy. Dysplasia, dystrophy, or myocarditis? Circulation 94:983-991

32. Thiene G, Basso C, Calabrese F et al (2005) Twenty years of progress and beckoning frontiers in cardiovascular pathology: Cardiomyopathies. Cardiovasc Pathol 14:165-169

33. Kaplan SR, Gard JJ, Protonotarios N (2004) Remodeling of myocyte gap junctions in arrhythmogenic right ventricular cardiomyopathy due to a deletion in plakoglobin (Naxos disease). Heart Rhythm 1:3-11

34. Sen-Chowdhry S, Syrris P, McKenna WJ (2005) Genetics of right ventricular cardiomyopathy. J Cardiovasc Electrophysiol 16:927-935

35. Valente M, Calabrese F, Thiene G et al (1998) In vivo evidence of apoptosis in arrhythmogenic right ventricular cardiomyopathy. Am J Pathol 152:470-484

36. Corrado D, Basso C, Thiene G et al (1997) Spectrum of clinicopathologic manifestations of arrhythmogenic right ventricular cardiomyopathy/dysplasia: A multicenter study. J Am Coll Cardiol 30:1512-1520

37. Harvey AM, Battersby IA, Faena M et al (2005) Arrhythmogenic right ventricular cardiomyopathy in two cats. J Small Anim Pract 46:151-156

38. Harpster NK (1983) Boxer cardiomyopathy. In: Kirk RW (ed) Current veterinary therapy in small animal practice. WB Saunders, Philadelphia, pp 329-337

39. Bright JM, McEntee M (1995) Isolated right ventricular cardiomyopathy in a dog. J Am Vet Med Assoc 207:64-66

40. Fernandez Del Palacio MJ, Bernal LJ et al (2001) Arrhythmogenic right ventricular dysplasia/cardiomyopathy in a Siberian husky. J Small Anim Pract 42:137-142

41. Simpson KW, Bonagura JD, Eaton KA (1994) Right ventricular cardiomyopathy in a dog. J Vet Int Med 8:306-309

42. Mohr AJ, Kirberger RM (2000) Arrhythmogenic right ventricular cardiomyopathy in a dog. J S Afr Vet Assoc 71:125-130

43. Spier AW, Meurs KM (2004) Evaluation of spontaneous variability in the frequency of ventricular arrhythmias in boxers with arrhythmogenic right ventricular cardiomyopathy. J Am Vet Med Assoc 224:538-541

44. Kraus MS, Moïse NS, Rishniw M et al (2002) Morphology of ventricular arrhythmias in the boxer described by 12-lead electrocardiography with pace mapping comparison. J Vet Int Med 16:153-158

45. Spier AW, Meurs KM (2004) Assessment of heart rate variability in boxers with arrhythmogenic right ven-

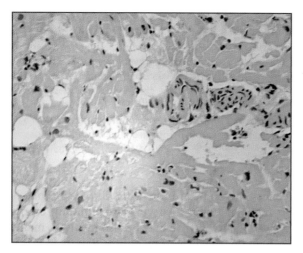

Fig. 9.1 • Endomyocardial biopsy from a patient with ARVC/D. Inflammatory cell infiltration is mainly represented by activated T-lymphocytes IHC for CD25. Original magnification ×50

Animal Models

Spontaneous animal models of ARVC/D found in domestic cats [30, 31] and boxer dogs [32] have been described. The combined clinical profile (sudden death, ventricular arrhythmias of suspected RV origin, and syncope) and pathological abnormalities (RV chamber enlargement and aneurysms, RV myocyte loss and fatty replacement, myocarditis, and apoptosis) provide compelling evidence for spontaneous heart disease in animals closely resembling the human condition of ARVC/D. The frequent occurrence of myocarditis and apoptosis also in animal models has suggested that both these processes are involved in the pathogenesis of ARVC/D.

Viral Studies

The presence of myocardial inflammation in more than two-thirds of cases has suggested that some pathologic features of ARVC/D may be considered a sequela of infective myocarditis [33]. Thus, fibrofatty infiltration may, in part, be viewed as a healing phenomenon in the setting of chronic myocarditis. Enterovirus was first investigated on the basis of an experimental model in which a BALB/C mice infected with Coxsackievirus B3 developed selective right ventricular myocardial cell death, acute mononuclear cell infiltration, and right ventricular aneurysm formation [34]. Several researchers have evaluated ARVC/D patients for the presence of enteroviral genome in the myocardium [17, 35-40] and controversial results have been reported, possibly reflecting different patient selection (Table 9.2).

In 1997, Heim et al. [37] reported the identification of enterovirus RNA in endomyocardial biopsies obtained from two male patients (15 and 26 years old, respectively) by use of *in situ hybridization*. One of these patients had a strong family history of ARVC/D. In both of these patients, fibrosis was identified in the myocardium, supporting the hypothesis that ARVC/D is a sequela of enterovirus myocarditis.

In another study involving eight patients, enteroviral RNA was identified in myocardial specimens with homology to coxsackievirus type B found in three subjects [17]. A negative study of viral genome was reported by Calabrese et al. in which there was a high rate of familial ARVC/D cases (50%) and only enteroviral genome was evaluated [38].

Table 9.2 • Molecular investigation in ARVC/D

First Author, year [Ref]	Sex	Mean age yrs	Family history	Methods	Viruses screened	Molecular finding
Kearney, 1995 [35]	2F	Not specified	Yes (2 cases)	PCR	EV, RSV, INVA-B, AV, CMV, HSV, EBV	None
Heim, 1997 [36]	4M, 2F	51	Not specified	N-PCR	EV	3 EV
Heim, 1997 [37]	2M	20	Yes (1 case)	ISH	EV	2 EV
Grumbach, 1998 [17]	4M, 4F	44	No	PCR	EV	3 EV
Calabrese, 2000 [38]	11M, 9F	40	Yes (9 cases)	PCR	EV	None
Bowles, 2002 [39]	7M, 12F	19	No	PCR	EV, RSV, INVA-B, AV, CMV, HSV, PV, EBV	5 EV, 2 AV
Chimenti, 2004 [40]	5M, 4F	29	No	PCR	EV, INV A-B, AV, CMV, HSV, PV, EBV, HCV	None

AV, Adenovirus; *CMV*, Cytomegalovirus; *EBV*, Ebstein Barr Virus; *EV*, Enterovirus; *HCV*, *F*, female; Hepatitis C Virus; *HSV*, Herpes Simplex Virus; *INV A-B*, Influenza virus A and B; *ISH*, in situ hybridization; *M*, male; *yrs*, years; *N-PCR*, nested-PCR; *PCR*, polimerase chain reaction; *PV*, Parvovirus B 19; *RSV*, Respiratory Syncitial virus

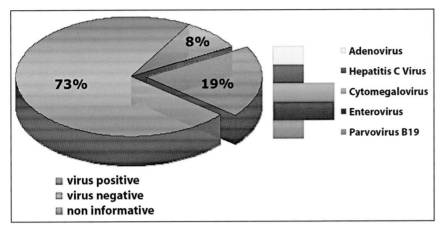

Fig. 9.2 • Viral genomes frequency in 36 endomyocardial biopsies from clinical and histological proven ARVC/D cases. Viral positivity was found in 7 (19%) of 36 cases

The role of other cardiotrophic viruses was reported by Bowles et al. [39]. The study involved 12 ARVC/D patients, who were considered sporadic cases after a pedigree analysis and a clinical screening of family members. Viruses were detected in 58% (7 out of 12): including enterovirus in five and adenovirus type 5 in two patients, respectively.

The presence of viruses and their role in ARVC/D patients was investigated by Chimenti et al. [40]. They studied 30 patients who were diagnosed with ARVC/D on the basis of having either two major criteria or one major plus at least two minor criteria [41]. At histology, ARVC/D was confirmed in nine patients, whereas the remaining met the Dallas criteria for myocarditis. The molecular investigation detected viral genome in four patients with myocarditis and in none with ARVC/D.

In Italy, our recent experience using molecular viral screening, both PCR and RT-PCR, confirmed the presence of different viral genomes in seven (19%) of 36 cases with clinical and histological evidence of ARVC/D (unpublished data) (Fig. 9.2).

Pathogenesis

Virus and Myocyte Death

Over the past two decades, the use of molecular-based studies have enabled viral genomes to be analyzed in the hearts of human subjects with cardiac dysfunction. Bowles and colleagues were the first to identify coxsackievirus in myocardial specimens of patients with myocarditis and dilated cardiomyopathy (DCM) using molecular techniques [42, 43]. Towbin and colleagues later showed the high incidence of adenovirus in myocarditis and DCM [44-48] as well as par-

vovirus B19 [49]. Viruses cause myocyte damage either by direct cytopathic effects or indirectly by immune-mediated mechanisms. Apoptosis is the principal type of cell death involved in the progressive myocyte loss of ARVC/D and evidence supporting this view has been collected both at autopsy [19] and from biopsy material [20]. The biochemical mechanisms involved in the high rate of apoptosis observed in ARVC/D are poorly understood. Overexpression of caspase CPP32, a cysteine protease required for apoptosis, has been observed in the RV of ARVC/D patients [1]. Interestingly, the presence of apoptosis was found in the early and acute symptomatic phase of the disease [20]. Apoptosis is involved in the pathogenesis of several viral infections in a dual fashion, as viruses have both apoptosis-inducing and apoptosis-suppressing functions during their replication in host cells [50]. Myocardial apoptosis might be directly associated with the viral presence or be mediated by inflammation (i.e., activation of the Fas receptor pathway, release of apoptotic cytokines) [51]. Perforin, granzyme B, or other cytotoxic-T-related products can, by themselves or by activating effector caspases, induce apoptosis [52]. Perforin-containing cells have been detected in the myocardium after coxsackievirus infection [53] and circumstantial evidence has indicated that perforin is involved in coxsackievirus-induced myocarditis [54].

Cytotoxic T lymphocytes have been frequently observed in samples from patients with ARVC/D and the association of this lymphocyte subset with apoptotic myocyte is a frequent event (Fig. 9.3).

Although apoptotic myocyte death is believed by many to be the main mechanism of myocardial loss, the association of necrotic cell death cannot be excluded. Enteroviral protease 2A directly cleaves human dystrophin in the hinge 3 region of this large cytoskeletal protein, leading to functional dystrophin impairment and loss of sarcolemmal integrity [55].

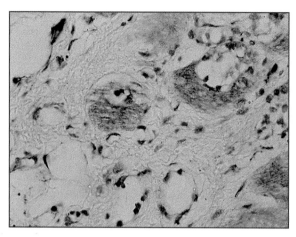

Fig. 9.3 • Endomyocardial biopsy from patient with ARVC/D. Double staining showing a strict relation of CD8 T lymphocyte (cytoplasm marked in brown) and apoptotic myocytes (marked in blue) TUNEL/IHC for CD8, original magnification, ×100

Table 9.3 • Familial ARVC/D and myocarditis

Author	N. patients
Sabel et al., 1990 [56]	2
Hisaoka et al., 1990 [57]	2
Pinamonti et al., 1996 [16]	2
D'Amati et al., 1998 [58]	2

Causative Role of Viruses

In familial cases of ARVC/D, autosomal dominant inheritance with variable penetrance has been reported and accounts for nearly 30%-50% of cases. In the remaining cases the disorder is believed to be related to an acquired etiology. As reported above, different cardiotropic viruses have been detected in myocardial samples from patients with ARVC/D. However, a small number of cases have been reported (Table 9.2), and therefore the incidence of viral forms of ARVC/D, as well as the prevalence of cardiotropic viruses in the disease, remain to be established. As in chronic forms of inflammatory cardiomyopathy (dilated cardiomyopathy), viruses could be the cause of slow, progressive myocyte damage. Relatively small viral loads during chronic latent infections appear to be able to sustain significant viral transcriptional activity over long periods of time and could result in recurrent bouts of apoptosis with progressive cell death and myocardial disappearance, followed by fibrofatty replacement. The interruption of myocyte-to-myocyte continuity due to fibro-fatty replacement subsequently can result in electrical signs and symptoms of the disease.

Contributing Role of Viruses

The inflammatory/infective theory does not exclude genetic aspects, although viral infections occur more rarely in familial cases. Myocarditis was found in members of the same family with ARVC/D leading to

the hypothesis of genetic predisposition to viral infection (Table 9.3) [16, 56-58]. A more complete comprehension of disease pathogenesis can only be drawn if both genetic and environmental factors are considered. In this genome-environment interaction, viral infections may play a *primary* or *secondary* role, both crucial conditions for the development and progression of the disease.

Primary Role

Many DNA and RNA viruses, following infection, can cause genetic alterations in somatic genes. These genetic alterations, referred to as mutations, may include deletions, chromosomal translocations, inversions, or point mutations. These genomic modifications could occur during viral integration to the host genome or play a role during subsequent steps of viral replication [59, 60].

These aspects are well known in the study of neoplastic disorders. Many oncogenic viruses are able to cause genetic alteration responsible for structural cellular changes promoting malignant transformation. Among structural proteins, cellular junctions are frequently altered during viral infections. The alteration of structural junction proteins after viral infection is one of the first and principal mechanisms responsible for virus-induced cell dysfunction and viral immortalization.

Thus, viral infections could play a primary contributing role in the acquired forms of ARVC/D, affecting the desmosome primarily by direct disruption.

Secondary Role

Genome-environment interaction is the basis of many complex disorders. In the setting of cardiovascular diseases, DCM represents a typical example [43-49, 61]. Recent research suggests that cardiotropic viruses are important environmental factors in the pathogenesis of "idiopathic" cases and that DCM more frequently results from interactions between genetic and environmental factors, whereas "pure" genetic forms may be uncommon. Genetic background could influence viral interaction at different levels: virus uptake, migration, and antiviral immunity. In other words, genetic defects of different types could be responsible for increased individual viral susceptibility (Fig. 9.4).

The majority of known cardiotropic viruses are taken up into the cell by receptor-mediated endocytosis and then further transported into the nucleus. The expression of viral receptors on target cells favor virus entry and migration. Overexpression of a common receptor for both coxsackievirus and adenovirus was detected in human DCM but not in other cardiomyopathies [62, 63] and is believed to potentially influence the pathogenesis of DCM.

Genetic abnormalities of immune pathways can also significantly alter the disease course in viral infection. Mice are protected from coxsackievirus B3 myocarditis by gene-targeted knockout of p56Lck, the Src family kinase essential for T-cell activation

[64]. On the other hand, coxsackievirus B3 infection of INF-β deficient mice results in higher mortality as compared to controls [65].

Genetically altered structural proteins of cardiomyocytes could favor viral infection and could themselves represent a target for the viruses, which then cause a progression of the disease. Experimental studies have demonstrated the extent to which such mutations may aggravate the cardiac damage caused by the virus. Coxsackievirus B3 infection, for example, has been shown to grossly decrease cardiac function in dystrophin-deficient mice via enteroviral protease 2A-mediated cleavage of dystrophin [55, 66].

In complex genetic disorders with heterogenecity of phenotypes, a comprehensive picture of the pathogenesis can only be drawn if both genetic and environmental factors are considered. Broadened understanding of the pathogenesis may crucially modify the clinical risk assessment and treatment of these patients.

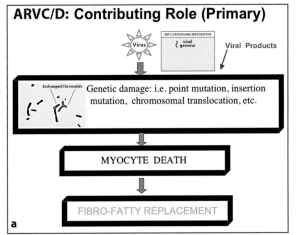

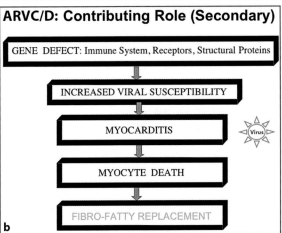

Fig. 9.4 • Diagrams showing possible pathogenetic role of viral infection on genetic substrate: (**a**) contributing role primary, (**b**) contributing role secondary

Conclusions

Different types of viral genomes are present in myocardial samples from some patients with ARVC/D. Multicenter studies, enrolling a large series of patients, are necessary to establish the incidence and prevalence of viral forms in the disease.

A variety of approaches are needed to obtain further insight into genome-environment interactions. In particular, transgenic animal models for known ARVC/D-associated gene mutations could facilitate the knowledge of pathogenetic mechanisms responsible for progressive myocyte damage.

References

1. Nava A, Rossi L, Thiene G (eds) (1997) Arrhythmogenic right ventricular cardiomyopathy/dysplasia. Elsevier, Amsterdam
2. Thiene G, Nava A, Corrado D et al (1988) Right ventricular cardiomyopathy and sudden death in young people. N Engl J Med 318:129-133
3. Corrado D, Thiene G, Nava A et al (1990) Sudden death in young competitive athletes: Clinicopathologic correlation in 22 cases. Am J Med 89:588-596
4. Towbin JA, Bowles NE (2002) The failing heart. Nature 415: 227-233
5. McKoy G, Protonotarios N, Crosby A et al (2000) Identification of a deletion in plakoglobin in arrhythmogenic right ventricular cardiomyopathy with palmoplantar keratoderma and woolly hair (Naxos disease). Lancet 355:2119-2124

6. Rampazzo A, Nava A, Malacrida S et al (2002) Mutation in human desmoplakin domain binding to plakoglobin causes a dominant form of arrhythmogenic right ventricular cardiomyopathy. Am J Hum Genet 71:1200-1206

7. Gerull B, Heuser A, Wichter T et al (2004) Mutations in the desmosomal protein plakophilin-2 are common in arrhythmogenic right ventricular cardiomyopathy. Nat Genet 36:1162-1164

8. Beffagna G, Occhi G, Nava A et al (2005) Regulatory mutations in transforming growth factor-β3 gene cause arrhythmogenic right ventricular cardiomyopathy type 1. Cardiovasc Res 65:366-373

9. Pilichou K, Nava A, Basso C et al (2006) Mutations in desmoglein-2 gene are associated with arrhythmogenic right ventricular cardiomyopathy. Circulation 113:1171-1179

10. Syrris P, Ward D, Evans S et al (2006) Arrhythmogenic right ventricular dysplasia/cardiomyopathy associated with mutations in the desmosomal gene desmocollin-2. Am J Hum Genet 79:978-984

11. Ananthasubramaniam K, Khaja F (1998) Arrhythmogenic right ventricular dysplasia/cardiomyopathy: Review for the clinician. Prog Cardiovasc Dis 41:237-246

12. Basso C, Thiene G, Corrado D et al (1996) Arrhythmogenic right ventricular cardiomyopathy. Dysplasia, dystrophy or myocarditis? Circulation 94:983-991

13. Miani D, Pinamonti B, Bussani R et al (1993) Right ventricular dysplasia: A clinical and pathological study of two families with left ventricular involvement. Br Heart J 69:151-157

14. Fontaine G, Fontaliran F, Lascault G et al (1990) Congenital and acquired right ventricular dysplasia. Arch Mal Coeur Vaiss 83:915-290

15. Thiene G, Corrado D, Nava A et al (1991) Right ventricular cardiomyopathy: Is there evidence of an inflammatory aetiology? Eur Heart J 12:22-25

16. Pinamonti B, Miani D, Sinagra G et al (1996) Familial right ventricular dysplasia with biventricular involvement and inflammatory infiltration. Heart 76:66-69

17. Grumbach IM, Heim A, Vonhof S et al (1998) Coxsackievirus genome in myocardium of patients with arrhythmogenic right ventricular dysplasia/cardiomyopathy. Cardiology 89:241-245

18. Williams GT, Smith CA (1993) Molecular regulation of apoptosis: Genetic controls on cell death. Cell 74:777-779

19. Mallat Z, Tedgui A, Fontaliran F et al (1996) Evidence of apoptosis in arrhythmogenic right ventricular dysplasia. N Engl J Med 335:1190-1196

20. Valente M, Calabrese F, Thiene G et al (1998) In vivo evidence of apoptosis in arrhythmogenic right ventricular cardiomyopathy. Am J Pathol 152:479-484

21. D'Amati G, di Gioia CR, Giordano C et al (2000). Myocyte transdifferentiation: A possible pathogenetic mechanism for arrhythmogenic right ventricular cardiomyopathy. Arch Pathol Lab Med 124:287-290

22. Corrado D, Basso C, Thiene G et al (1997) Spectrum of clinicopathologic manifestations of arrhythmogenic right ventricular cardiomyopathy/dysplasia: A multicenter study. J Am Coll Cardiol 30:1512-1520

23. Orth T, Herr W, Spahn T et al (1997) Human parvovirus B19 infection associated with severe acute perimyocarditis in a 34-year-old man. Eur Heart J 18:524-525

24. Nilsson K, Lindquist O, Påhlson C (1999) Association of *Rickettsia helvetica* with chronic perimyocarditis in sudden cardiac death. Lancet 354:1169-1173

25. Ristic AD, Maisch B, Hufnagel G et al (2000) Arrhythmias in acute pericarditis. An endomyocardial biopsy study. Herz 25:729-733

26. Pankuweit S, Moll R, Baandrup U et al (2003) Prevalence of the parvovirus B19 genome in endomyocardial biopsy specimens. Hum Pathol 34:497-503

27. Lobo FV, Heggtveit HA, Butany J et al (1992) Right ventricular dysplasia: Morphological findings in 13 cases. Can J Card 8:261-268

28. Fornes P, Ratel S, Lecomte D (1998) Pathology of arrhythmogenic right ventricular cardiomyopathy/dysplasia – An autopsy study of 20 forensic cases. J Forensic Sci 43:777-783

29. Burke AP, Farb A, Tashko G et al (1998) Arrhythmogenic right ventricular cardiomyopathy and fatty replacement of the right ventricular myocardium: Are they different diseases? Circulation 97:1571-1580

30. Fox PR, Maron BJ, Basso C et al (2000) Spontaneously occurring arrhythmogenic right ventricular cardiomyopathy in the domestic cat: A new animal model similar to the human disease. Circulation 102:1863-1870

31. Harvey AM, Battersby IA, Faena M et al (2005) Arrhythmogenic right ventricular cardiomyopathy in two cats. J Small Anim Pract 46:151-156

32. Basso C, Fox PR, Meurs KM et al (2004) Arrhythmogenic right ventricular cardiomyopathy causing sudden cardiac death in boxer dogs: A new animal model of human disease. Circulation 109:1180-1185

33. Calabrese F, Basso C, Carturan E et al (2006) Arrhythmogenic right ventricular cardiomyopathy/dysplasia: Is there a role for viruses? Cardiovasc Pathol 15:11-17

34. Matsumori A, Kawai C. (1980) Coxsackie virus B3 perimyocarditis in BALB/c mice: Experimental model of chronic perimyocarditis in the right ventricle. J Pathol l131:97-106

35. Kearney DL, Towbin JA, Bricker JT et al (1995) Familial right ventricular dysplasia (cardiomyopathy). Pediatr Pathol Lab Med 15:181-189

36. Heim A, Grumbach I, Hake S et al (1997) Enterovirus heart disease of adults: A persistent, limited organ infection in the presence of neutralizing antibodies. J Med Virol 53:196-204

37. Heim A, Grumbach I, Stille-Siegener M et al (1997) Detection of enterovirus RNA in the myocardium of a patient with arrhythmogenic right ventricular cardiomyopathy by in situ hybridization. Clin Infect Dis 25:1471-1472

38. Calabrese F, Angelini A, Thiene G et al (2000) No detection of enteroviral genome in the myocardium of patients with arrhythmogenic right ventricular cardiomyopathy. J Clin Pathol 53:382-387

39. Bowles NE, Ni J, Marcus F et al (2002) The detection of cardiotropic viruses in the myocardium of patients

with arrhythmogenic right ventriculardysplasia/cardiomyopathy. J Am Coll Cardiol 39:892-895

40. Chimenti C, Pieroni M, Maseri A et al (2004) Histologic findings in patients with clinical and instrumental diagnosis of sporadic arrhythmogenic right ventricular dysplasia. J Am Coll Cardiol 43:2305-2313

41. McKenna WJ, Thiene G, Nava A et al (1994) Diagnosis of arrhythmogenic right ventricular dysplasia/cardiomyopathy. Task Force of the Working Group Myocardial and Pericardial Disease of the European Society of Cardiology and of the Scientific Council on Cardiomyopathies of the International Society and Federation of Cardiology. Br Heart J 71:215-218

42. Bowles NE, Richardson PJ, Olsen EG et al (1986) Detection of Coxsackie-B-virus-specific RNA sequences in myocardial biopsy samples from patients with myocarditis and dilated cardiomyopathy. Lancet 1:1120-1123

43. Bowles NE, Rose ML, Taylor P et al (1989) End-stage dilated cardiomyopathy: Persistence of enterovirus RNA in myocardium at cardiac transplantation. Circulation 80:1128-1136

44. Towbin JA, Griffin LD, Martin AB et al (1994) Intrauterine adenoviral myocarditis presenting a nonimmune hydrops fetalis: Diagnosis by polymerase chain reaction. Ped Inf Dis 13:144-150

45. Martin AB, Webber S, Fricker FJ et al (1994) Acute myocarditis: Rapid diagnosis by polymerase chain reaction (PCR) in children. Circulation 90:330-339

46. Griffin L, Kearney D, Ni J et al (1995) Analysis of formalin-fixed and frozen myocardial autopsy samples for viral genome in childhood myocarditis and dilated cardiomyopathy with endocardial fibroelastosis using polymerse chain reaction (PCR). Cardiovasc Pathol 4:3-11

47. Bowles NE, Ni J, Kearney DL et al (2003) Detection of viruses in myocardial tissues by polymerase chain reaction: Evidence of adenovirus as a common cause of myocarditis in children and adults. J Am Coll Cardiol 42:466-472

48. Pauschinger M, Bowles NE, Fuentes-Garcia FJ et al (1999) Detection of adenoviral genome in the myocardium of adult patients with idiopathic left ventricular dysfunction. Circulation 99:1348-1354

49. Schowengerdt KO, Ni J, Denfield SW et al (1996) Diagnosis, surveillance, and epidemiologic evaluation of viral infection in pediatric cardiac transplant recipients using the polymerase chain reaction (PCR). J Heart Lung Transplant 15:111-123

50. Teodoro JG, Branton PE (1997) Regulation of apoptosis by viral gene products. J Virol 71:1739-1746

51. Kerr JFR, Wyllie AH, Currie AR (1972) Apoptosis: A basic biological phenomenon with wide-ranging implications in tissue kinetics. Br J Cancer 26:239-257

52. Talanian RV, Yang X, Turbov J et al (1997) Granule-mediated killing: Pathways for granzyme B-initiated apoptosis. J Exp Med 186:1323-1331

53. Seko Y, Shinkai Y, Kawasaki A et al (1991) Expression of perforin in infiltrating cells in murine hearts with acute myocarditis caused by coxsackievirus B3. Circulation 84:788-795

54. Seko Y, Shinkai Y, Kawasaki A et al (1993) Evidence of perforin-mediated cardiac myocyte injury in acute murine myocarditis caused by Coxsackie virus B3. J Pathol 170:53-58

55. Badorff C, Berkely N, Mehrotra S et al (2000) Enteroviral protease 2A directly cleaves dystrophin and is inhibited by a dystrophin-based substrate analogue. J Biol Chem 275:11191-11197

56. Sabel KG, Blomstrom-Lundqvist C, Olsson SB et al (1990) Arrhythmogenic right ventricular dysplasia in brother and sister: Is it related to myocarditis? Pediatr Cardiol 11:113-116

57. Hisaoka T, Kawai S, Ohi H et al (1990) Two cases of chronic myocarditis mimicking arrhythmogenic right ventricular dysplasia. Heart Vessels 5:51-54

58. D'Amati G, Fiore F, Giordano C et al (1998) Pathologic evidence of arrhythmogenic cardiomyopathy and myocarditis in two siblings. Cardiovasc Pathol 7:39-46

59. Kasai Y, Takeda S, Takagi H (1996) Pathogenesis of hepatocellular carcinoma: A review from the viewpoint of molecular analysis. Semin Surg Oncol 12:155-159

60. Wentzensen N, Vinokurova S, von Knebel Doeberitz M (2004) Systematic review of genomic integration sites of human papillomavirus genomes in epithelial dysplasia and invasive cancer of the female lower genital tract. Cancer Res 64:3878-3884

61. Calabrese F, Thiene G (2003) Myocarditis and inflammatory cardiomyopathy: Microbiological and molecular biological aspects. Cardiovasc Res 60:11-25

62. Noutsias M, Fechner H, de Jonge H et al (2001) Human coxsackie-adenovirus receptor is colocalized with integrins alpha(v)beta(3) and alpha(v)beta(5) on the cardiomyocyte sarcolemma and upregulated in dilated cardiomyopathy: Implications for cardiotropic viral infections. Circulation 104:275-280

63. Fechner H, Noutsias M, Tschoepe C et al (2003) Induction of coxsackievirus-adenovirus-receptor expression during myocardial tissue formation and remodeling: Identification of a cell-to-cell contact-dependent regulatory mechanism. Circulation 107:876-882

64. Liu P, Aitken K, Kong YY et al (2000) The tyrosine kinase p56lck is essential in coxsackievirus B3-mediated heart disease. Nat Med 6:429-434

65. Deonarain R, Cerullo D, Fuse K et al (2004) Protective role for interferon-beta in coxsackievirus B3 infection. Circulation 110:3540-3543

66. Xiong D, Lee GH, Bardoff C et al (2002) Dystrophin deficiency markedly increases enterovirus-induced cardiomyopathy: A genetic predisposition to viral heart disease. Nat Med 8:872-877

CHAPTER 10

DIAGNOSIS: TASK FORCE CRITERIA INCLUDING MODIFICATIONS FOR FAMILY MEMBERS

Deirdre Ward, Petros Syrris, Srijita Sen-Chowdhry, William J. McKenna

Introduction

Arrhythmogenic right ventricular cardiomyopathy/dysplasia (ARVC/D) is a heart muscle disorder associated with the occurrence of ventricular arrhythmias arising from the right ventricle in the presence of subtle or diffuse morphological changes [1-4]. Histologically the condition is characterized by myocyte loss with fatty or fibrofatty replacement [5]. The reclassification of cardiomyopathies by the World Health Organization/International Society and Federation of Cardiology Task Force on the Definition and Classification of Cardiomyopathies in 1995 defined ARVC/D as being "characterized by progressive fibrofatty replacement of the right ventricular myocardium, initially with typical regional, and later global, right and some left ventricular involvement, with relative sparing of the septum. Familial disease is common, with autosomal dominant inheritance and incomplete penetrance; a recessive form is described. Presentation with arrhythmias and sudden death is common, particularly in the young" [6].

The original theory that this is a dysplastic process, with partial or complete congenital absence of ventricular myocardium, has been largely disproved by clinical and pathological evidence demonstrating the acquired and progressive nature of the condition [3, 5-13]. One case of antenatal detection of right ventricular structural abnormalities associated with ventricular ectopy of right ventricular origin has been reported [14]. This may reflect a different disorder, sometimes known as Uhl's anomaly, characterized by congenital absence, total or subtotal, of right ventricular myocardium [15]. A genetic basis for classical "acquired" ARVC/D has been identified, with predominantly autosomal dominant transmission. The genes identified have demonstrated ARVC/D to be, for the most part, a disease of the desmosome [16-21]. Some autosomal recessive forms of desmosomal disease have been characterized [22, 23], as well as some non-desmosomal forms associated with effort-induced polymorphic ventricular tachycardia [24] and transcriptional abnormalities [25]. To date, however, gene mutations are only identified in 40% of cases [21] suggesting that the other 60% of cases may be comprised of incorrect diagnoses, other cell adhesion gene mutations or phenocopies of ARVC/D.

The first case series published in 1982 described clinical findings in 24 adults, the majority of whom presented with symptomatic ventricular tachycardia [1]. There was a high preponderance of male patients (ratio to females 2.7:1) and onset of symptoms was typically in the fourth decade of life although the age range was broad (13-59 years). Those clinical findings reflect the investigations available at the time. On chest x-ray, the cardiothoracic ratio exceeded 50% in 72% of patients. The most frequent finding on ECG was right precordial T-wave inversion (V1 to V4), present in over 85% of those who had documented ventricular tachycardia. Incomplete or complete right bundle branch block was present in over one third of all patients. Postexcitation waves (Epsilon waves) were seen on the resting ECG in almost one third of patients, and confirmed on signal-averaged ECG. An additional one third of patients had late potentials on signal-averaged ECG but no indication of this on the ECG. Over 90% of patients had documented spontaneous ventricular tachycardia, and in all but one of these the morphology was confirmed as left bundle branch block, consistent with a right ventricular origin. Formal electrophysiological studies were performed in most patients, and almost invariably ventricular tachycardia was induced, usually with the same morphology as the spontaneously occurring arrhythmia. Conventional 2D echo only became available towards the latter part of the follow-up in this study, so only one third of patients underwent such evaluation. The patients with arrhythmia who had 2D echo showed increased RV:LV ratios, and most had right ventricular wall motion abnormalities, although one had left posterior wall involvement. At cardiac catheterization, most patients had normal hemodynamics, although in some cases the right atrial a-wave amplitude was increased. Right ventricular angiography demonstrated global enlargement in most, and wall motion abnormality in some. Cardiac morphological abnormalities were confirmed by direct visualization in half of the patients (mostly at the time of surgery for intractable ventricular arrhythmia resistant to medical therapy). The authors first described the high frequency of structural abnormalities at the 3 points of the "triangle of dysplasia" (the pulmonary infundibulum, the apex, and the inferior wall or subtricuspid region). They noted that in two of their patients with ventricular tachycardia, clinical investigations had not confirmed the diagnosis, but subsequent pathology review of tissue removed at surgery identified features typical of ARVC/D.

As one would expect with any newly described condition, the cases presented represent the more severe end of the spectrum of disease expression. Indeed the Authors reviewed available information on an additional 34 adult cases reported in the literature; less than half of these had documented ventricular tachycardia. Their prevalence (90%) is unusually high, and may have reflected referral bias as they have a special interest in arrhythmias. Only one of their 24 patients was thought to have a familial form of the disease.

In the ensuing years, more cases of ARVC/D were reported and a heterogeneous pattern of disease expression emerged. In the Veneto region of Italy ARVC/D emerged as a significant cause of sudden death in the young. In 20% of sudden deaths occurring in people under age 35 years, features of ARVC/D were detected at postmortem evaluation. In almost half of these there were no prior reported symptoms, and despite history of palpitation and/or syncope in the others, the diagnosis had not been suspected prior to their death [3]. Additionally, in a study of sudden deaths in young athletes conducted over a 10-year period, over a quarter of cases had a postmortem diagnosis of ARVC/D [4]. Other milder phenotypes were emerging, with patients initially diagnosed as having idiopathic ventricular arrhythmia with "normal hearts," with subsequent detailed echo or angiographic studies showing evidence of regional or segmental right and/or left ventricular structural or dynamic abnormalities [26]. Familial disease was also being identified at a higher frequency with disease identified in identical and nonidentical twins [27] and up to 30% in one case series [26].

Task Force Criteria

In many of these individuals, the clinical findings were more subtle than those reported by Marcus et al. [1], and yet they appeared to be affected by a variant of

the same condition. In some of those identified at postmortem, clinical findings antemortem had perhaps not been recognized or interpreted appropriately, and opportunities to institute potentially life-saving measures were missed. The gold standard for making a diagnosis of ARVC/D is accepted as the demonstration of transmural fibrofatty replacement of right ventricular myocardium, determined at either postmortem or surgery. This definition presents an obvious limitation in normal clinical practice. Even using endomyocardial biopsies as a diagnostic tool, by definition the sample is not transmural and it is usually taken from the interventricular septum, not recognized as part of the triangle of dysplasia; as such, absence of characteristic changes would not exclude the diagnosis. Reliance on an invasive and potentially high risk procedure as a sole diagnostic tool, given the known morphological abnormalities encountered in the right ventricle, is not practical for screening in large populations. The other features documented in patients with ARVC/D are variably lacking in specificity for the condition. As a result of these difficulties in clinically diagnosing ARVC/D, a Task Force of experienced clinicians in the field of cardiomyopathy was convened under the auspices of the European Society of Cardiology (Working Group on Myocardial and Pericardial Diseases) and the International Society and Federation of Cardiology (Scientific Council). The remit of this Task Force was to agree criteria on clinical evaluation that would delineate the spectrum of disease that justifiably can be called right ventricular dysplasia in clinical practice [28].

Based on the contemporaneously available evidence, the Task Force looked at clinical criteria in six different groupings. Diagnostic criteria were assigned major or minor status according to their specificity for the condition. A diagnosis of ARVC/D was to be considered fulfilled by the presence of different groups of two major criteria, one major and two minor criteria, or four minor criteria (Table 10.1).

Right ventricular morphological abnormalities, as defined by echocardiography, angiography, magnetic resonance imaging or nuclear scintigraphy, are perhaps the most difficult to standardize. The identification of regional wall motion abnormalities still to this day requires a subjective judgement, and is therefore open to over- and under-reporting. The measurement of right ventricular volumes, dimensions, and ventricular function is problematic, as the structure of the right ventricle is not amenable to the same mathematical assumptions which permit analogous measurements in the left ventricle. Definition of the normal reference range for the right ventricle in each of these parameters is based on a relatively

Table 10.1 • Task force criteria for diagnosis of ARVC/D. Adapted from [28]

I. Global and/or regional dysfunction and structural alterations*	IV. Depolarisation/conduction abnormalities
Major:	*Major:*
Severe dilatation and reduction in systolic function of RV with no (or only mild) impairment of LV	Epsilon waves or localised prolongation of the QRS complex in V1-V3 (>110 ms)
Localised RV aneurysms (akinetic or dyskinetic areas with diastolic bulging)	*Minor:*
Severe segmental dilatation of the RV	Late potentials demonstrated on signal averaged ECG
Minor:	
Mild global RV dilatation and /or reduction in ejection fraction with normal LV	
Mild segmental dilatation of RV	
Regional RV hypokinesia	
II. Tissue characterisation of walls	**V. Arrhythmias**
Major:	*Minor:*
Fibrofatty replacement of myocardium demonstrated on endomyocardial biopsy	Sustained and non-sustained ventricular tachycardia with left bundle branch block morphology (documented on ECG, Holter or exercise testing)
	Frequent ventricular extrasystoles (>1000 over 24 hrs Holter monitoring)
III. Repolarisation abnormalities	**VI. Family history**
Minor:	*Major:*
Inverted T-waves in right precordial leads (V2 and V3) (individuals >12 years of age; in the absence of right bundle branch block)	Familial disease confirmed at necropsy or surgery
	Minor:
	Family history of premature sudden death (<35 years) due to suspected right ventricular dysplasia
	Family history of clinical diagnosis based on the present criteria

ECG, electrocardiogram; *LV*, left ventricle; *RV*, right ventricle
* Morphological changes in I as detected by echocardiography, angiography, cardiac magnetic resonance imaging or radionuclide scintigraphy

small study of 41 patients using multiple tomographic planes to overcome the difficulties relating to structure [29]. Dilation of a segment or the whole right ventricle was defined as being mild if measured dimensions were 2-3 standard deviations, and severe if ≥3 standard deviations greater than normal, based on evidence from studies of ARVC/D patients evaluated by echocardiography and/or angiography [8, 30-33]. In an effort to improve the specificity of the criteria it was stipulated that the finding of morphological or functional abnormalities of the right ventricle must be in the absence of any more than mild left ventricular systolic impairment. This was in an effort to avoid inclusion of dilated cardiomyopathy with right ventricular involvement under the diagnostic umbrella of ARVC/D. When these criteria were written, dilated cardiomyopathy and ARVC/D were considered to be entirely distinct entities, although evidence of considerable overlap in phenotypic presentation has come to light, mostly in the last decade [17, 18, 34-37]. By definition, therefore, the

diagnostic criteria allow for only mild left ventricular involvement, which does not reflect currently available information on the prevalence of left ventricular involvement in ARVC/D.

Endomyocardial biopsy findings of fibrofatty replacement are rarely diagnostic, although this was given major status as a diagnostic criterion as it would strongly support any findings on the other clinical investigations. Specific histomorphometric parameters of myocytes, interstitium, fibrous and fatty tissue were evaluated on biopsy samples by the Padua Group, and threshold values of <45% area of myocytes, >40% fibrous, and >3% fatty tissue were defined as diagnostic of ARVC/D with 67% sensitivity and over 90% specificity for at least one parameter [38].

Repolarization abnormalities on ECG, consisting of T-wave inversion in the right precordial leads (beyond V1 to include V2 and V3) was quite a consistent finding in earlier reported case series (over 85% as reported by Marcus et al. [1]). Subsequent case series have described a variable prevalence of right precor-

tailed understanding of the natural history of the condition would promote evolution of the criteria to allow a more succinct clinical or genetic diagnosis. Some of the limitations of the criteria are detailed above.

Task Force Criteria Revisited

Even before the publication of the Task Force criteria in 1994, study of relatives of probands diagnosed with ARVC/D identified features of disease which were not as marked as in the proband, suggesting considerable heterogeneity of disease expression, even within relatives carrying the same gene mutation. There was evidence supporting both incomplete and age-related penetrance [53]. From the Veneto region of Italy we have evidence on postmortem of ARVC/D in athletes who did not fulfill the diagnostic criteria antemortem. This so-called concealed phase of ARVC/D is problematic, as fatal arrhythmias can occur in the absence of gross morphological changes [3-5]. Since the publication of the Task Force criteria in 1994, the identification of specific gene mutations responsible for ARVC/D has provided evidence of gene carriers with some features of ARVC/D which are insufficient to fulfill the Task Force criteria. Logic dictates that these subjects have at least a "forme fruste" of ARVC/D and data is still lacking as to whether the natural history for those with incomplete penetrance differs substantially from those who fulfill classical Task Force criteria for ARVC/D.

Previous evaluation of relatives of patients with hypertrophic and dilated cardiomyopathy has shown that some have phenotypic abnormalities which, while nondiagnostic, are indicative of disease expression [54, 55]. Hamid et al. evaluated family members of ARVC/D probands to determine if reliance on Task Force criteria to diagnose ARVC/D would result in significant underreporting in the setting of family screening [56]. They evaluated almost 300 relatives of 67 probands (a mean of 4.4 subjects per family). Features of ARVC/D

fulfillling diagnostic criteria were identified in 10% of relatives, suggesting familial disease in 28% of probands. This is somewhat less than what reported elsewhere of up to 50% familial disease [57]. However a further 11% of relatives had isolated minor criteria on clinical evaluation. These included T-wave inversion of right precordial leads in 41% and a positive signal-averaged ECG in almost one third. A small proportion had an excess of 200 ventricular ectopics on 24-h Holter monitoring (2%). These "nondiagnostic" cases, if accepted by logic to be affected in the context of a definitely affected relative and 50% gene transmission, would bring the total proportion of familial disease to 50%, which is similar to the findings in dilated cardiomyopathy (when isolated left ventricular enlargement or depressed fractional shortening are included) [55] and in hypertrophic cardiomyopathy (when isolated ECG abnormalities or mild hypertrophy on echo are included) [54]. The authors therefore propose a modification of the Task Force criteria, which could be used as a diagnostic tool, but only in first degree relatives of a patient with confirmed ARVC/D (Table 10.2). In this context, the presence of any one of right precordial T-wave inversion, late potentials on signal-averaged ECG, ventricular tachycardia with LBBB morphology, or minor functional or morphological changes of the right ventricle on imaging should be considered diagnostic for familial ARVC/D. In addition, they proposed that the arbitrary threshold value of 1,000 ventricular ectopics in a 24-h period be reduced to 200 ventricular ectopics, which would appear to be indicative of familial disease expression (Table 10.2).

As with the Task Force criteria, these proposed modified criteria require validation in prospectively evaluated familial ARVC/D. With the increasing number of disease-causing genes identified, there has been some evidence of improved diagnostic yield incorporating both diagnostic criteria. Bauce et al. described the findings in probands and relatives with four novel desmoplakin mutations [18]. Applying

Table 10.2 · Proposed modification of Task Force criteria for the diagnosis of familial ARVC/D. Adapted and reproduced from [56] with permission from the BMJ Publishing Group

Proven ARVC/D in a first-degree relative plus one of the following	
I. ECG: T-wave inversion in the right precordial leads (V2 and V3)	**II. Signal averaged ECG:** Demonstration of late potentials
III. Arrhythmia: Ventricular tachycardia with left bundle branch block morphology (documented on ECG, Holter monitoring or during exercise testing) >200 ventricular extrasystoles over 24 hours (Holter monitor)	**IV. Structural or functional abnormality of the right ventricle:** Mild global RV dilatation of the RV and/or reduction in ejection fraction with normal LV Mild segmental dilatation of the RV Regional RV hypokinesia

ARVC/D, Arrhythmogenic Right Ventricular Cardiomyopathy/Dysplesia; *ECG,* electrocardiogram; *LV,* left ventricle; *RV,* right ventricle

Task Force criteria, only 54% of gene carriers achieved the threshold for a diagnosis of ARVC/D. However, two thirds of mutation carriers were found to have some abnormality on ECG or echo. One of these with a nonspecific ECG abnormality alone died suddenly shortly after evaluation. Applying the modified criteria of Hamid et al. [56], an additional 15% of relatives could be considered affected, bringing gene penetrance for desmoplakin to almost 70%.

Our experience with plakophilin-2 mutations is similar. In eleven probands and their relatives we identified 66% of gene carriers who fulfillled Task Force criteria. Extending the diagnosis to those who fulfill the proposed modified criteria suggests gene penetrance for these families approaches 100% [20].

While these data support the benefit in modifying diagnostic criteria for familial disease, genotype phenotype studies have also highlighted limitations of the proposed system. This is perhaps not unexpected, given the nonspecific nature of most of the diagnostic criteria, as previously discussed. In two relatives without plakophilin-2 mutations, clinical evaluation had identified right ventricular enlargement in one, and high volume ventricular ectopy in another, but no other clinical features of ARVC/D in either. This had led to the clinical suspicion of gene carrier status, which was subsequently proved not to be the case [20]. Also, in evaluating families with desmoglein-2 mutations, we identified a mother and daughter whose only abnormal finding was late potentials on signal-averaged ECG. As

their father/grandfather had died suddenly at the age of 54, it was assumed that this was likely related to ARVC/D (as his nephew had died with postmortem pathological confirmation of ARVC/D). It was subsequently confirmed that the 54-year-old man died as a result of myocardial infarction, with fresh coronary thrombosis identified at postmortem, and the disease both clinically and genetically segregated with the other side of the proband's family. Therefore exclusive use of Task Force criteria has been shown to result in false negative diagnoses, and exclusive application of the proposed modified criteria within the context of familial ARVC/D will result in false positive diagnoses.

A further limitation of both criteria is the exclusion of left ventricular disease as an indicator of disease expression. Indeed, the Task Force criteria by definition exclude those with more than mild reduction in left ventricular systolic function. Many case series over the last 20 years have described varying proportions of patients exhibiting signs of left ventricular involvement. These range from 16% [42] to 27% [18], and if only those with Task Force criteria disease expression are considered, for desmoplakin the prevalence is over 40%. A review of pathological findings of 47 patients whose hearts were examined at autopsy or cardiac transplantation found that 76% had evidence of left ventricular involvement, either microscopically or macro- and microscopically, and these patients had a higher incidence of clinical complications (arrhythmias and heart failure) [34] (Fig. 10.3).

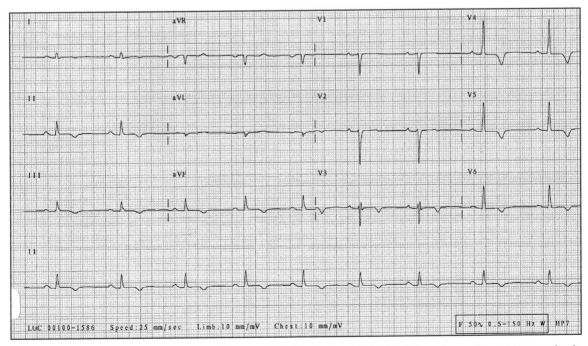

Fig. 10.3 • ECG from the patient whose Signal Averaged ECG is displayed in Fig. 10.2. There is poor R-wave progression in the right precordial leads, but T-wave inversion is only evident in the inferior leads and V3 to V6

We have recently published our findings related to a large family with a novel desmoplakin mutation [17]. On evaluating nine living relatives of a proband with isolated left ventricular fibrofatty change on postmortem, only four of these mutation carriers fulfilled Task Force criteria for a diagnosis of ARVC/D. Left ventricular disease was noted to be a prominent feature, both on imaging and in evidence of left precordial variants of the ECG patterns associated with ARVC/D. By modifying the Task Force criteria to include left ventricular rather than right ventricular abnormalities, the penetrance of this mutation was 93%, and the one patient who did not fulfill left ventricular Task Force criteria actually fulfilled right ventricular traditional criteria.

Conclusions

This highlights the challenge in evolving the current diagnostic criteria to encompass all aspects of this genetically and clinically heterogeneous condition. The optimal diagnostic criteria likely lie between these three models, although the gold standard should be based on genetic identification where possible.

Acknowledgements

We gratefully acknowledge support of our overall research work from: EC 5th Framework Program Research & Technology Development #QLG1-CT-2000-01091 and a British Heart Foundation Program Grant PG/03/036/15247. Drs. Ward and Sen – Chowdhry were supported by British Heart Foundation Junior Research Fellowships.

References

1. Marcus FI, Fontaine GH, Guiraudon G et al (1982) Right ventricular dysplasia: A report of 24 adult cases. Circulation 65:384-398
2. Fontaine G, Guiraudon G, Frank R et al (1982) Arrhythmogenic right ventricular dysplasia and Uhl's disease. Arch Mal Coeur Vaiss 75:361-371
3. Thiene G, Nava A, Corrado D et al (1988) Right ventricular cardiomyopathy and sudden death in young people. N Engl J Med 318:129-133
4. Corrado D, Thiene G, Nava A et al (1990) Sudden death in young competitive athletes: Clinicopathologic correlations in 22 cases. Am J Med 89:588-596
5. Basso C, Thiene G, Corrado D et al (1996) Arrhythmogenic right ventricular cardiomyopathy. Dysplasia, dystrophy, or myocarditis? Circulation 94:983-991
6. Richardson P, McKenna W, Bristow M et al (1996) Report of the 1995 World Health Organization/International Society and Federation of Cardiology Task Force on the Definition and Classification of cardiomyopathies. Circulation 93:841-842
7. Nava A, Scognamiglio R, Thiene G et al (1987) A polymorphic form of familial arrhythmogenic right ventricular dysplasia. Am J Cardiol 59:1405-1409
8. Daliento L, Rizzoli G, Thiene G et al (1990) Diagnostic accuracy of right ventriculography in arrhythmogenic right ventricular cardiomyopathy. Am J Cardiol 66:741-745
9. Baandrup U, Florio RA, Rehahn M et al (1981) Critical analysis of endomyocardial biopsies from patients suspected of having cardiomyopathy. II: Comparison of histology and clinical/haemodynamic information. Br Heart J 45:487-493
10. Fitchett DH, Sugrue DD, MacArthur CG et al (1984) Right ventricular dilated cardiomyopathy. Br Heart J 51:25-29
11. Thiene G, Corrado D, Nava A et al (1991) Right ventricular cardiomyopathy: Is there evidence of an inflammatory aetiology? Eur Heart J 12:22-25
12. Morgera T, Salvi A, Alberti E et al (1985) Morphological findings in apparently idiopathic ventricular tachycardia. An echocardiographic haemodynamic and histologic study. Eur Heart J 6:323-334
13. Bonacina E, Recalcati F, Mangiavacchi M et al (1989) Interstitial myocardial lipomatosis: A morphological study on endomyocardial biopsies and diseased hearts surgically removed for heart transplantation. Eur Heart J 10:100-102
14. Rustico MA, Benettoni A, Fontaliran F et al (2001) Prenatal echocardiographic appearance of arrhythmogenic right ventricle dysplasia: A case report. Fetal Diagn Ther 16:433-436
15. Uhl HS (1952) A previously undescribed congenital malformation of the heart: Almost total absence of the myocardium of the right ventricle. Bull Johns Hopkins Hosp 91:197-209
16. Rampazzo A, Nava A, Malacrida S et al (2002) Mutation in human desmoplakin domain binding to plakoglobin causes a dominant form of arrhythmogenic right ventricular cardiomyopathy. Am J Hum Genet 71:1200-1206
17. Norman M, Simpson M, Mogensen J et al (2005) Novel mutation in desmoplakin causes arrhythmogenic left ventricular cardiomyopathy. Circulation 112:636-642
18. Bauce B, Basso C, Rampazzo A et al (2005) Clinical profile of four families with arrhythmogenic right ventricular cardiomyopathy caused by dominant desmoplakin mutations. Eur Heart J 26:1666-1675
19. Gerull B, Heuser A, Wichter T et al (2004) Mutations in the desmosomal protein plakophilin-2 are common in arrhythmogenic right ventricular cardiomyopathy. Nat Genet 36:1162-1164
20. Syrris P, Ward D, Asimaki A et al (2006) Clinical expression of plakophilin-2 mutations in familial arrhythmogenic right ventricular cardiomyopathy. Circulation 113:356-364

21. Pilichou K, Nava A, Basso C et al (2006) Mutations in desmoglein-2 gene are associated with arrhythmogenic right ventricular cardiomyopathy. Circulation 113:1171-1179

22. McKoy G, Protonotarios N, Crosby A et al (2000) Identification of a deletion in plakoglobin in arrhythmogenic right ventricular cardiomyopathy with palmoplantar keratoderma and woolly hair (Naxos disease). Lancet 355:2119-2124

23. Norgett EE, Hatsell SJ, Carvajal-Huerta L et al (2000) Recessive mutation in desmoplakin disrupts desmoplakin-intermediate filament interactions and causes dilated cardiomyopathy, woolly hair and keratoderma. Hum Mol Genet 9:2761-2766

24. Bauce B, Rampazzo A, Basso C et al (2002) Screening for ryanodine receptor type 2 mutations in families with effort-induced polymorphic ventricular arrhythmias and sudden death: Early diagnosis of asymptomatic carriers. J Am Coll Cardiol 40:341-349

25. Beffagna G, Occhi G, Nava A et al (2005) Regulatory mutations in transforming growth factor-beta3 gene cause arrhythmogenic right ventricular cardiomyopathy type 1. Cardiovasc Res 65:366-373

26. Nava A, Thiene G, Canciani B et al (1992) Clinical profile of concealed form of arrhythmogenic right ventricular cardiomyopathy presenting with apparently idiopathic ventricular arrhythmias. Int J Cardiol 35:195-206

27. Buja G, Nava A, Daliento L et al (1993) Right ventricular cardiomyopathy in identical and nonidentical young twins. Am Heart J 126:1187-1193

28. McKenna WJ, Thiene G, Nava A et al (1994) Diagnosis of arrhythmogenic right ventricular dysplasia/cardiomyopathy. Task Force of the Working Group Myocardial and Pericardial Disease of the European Society of Cardiology and of the Scientific Council on Cardiomyopathies of the International Society and Federation of Cardiology. Br Heart J 71:215-218

29. Foale R, Nihoyannopoulos P, McKenna W et al (1986) Echocardiographic measurement of the normal adult right ventricle. Br Heart J 56:33-44

30. Robertson JH, Bardy GH, German LD et al (1985) Comparison of two-dimensional echocardiographic and angiographic findings in arrhythmogenic right ventricular dysplasia. Am J Cardiol 55:1506-1508

31. Blomstrom-Lundqvist C, Beckman-Suurkula M, Wallentin I et al (1988) Ventricular dimensions and wall motion assessed by echocardiography in patients with arrhythmogenic right ventricular dysplasia. Eur Heart J 9:1291-1302

32. Drobinski G, Verdiere C, Fontaine GH et al (1985) Angiocardiographic diagnosis in right ventricular dysplasia. Arch Mal Coeur Vaiss 78:544-551

33. Daubert C, Descaves C, Foulgoc JL et al (1988) Critical analysis of cineangiographic criteria for diagnosis of arrhythmogenic right ventricular dysplasia. Am Heart J 115:448-459

34. Corrado D, Basso C, Thiene G et al (1997) Spectrum of clinicopathologic manifestations of arrhythmogenic right ventricular cardiomyopathy/dysplasia: A multicenter study. J Am Coll Cardiol 30:1512-1520

35. d'Amati G, Leone O, di Gioia CR et al (2001) Arrhythmogenic right ventricular cardiomyopathy: Clinicopathologic correlation based on a revised definition of pathologic patterns. Hum Pathol 32:1078-1086

36. Lindstrom L, Nylander E, Larsson H et al (2005) Left ventricular involvement in arrhythmogenic right ventricular cardiomyopathy – A scintigraphic and echocardiographic study. Clin Physiol Funct Imaging 25:171-177

37. Pinamonti B, Salvi A, Silvestri F et al (1989) Left ventricular involvement in right ventricular cardiomyopathy. Eur Heart J 10:20-21

38. Angelini A, Thiene G, Boffa GM et al (1993) Endomyocardial biopsy in right ventricular cardiomyopathy. Int J Cardiol 40:273-282

39. Fontaine G, Umemura J, Di Donna P et al (1993) Duration of QRS complexes in arrhythmogenic right ventricular dysplasia. A new non-invasive diagnostic marker. Ann Cardiol Angeiol (Paris) 42:399-405

40. Peters S, Trummel M (2003) Diagnosis of arrhythmogenic right ventricular dysplasia-cardiomyopathy: Value of standard ECG revisited. Ann Noninvasive Electrocardiol 8:238-245

41. Pinamonti B, Sinagra G, Salvi A et al (1992) Left ventricular involvement in right ventricular dysplasia. Am Heart J 123:711-724

42. Nava A, Bauce B, Basso C et al (2000) Clinical profile and long-term follow-up of 37 families with arrhythmogenic right ventricular cardiomyopathy. J Am Coll Cardiol 36:2226-2233

43. Dalal D, Nasir K, Bomma C et al (2005) Arrhythmogenic right ventricular dysplasia: A United States experience. Circulation 112:3823-3832

44. Fontaine G, Fontaliran F, Hebert JL et al (1999) Arrhythmogenic right ventricular dysplasia. Annu Rev Med 50:17-35

45. Turrini P, Corrado D, Basso C et al (2001) Dispersion of ventricular depolarization-repolarization: A non-invasive marker for risk stratification in arrhythmogenic right ventricular cardiomyopathy. Circulation 103:3075-3080

46. Breithardt G, Borggrefe M, Karbenn U (1990) Late potentials as predictors of risk after thrombolytic treatment? Br Heart J 64:174-176

47. Breithardt G, Borggrefe M, Martinez-Rubio A et al (1990) Identification of patients at risk of ventricular tachyarrhythmias after myocardial infarction. Cardiologia 35:19-22

48. Blomstrom-Lundqvist C, Hirsch I, Olsson SB et al (1988) Quantitative analysis of the signal-averaged QRS in patients with arrhythmogenic right ventricular dysplasia. Eur Heart J 9:301-312

49. Leclercq JF, Coumel P (1993) Late potentials in arrhythmogenic right ventricular dysplasia. Prevalence, diagnostic and prognostic values. Eur Heart J 14:80-83

50. Oselladore L, Nava A, Buja G et al (1995) Signal-averaged electrocardiography in familial form of arrhyth-

mogenic right ventricular cardiomyopathy. Am J Cardiol 75:1038-1041

51. Turrini P, Angelini A, Thiene G et al (1999) Late potentials and ventricular arrhythmias in arrhythmogenic right ventricular cardiomyopathy. Am J Cardiol 83:1214-1219

52. Gaita F, Giustetto C, Di Donna P et al (2001) Long-term follow-up of right ventricular monomorphic extrasystoles. J Am Coll Cardiol 38:364-370

53. Nava A, Thiene G, Canciani B et al (1988) Familial occurrence of right ventricular dysplasia: A study involving nine families. J Am Coll Cardiol 12:1222-1228

54. McKenna WJ, Spirito P, Desnos M et al (1997) Experience from clinical genetics in hypertrophic cardiomyopathy: Proposal for new diagnostic criteria in adult members of affected families. Heart 77:130-132

55. Baig MK, Goldman JH, Caforio AL et al (1998) Familial dilated cardiomyopathy: Cardiac abnormalities are common in asymptomatic relatives and may represent early disease. J Am Coll Cardiol 31:195-201

56. Hamid MS, Norman M, Quraishi A et al (2002) Prospective evaluation of relatives for familial arrhythmogenic right ventricular cardiomyopathy/dysplasia reveals a need to broaden diagnostic criteria. J Am Coll Cardiol 40:1445-1450

57. Corrado D, Basso C, Thiene G (2000) Arrhythmogenic right ventricular cardiomyopathy: Diagnosis, prognosis, and treatment. Heart 83:588-595

| CHAPTER 11 | STRENGTHS AND WEAKNESSES OF THE TASK FORCE CRITERIA – PROPOSED MODIFICATIONS |

Frank I. Marcus, Duane Sherrill

Introduction

The diagnosis of ARVC/D is readily apparent when patients have the typical features including ECG changes and morphological abnormalities limited to the right ventricle. Since the right ventricular structure and contractile pattern is asymmetrical it can be difficult to differentiate normal from mild abnormalities of this complex ventricular chamber [1, 2]. This may cause uncertainty in differentiating ARVC/D from normal variants or from idiopathic ventricular tachycardia arising from the right ventricular outflow tract, a condition that is not hereditary and has a good prognosis [3-6]. These problems were recognized in the decade after the clinical profile of ARVDC/D was first described [7]. To address these uncertainties a Task Force was assembled that proposed diagnostic criteria for ARVC/D. The Task Force agreed that there was no single test that is sufficiently specific and sensitive to be used to establish this diagnosis. Therefore, major and minor criteria were selected and it was proposed that the diagnosis of ARVC/D be made using combinations of these criteria [8] (Table 11.1). The

Table 11.1 • Task Force criteria for diagnosis of ARVC/D

	Major	Minor
I. Global and/or regional dysfunction and structural alterations*	Severe dilatation and reduction of right ventricular ejection fraction with no (or only mild) LV impairment Localized right ventricular aneurysms (akinetic or dyskinetic areas with diastolic bulging) Severe segmental dilatation of the right ventricle	Mild global right ventricular dilatation and/or ejection fraction reduction with normal left ventricle Mild segmental dilatation of the right ventricle Regional right ventricular hypokinesia
II. Tissue characterization of wall	Fibrofatty replacement of myocardium on endomyocardial biopsy	
III. Repolarization abnormalities		Inverted T waves in right precordial leads (V2 and V3) (people aged >12 years, in absence of right bundle branch block)
IV. Depolarization/conduction abnormalities	Epsilon waves or localized prolongation (>110ms) of the QRS complex in right precordial leads (V1-V3)	Late potentials (signal-averaged ECG)
V. Arrhythmias	Arrhythmias listed below plus T wave abnormalities-see III Repolarization abnormalities	Left bundle branch block type ventricular tachycardia (sustained and nonsustained) (ECG, Holter, exercise testing) Frequent ventricular extrasystoles (>1000/24 hours) (Holter)
VI. Family history	Familial disease confirmed at necropsy or surgery	Family history of premature sudden death (<35 years) due to suspected right ventricular dysplasia Familial history (clinical diagnosis based on present criteria)

* Detected by echocardiography, angiography, magnetic resonance imaging, or radionuclide scintigraphy. *ECG*, electrocardiogram; *LV*, left ventricle.
Reproduced from [8] with permission from BMJ Publishing Group. The diagnosis of ARVC/D would be fulfilled by the presence of two major, or one major plus two minor criteria or four minor criteria from different groups

strength of these guidelines is that they have been extremely useful in providing standardized criteria to establish the diagnosis of ARVC/D. Since the guidelines were published, there has been a large accumulation of experience in the diagnosis of ARVC/D as well as improvements in diagnostic imaging techniques including 2D echocardiography, MRI, and angiography.

When one attempts to classify patients suspected of having this condition, certain limitations of the Task Force criteria become evident since some are qualitative and subjective.

In general the major limitations of the Task Force criteria relate to the definition or quantification of the various categories. In the original report it was stated that dilatation of the right ventricle or segments of the right ventricle was defined by echocardiography or angiography. Mild dilatation was assessed as 2-3 standard deviations (SD) from normal and >3 SD would be as categorized as severe dilatation. There was no definition of moderate dilatation. Yoerger et al. [9] performed an analysis of 2D echocardiograms in 29 probands who were diagnosed with ARVC/D independent of the echocardiogram. The echocardiograms were done according to a specific protocol (Table 11.2). They found that the RV fractional area change (FAC) was significantly decreased in probands vs. control patients (27.2±16 mm vs. 41.0±7.1 mm p=0.0003) and that the right ventricular outflow tract was the most commonly enlarged dimension in the ARVC/D probands (37.9±6.6mm) vs. control patients (26.2±4.9 mm p=<0.0001) (Table 11.2).

These data and the original Task Force definition of mild enlargement as >2 and <3 SD and ≥3 SD as severe have been calculated and are presented in Table 11.3. Normal values and cut-off values are not available from a large population database for these right ventricular echocardiogram-derived dimensions based on gender or adjusted for body surface area. When information from a large database of normals is forthcoming, the calculated values for right ventricular enlargement may require adjustment.

Evaluation of global right ventricular function that is mildly impaired constitutes a minor criterion. In a study of echocardiography in 15 patients with ARVC/D and in a control group of 25 healthy subjects, interobserver agreement for subjective assessment of regional wall motion in patients was moderate as evaluated by the weighted Kappa test (Kw) (Kw=0.47) but poor in the normal subjects (Kw<0.2) [1]. Since mild segmental dilatation of the right ventricle is considered a minor criterion, this evaluation could affect whether the patient would be designated as having the disease by meeting the Task Force criteria.

Although the information and calculations presented in Table 11.3 correspond with the definitions of mild and severe right ventricular enlargement presented in the original Task Force document, this categorization of using a fixed deviation from the standard may not be an optimal way of differentiating mild from moderate and severe abnormalities since it does not take into account the sensitivity and specificity of these arbitrary cut-off points.

Table 11.2 • Quantitative echocardiographic measurements of the right ventricle in 29 normal subjects and 29 ARVC/D probands

Right Heart Dimensions	Normal* Controls (± SD)	Normal * Controls Indexed to BSA	ARVC/D Probands (± SD)	ARVC/D Probands Indexed to BSA
RVOT-PLAX diastole (mm)	26.2±4.9	14.4±2.4	37.9±6.6	21.0±4.1
RVOT-PSAX diastole (mm)	31.1±4.7	17.0±2.6	38.9±4.7	21.5±3.0
RVOT/Aortic valve ratio	1.04±0.2	0.57±0.14	1.28±0.2	0.71±0.16
RV medial-lateral Apical 4 Chamber diastole (mm)	25.1±4.0	13.7±2.3	34.0±8.9	18.7±4.8
RV LAX length-Apical 4 Chamber diastole (mm)	76.1±7.6	41.8±3.4	79.2±15.6	43.7±9.2
RV End Diastolic Area (cm^2)	17.9±3.5	9.8±1.3	25.2±7.7	13.8±4.1
RV End Systolic Area (cm^2)	10.5±2.3	5.7±0.9	18.9±8.4	10.3±4.4
RV FAC (%)	41±7		27.2±16	

BSA, body surface, area; *FAC*, fractional area change; *PLAX*, parasternal long axis; *PSAX*, parasternal short axis; *RV*, right ventricle; *RVOT*, right ventricular outflow tract; *SD*, standard deviation. Data are presented as mean ±1 standard deviation
* Normal controls are age and sex matched to the ARVC/D probands
Modified from [9]

Table 11.3 • Calculated data to define mild and severe RV dilatation and dysfunction by echocardiography

	Men		Women	
	Raw cut-off	BSA cut-off	Raw cut-off	BSA cut-off
RV EDV (ml)				
2 SD from normal mean RV EDV	208	102	161	88
3 SD from normal mean RV EDV	239	116	185	99
RV ESV (ml)				
2 SD from normal mean RV ESV	88	44	60	34
3 SD from normal mean RV ESV	105	52	73	40
RV 4CH EDD (mm)				
2 SD from normal mean RV 4CH EDD	50	25	47	28
3 SD from normal mean RV 4CH EDD	55	28	52	31
RVEF				
2 SD from normal mean RVEF	0.42		0.49	
3 SD from normal mean RVEF	0.32		0.39	

* Data derived using a fast gradient echo cine MRI acquired in the short axis plane. There were 425 normal subjects; 191 men; The mean age was 61±10 years. Ref. from John Hopkins Database, Tandri et al. [10]
** BSA, body surface area; ChL, chamber length; EDD, end diastolic dimension; EDV, end diastolic volume; EF, ejection; ESV, end systolic volume; RV, right ventricle; SD, standard deviation; sa, short axis

In the Task Force document it was stated that experience with magnetic resonance imaging (MRI) and computed tomography (CT) in the diagnosis of right ventricular dysplasia was limited and required further evaluation. The MRI should be particularly valuable for accurately calculating right ventricular end diastolic and systolic volumes since the volumes are derived from a 3D model, thus distinguishing normal from abnormal. Descriptive measures are presented in Table 11.4 and were obtained from 425 normal subjects from the Johns Hopkins Hospital database under the direction of Bluemke et al. [10]. As one can see, these volume measurements as well as dimensions of the right ventricle are significantly different for men and women. The normal cut-off values for these measurements are listed in Table 11.4. This data from normal subjects can be compared with measurements from probands with ARVC/D in whom the diagnosis is made by Task Force criteria not including the MRI data. As previously mentioned, using these cut-off values to categorize the degree of abnormality based on standard deviation from the mean may not be an ideal way to categorize the various degrees of functional and structural abnormalities since it does not take

Table 11.4 • Quantitative data for gender specific raw, and BSA-adjusted RV variables by Cine MR

Parameter	Cut-off	BSA Indexed Cut-off
RV Global Dilation		
Mild is >2 SD from normal mean RVED area	>25 cm^2	12 cm^2/m^2
Severe is >3 SD from normal mean RVED Area	>28 cm^2	14 cm^2/m^2
RV segmental dilation	>36 mm	19 mm/m^2
Mild is >2 SD from normal mean RVOT (plax dia)	>41 mm	22 mm/m^2
Severe is >3 SD from normal mean RVOT (plax dia)	>41 mm	22 mm/m^2
Mild is >2 SD from normal mean RVOT (sax dia)	>33 mm	18 mm/m^2
Severe is >3 SD from normal mean RVOT (sax dia)	>37 mm	21 mm/m^2
Mild is >2 SD from normal mean RVML (4ch dia)	<27%	
Severe is 3>SD from normal mean RVML (4ch dia)	<20%	
Reduction in RVEF		
Mild is <2 SD from normal mean RVFAC		
Severe is <3 SD from normal mean RVFAC		

RVOT (plax dia), RVOT parasternal long axis diameter; RVOT (sax dia), RVOT short axis diameter: RVML (4ch dia), RV medial lateral apical 4 chamber diameter; RVED, right ventricular end diastolic; RVFAC, RV fractional area change; RVOT, right ventricular outflow tract; SD, standard deviation

Table 11.5 • Quantitative angiographic measurements of the right ventricle

Author Ref No.	Views	N.	RVEF (%)	RV-EDV Index (ml/m²)	RVESV Index (ml/m²)	RVSV Index (ml/m²)
Baudouy [12]	30° RAO, 60° LAO	20	55±4	70.±7	32±4	
Chiddo [13]	20°RAO	16	55±5	80±8		
Chioin [14]	AP, LAT	22	60±6	94±15	37±9	57±11
Daliento [15]	Not specified	18	60	95	38	
Daubert [16]	30 RAO, 60 LAO	10	59±6	79±10	32±6	47±8
Ferlinz1 [17]	30 RAO, 60° LAO	10		74±16	26±6	
Genzler [18]	AP, LAT	9	51±8	81±12	39±9	
Hebert [19]	45°RAO 45°LAO	11	58±5	82±21	35±11	46±13
			Total			
*Mean ±1SD		N=116	57±5	74±12	34±7	50±11
*Mild 1-2 SD			<52%	>86	>41	>61
Moderate to severe >2SD			>48%	>98	>48	>72

Mean ±1 SD of the pooled standard deviations; *AP*, antero posterior; *LAO*, left anterior oblique; *LAT*, lateral; *RAO*, right anterior oblique; *RV-EDV*, right ventricular - end diastolic volume; *RVEF*, right ventricular ejection fraction; *RVESV*, right ventricular end systolic volume; *RVSV*, right ventricular systolic volume; *SD*, standard deviation

into consideration the sensitivity as well as specificity of these measurements.

Angiographic evaluation of right ventricular wall motion is considered to be the best available method for analysis of regional wall motion abnormalities. The study is obtained in several projections including the PA, lateral, 30° RAO, and 60° LAO views. Since the right ventricle does not contract symmetrically, it requires considerable experience to determine abnormal wall motion in any one segment. A computer-based method for quantitative analysis of the regional wall motion of the right ventricle as well as volumes is being developed and this should greatly aid in the quantitation of the above parameters [11]. Ventricular volume by angiography is less accurate than that by MRI because it is based on a single or 2D view of the right ventricle whereas the MRI volume is based on a 3D analysis. The available data from the literature for the normal right ventricular angiographic measurements are listed in Table 11.5 [12-19].

Tissue Characterization of Walls

This major criterion for the diagnosis of ARVC/D is that of fibrofatty replacement of myocardium on endomyocardial biopsy. Fatty tissue may be a normal component of the right ventricular free wall [20-23]. The definition of "fibrofatty replacement" was not provided in the original Task Force criteria. The major problem with the pathological evaluation from myocardial biopsy relates to the fact that, in ARVC/D, the pathology may be spotty, and biopsies may not be obtained from the affected region. Importantly, the most common site for right ventricular biopsy is the septum and the septum is seldom involved in ARVC/D. Fortunately, the risk of perforation due to biopsy of the free wall of the right ventricle is small when performed according to strict guidelines, including avoiding biopsy of the thin wall dysfunctional regions [24-25]. Biopsies are obtained from adjacent regions.

Angelini et al. [26] proposed that diagnostic values for ARVC/D in right ventricular endomyocardial biopsies are the presence of <45% myocytes, >40% fibrous tissue, and >3% fatty tissue. The normal amount of myocytes is 80%-85%. These measurements are based on analysis of endomyocardial biopsies from 30 patients with ARVC/D, 29 patients with dilated cardiomyopathy, and 30 controls. The following criteria have been utilized to evaluate right ventricular biopsy samples in the ARVC/D North American Multidisciplinary Study of Right Ventricular Dysplasia. If there are <45% myocytes due to replacement by either fibrous tissue or fatty tissue, the biopsy is consistent with ARVC/D. If the residual myocardium is between 45%-70%, findings are classified as indeterminate; finally if the residual myocardium exceeds 70%, the biopsy is considered negative. Sensitivity and specificity of these criteria are undergoing evaluation in the above registry.

Repolarization Abnormalities

These are listed as minor criteria and consist of inverted T waves in the right precordial leads V_1, V_2, and V_3 in individuals aged 12-45 years (in the absence of right bundle branch block, or RBBB). A review of the literature indicates that T-wave inversion beyond V_3 and otherwise healthy individuals between age 19 and 45 is relatively specific for this disease [27]. This pattern occurs in only 3% of healthy/normal women and 1% of men in this age category. It has been observed that there may be T-wave lability from one ECG recording to another. It is not known whether this change is due to different lead placement or to a physiological change.

Depolarization/Conduction Abnormalities

Under this category, major criteria are the presence of epsilon waves or localized prolongation (>110 msec) of the QRS complex in the right precordial leads, V_1-V_3. The definition of epsilon waves was not provided in the Task Force publication. It is proposed that epsilon waves be defined as reproducible low-amplitude, low-frequency waves observed in leads V_1-V_3 after the end of QRS complex, usually before the onset of the T waves. The identification of the epsilon waves can be enhanced by recording the ECG signals with a high pass filter of 40 Hz at twice the usual gain to 20 mV/mm, and by increasing the recording speed to 50 mm per second [28, 29].

Localized prolongation of the QRS >110 msec in the right precordial leads is an indication of delayed conduction over the right ventricle (right ventricular parietal block). Additional parameters for measuring delayed conduction over the right ventricle, such as an S wave duration >55 msec, has been proposed as a sensitive marker of ARVC/D [30]. This finding requires further prospective confirmation.

Under this same category of depolarization/conduction abnormalities, minor criteria include the presence of late potentials as evaluated by the signal averaged electrocardiogram (SAECCG). The normal values of filter settings were not provided in the original Task Force publication. The SAECG should be performed using a 40-250 Hz filter with a noise level <0.3 µV. The standard normal values include a filtered QRS duration of <114 msec, duration of low amplitude signals of <40 µV (LAS 40) of <38 msec, and a root mean square amplitude of the last 40 msec of the QRS signal (RMS 40) of >20 µV. The presence of late potentials is defined as an abnormality in two of the three parameters. The above standard criteria for normals do not take into account the fact that there is a difference in the normal values of the SAECG in men and women and that the normal values also are dependent upon the type of equipment used, primarily relating to the fil-

Table 11.6 • Normal SAECG criteria according to equipment and gender

Equipment	Gender	f QRS ms	LAS ms	RMS µV
General Electric	M	≤124	≤42	≥16
(Marquette)	F	≤116	≤42	≥15
ART (Corazonix)	M	≤115	≤47	≥11
	F	≤107	≤43	≥13

tering system that may differ from one instrument to another. Based on results from the literature, normal values for SAECG based on equipment and gender are shown in Table 11.6 [31].

The Presence of Arrhythmias

These are a minor criterion and consist of >1000 premature ventricular beats of left bundle branch block morphology (LBBB) during a 24-h Holter monitor recording or sustained and nonsustained ventricular tachycardia recorded by electrocardiogram, Holter monitoring or exercise testing, as well as during an electrophysiological study. Attention must be directed to the morphology of the premature ventricular beats, particularly during Holter monitoring, since the recording leads may not be uniform from one instrument or center to another. The PVCs or VT should be revaluated to be certain that they are of LBBB configuration.

As mentioned above, ventricular arrhythmias are listed as a minor criterion. Modification of this criterion to a major criterion has been proposed consisting of a combination of right ventricular arrhythmias in conjunction with T wave abnormalities [32]. This combination may enhance the sensitivity of the Task Force criteria. This finding is based on a retrospective analysis of 24 patients with the obvious clinical diagnosis of ARVC/D and positive histology. The Task Force criteria for arrhythmias were present in only ten patients, thus resulting in a low sensitivity of only 42%. However a sensitivity of 100% was obtained if the negative T waves were designated as a major criterion when associated with LBBB ventricular tachycardia [32]. It seems reasonable that this combination should be utilized for the diagnosis of ARVC/D and should be incorporated as major criteria. This change should increase the sensitivity of the Task Force criteria without decreasing the specificity.

The final criterion for the diagnosis for ARVC/D is that of a family history of the disease. This consists of a major and minor category. The major category is that of familial disease confirmed at necropsy or surgery. The autopsy reports indicating the presence of

ARVC/D as a cause of death needs to be critically examined. Frequently this is based on the finding of no other cardiac pathology except that of fatty infiltration of the free wall of the right ventricle in an individual with sudden death. Infiltration of fat in the right ventricular myocardium in the absence of fibrosis can be seen frequently in normal hearts, especially in the anterior apical region [20, 21, 23]. Minimal requirements for the diagnosis of ARVC/D at autopsy should include the following [33]. There should be no other pathological findings to explain cardiac death by gross or microscopic examination. The right ventricle may be normal in size or moderately increased. The presence of right ventricular aneurysms should be considered pathognomonic. At histology the amount of myocardial loss is diagnostic. When there is predominantly fibrous replacement, the loss may be limited to the outer half of the right ventricular free wall. When there is predominately fatty replacement, the myocardial loss should be transmural, at least in the inflow or outflow tract. The presence of even a small amount of replacement-type fibrosis with myocyte nuclear abnormalities is essential for the diagnosis. Thinning of the right ventricular wall is indicative but not essential for the diagnosis. When fatty tissue replacement is predominant, the right ventricular wall thickness may be increased ("pseudohypertrophy").

A minor criterion is that of family history of premature sudden death due to suspected ARVC/D or a family history with a clinical diagnosis based on present criteria. Recently a modification of the Task Force criteria was proposed based on the findings that the phenotypic expression of the disease in family members may be less severe than in probands [34] (Table 11.7). If family members fulfill these criteria, these individuals may be considered as probably affected.

Conclusions

An unequivocal reference or gold standard on which to base the diagnosis of ARVC/D is that of gene identification to determine whether a patient or relative is a carrier of a genetic mutation associated with ARVC/D. To date ten genetic loci have been mapped for ARVC/D and six genes have been identified. The genetic abnormalities primarily involve defects in the adhesion molecules desmosomal proteins. A family member may be genetically affected but not have any phenotypic manifestations of the disease. It is important to be able to determine that an individual has the phenotypic expression of the disease since this finding may alter treatment and follow-up. The Task Force criteria are critical to this assessment.

Table 11.7 • Modified Task Force criteria for Familial ARVC/D*

Minor
I. Structural or functional abnormality of the right ventricle**
Mild global right ventricular dilatation and/or ejection fraction reduction with normal left ventricle
Mild segmental dilatation of the right ventricle
Regional right ventricular hypokinesia
Minor
III. Repolarization Abnormalities
Inverted T waves in right precordial leads (V_2 and V_3) in people aged >12 years, in absence of right bundle branch block
Minor
IV. Depolarization/Conduction Abnormalities
Late potentials on signal-averaged ECG
Minor
V. Arrhythmias
Left bundle branch block type ventricular tachycardia (sustained or nonsustained) by ECG, Holter, or exercise testing
Ventricular extrasystoles (>200/24 hours on Holter)***

*   From Hamid et al. [34]
** Detected by echocardiography, angiography, magnetic resonance imaging
*** Modified. Originally >1000/24h
The diagnosis of probable ARVC/D would be fulfilled by the presence of ARVC/D in a first degree relative meeting the Task Force criteria plus one of the minor criteria listed above
LV, left ventricle

In summary, the Task Force criteria are essential for standard classification of individuals who are affected with this condition. The strength of this classification is that it is usually specific. The weakness of the classification is that these criteria lack sensitivity for the diagnosis and are largely qualitative rather than quantitative. It is now necessary to update and modify these criteria.

Acknowledgements

This work was supported in part by Grant UO1-HL65594 from the National Heart, Lung, and Blood Institutes, National Institutes of Health, Bethesda, Maryland.

References

1. Lindstrom L, Wilkenshoff UM, Larsson N et al (2001) Echocardiographic assessment of arrhythmogenic right ventricular cardiomyopathy. Heart 86:31-38

2. Sievers B, Addo M, Franken U et al (2004) Right ventricular wall motion abnormalities found in healthy subjects by cardiovascular magnetic resonance imaging and characterized with a new segmental model. J Cardiovasc Magn Res 6:601-608

3. Kazmierczak J; De Sutter J, Tavernier R et al (1988) Electrocardiographic and morphometric features in patients with ventricular tachycardia of right ventricular origin. Heart 79:388-393

4. Gaita F, Giustetto C, Di Donna P et al (2001) Long-term follow-up of right ventricular monomorphic extrasystoles. J Am Coll Cardiol 38:364-370

5. O'Donnell D, Cox D, Bourke J et al (2003) Clinical and electrophysiological differences between patients with arrhythmogenic right ventricular dysplasia and right ventricular outflow tract tachycardia. Eur Heart J 24:801-810

6. Pinski SL (2000) The right ventricular tachycardias. J Electrocardiol 33:103-113

7. Marcus FI, Fontaine GH, Guiraudon G et al (1982) Right ventricular dysplasia: A report of 24 adult cases. Circulation 65:384-398

8. McKenna WJ, Thiene G, Nava A et al (1994) Diagnosis of arrhythmogenic right ventricular dysplasia/cardiomyopathy. Task Force of the Working Group Myocardial and Pericardial Disease of the European Society of Cardiology and of the Scientific Council on Cardiomyopathies of the International Society and Federation of Cardiology. Br Heart J 71:215-218

9. Yoerger D. Marcus F, Sherrill D et al (2005) Echocardiographic findings in patients meeting task force criteria for arrhythmogenic right ventricular cardiomyopathy dysplasia. New insights from the multicenter: Study of RV dysplasia. J Am Coll Card 45:860-865

10. Tandri H, Calkins H, Bluemke D et al Magnetic resonance and computer tomography imaging of arrhythmogenic right ventricular cardiomyopathy/dysplasia. Chapter 15

11. Indik J, Dallas, Ovitt T et al (2005) Do patients with right ventricular outflow tract ventricular arrhythmias have normal right ventricular wall motion? A quantitative analysis compared to normal subjects. Cardiology 104:10-15

12. Baudouy M, Guivarc H, Guarin I et al (1985) Méthode d'exploitation informatique de la cine-angiographie du ventricule droit. Arch Mal Coeur 78:386-392

13. Chiddo A, Locuratolo N, Gaglione A et al (1989) Right ventricular dysplasia: Angiographic study. Eur Heart J 10:42-45

14. Chioin R, Chirillo F, Pedon L et al (1989) Angiography of normal right ventricle. Cardiovasc Imag 1:45-51

15. Daliento L, Rizzoli G, Thiene G et al (1990) Diagnostic accuracy of right ventriculography in arrhythmogenic right ventricular cardiomyopathy. Am J Cardiol 66:741-745

16. Daubert C, Descaves C, Foulgoc JL et al (1988) Critical analysis of cineangiographic criteria for diagnosis of arrhythmogenic right ventricular dysplasia. Am Heart J 115:448-459

17. Ferlinz J (1977) Measurements of right ventricular volumes in man from single plane cineangiograms. A comparison to the biplane approach. Am Heart J 94:87

18. Genzler RD, Briselli MF, Gault JH (1974) Angiographic estimation of right ventricular volume in man. Circulation 50:324-330

19. Hebert JL, Chemla D, Gerard O et al (2004) Angiographic right and left ventricular function in arrhythmogenic right ventricular dysplasia. Am J Cardiol 93:728-733

20. Fontaine G, Fontaliran F, Zenati, O et al (1999) Fat in the heart a feature unique to the human species? Observational reflections on an unsolved problem. Acta Cardiol 54:189-194

21. Burke AP, Farb A, Tashko G et al (1998) Arrhythmogenic right ventricular cardiomyopathy and fatty replacement of the right ventricular myocardium: Are they different diseases? Circulation 97:1571-1580

22. Lobo FV (2001) Arrhythmogenic right ventricular cardiomyopathy/dysplasia: Issues in diagnosis. Pathology Case Reviews 6:287-296

23. Basso C, Thiene G (2005) Adipositas cordis, fatty infiltration of the right ventricle, and arrhythmogenic right ventricular cardiomyopathy. Just a matter of fat? Cardiovasc Pathol 14:37-41

24. Wichter T, Hindricks G, Lerch H et al (1994) Regional myocardial sympathetic dysinnervation in arrhythmogenic right ventricular cardiomyopathy: An analysis using ^{123}I-Meta iodobenzylguanidine scintigraphy. Circulation 89:667-683

25. Chimenti C, Pieroni M, Maseri A et al (2004) Histology findings in patients with clinical and instrumental diagnosis of sporadic arrhythmogenic right ventricular dysplasia. J Am Coll Cardiol 43:2305-2313

26. Angelini A, Basso C, Nava A et al (1996) Endomyocardial biopsy in right ventricular cardiomyopathy. Am Heart J 132:203-206

27. Marcus FI, Fontaine G (2005) Prevalence of T wave inversion beyond V_1 in young normal individuals and usefulness for the diagnosis of arrhythmogenic right ventricular cardiomyopathy/dysplasia. Am J Cardiol 95:1070-1071

28. Marcus FI, Fontaine G (1995) Arrhythmogenic right ventricular dysplasia/cardiomyopathy: A review. PACE 18:1298-1314

29. Turrini P, Angelini A, Thiene G et al (1999) Late potentials and ventricular arrhythmias in arrhythmogenic right ventricular cardiomyopathy. Am J Cardiol 83:1214-1219

30. Nasir K, Bomma C, Tandri H et al (2004) Electrocardiographic features of arrhythmogenic right ventricular dysplasia/cardiomyopathy according to disease severity: A need to broaden diagnostic criteria. Circulation 110-114:1527-1534

31. Marcus FI, Zareba W, Sherill D (2007) Evaluate of the normal values for signal-averaged electrocardiogram. J. Cardiovascular Electrophysiology 18:231-233

32. Baraka M, Fontaliran F, Frank R et al (1998) Value of task force criteria in the diagnosis of arrhythmogenic right ventricular dysplasia cardiomyopathy. Herzschr Elektrophys 9:163-168

33. Basso C, Thiene G, Corrado D et al (1996) Arrhythmogenic right ventricular cardiomyopathy: Dysplasia, dystrophy or myocarditis? Circulation 94:983-991

34. Hamid MS, Norman M, Quraishi A et al (2002) Prospective evaluation of relatives for familial arrhythmogenic right ventricular cardiodmyopathy/dysplasia reveals a need to broaden diagnostic criteria. J Am Coll Cardiol 40:1445-1450

CHAPTER 12

IDIOPATHIC RIGHT VENTRICULAR OUTFLOW TRACT TACHYCARDIA

Gianfranco Buja, Barbara Ignatiuk, Thomas Wichter, Domenico Corrado

Introduction

The right ventricular outflow tract (RVOT) is the most common site of origin of ventricular tachycardia (VT) occurring in patients with an apparently normal heart (idiopathic VT). However, it is also a focus of arrhythmias due to arrhythmogenic right ventricular cardiomyopathy/dysplasia (ARVC/D). These two conditions can be easily confused, especially if myocardial abnormalities are mild or minimal as in patients with ARVC/D in its early stage [1].

Idiopathic RVOT tachycardia is generally a benign condition with an excellent long-term prognosis and is not familial [2]. Occasionally, it can be very symptomatic and even invalidating, but is amenable to curative therapy with catheter ablation [3]. ARVC/D is an inherited and progressive cardiomyopathy characterized by right ventricular dysfunction due to fibrofatty replacement of the myocardium which predisposes to electrical instability that can precipitate ventricular tachycardia and sudden death [4-8]. Although catheter ablation has been reported as having good acute success rate in ventricular tachycardia, recurrences are common due to progression of the disease which predisposes to the occurrence of new arrhythmogenic foci [9, 10]. The defibrillator is the only effective protection against arrhythmic sudden death [11, 12].

Distinction between these two conditions is extremely important because it implies different management strategies. Differential diagnosis, however, may be challenging.

In this article, we review the available literature regarding definition, classification, pathophysiological mechanisms, clinical characteristics, and management of idiopathic RVOT VT. In addition, we discuss criteria to aid in the differentiation of idiopathic RVOT VT from VT due to ARVC/D.

Ventricular Tachyarrhythmias in Normal Hearts: Overview and Classification

VT is usually associated with structural cardiac disease. The most common anatomic substrate of ventricular arrhythmias is chronic ischemic heart disease. Other structural disorders associated with VT are valvular and congenital heart disease, cardiac tumors, myocarditis, and cardiomyopathies. Only approximately 10% of arrhythmias occur in the absence of structural heart disease assessed by clinical examination and imaging studies. Some of them may be caused by inherited cardiac diseases such as catecholaminergic polymorphic VT syndrome, long QT syndrome, and the Brugada syndrome [13].

VT occurring in subjects without any clinically demonstrable underlying cardiac abnormality is referred to as "idiopathic" [2]. The clinical manifestations range from nonsustained, asymptomatic VT to sustained arrhythmias, which rarely can cause hemodynamic compromise and cardiac arrest. It can be classified with respect to the site of origin, the morphologic features (QRS configuration and axis), evidence for catecholamine-dependence, as well as the response to programmed stimulation and to pharmacological agents (adenosine, verapamil, and propranolol) [14].

Probably due to an embryological origin [15], that differs from the other heart structures, 90% of idiopathic VT originate from the RVOT, whereas 10% arise from the left (LVOT). As an alternative, defective sympathetic innervation of these regions may be the underlying substrate predisposing to enhanced arrhythmogenicity [16]. Somatic cell mutation in the RVOT leading to increased concentration of intracellular cAMP in response to beta-adrenergic stimulation may also predispose to some forms of RVOT tachycardia [17].

Over the last two decades, the cellular mechanisms of idiopathic VT have been under investigation in experimental models and in humans. The potential electrophysiological mechanisms that have been proposed include triggered activity, re-entry, and abnormal automaticity.

According to current knowledge, idiopathic VT can be classified in three main categories based on cellular and electrophysiological mechanism (Table 12.1):
1. Adenosine-sensitive VT due to triggered activity (delayed afterdepolarizations);
2. Propranolol-sensitive (automatic);
3. Verapamil-sensitive (due to intrafascicular re-entry).

Currently, the cellular mechanism of idiopathic tachycardias from RVOT and LVOT is thought to be cyclic AMP-mediated triggered activity that is dependent on delayed afterdepolarizations. These tachycardias are characterized by sensitivity to adenosine [18, 19]. The mechanism of idiopathic outflow tract VT may be explained by adrenergic mediated automaticity (propranolol-sensitive tachycardias) in only a small number of patients. In contrast, re-entry is the most common mechanism of ventricular arrhythmias in structural cardiac disorders (myocardial infarction, congenital heart disease, and cardiomyopathies including ARVC/D). The mechanism of verapamil-sensitive-fascicular-tachycardia seems to be re-entry involving the fascicles of the left bundle branch. Re-entry involving Purkinje tissue in or adjacent to a left ventricular false tendon has been also proposed. This arrhythmia originates from the LV and has a distinct RBBB morphology with left-axis configuration (suggesting exit site from the left posterior fascicle) or with right-axis configuration (exit site from the left anterior fascicle).

Although RVOT and LVOT are anatomically separate, they have an embryologic origin from a common solitary outflow tract (Fig. 12.1) [15]. The myocardium of the outflow tract has different properties as compared with the atrial or ventricular myocardium. Myocardial cells of the outflow tract are reminiscent of early development. The outflow tract has a lower rate of proliferation, a more "primitive" contractile phenotype (poorly developed sarcomeric and sarcoplasmic reticular structures, persistent expression of smooth muscle alpha-actin), and slower impulse conduction consistent with its role as a sphincter in the embryonic heart tube [20]. Based on these common features, it has been suggested that RVOT and LVOT arrhythmias should be considered as a single entity, and classified together as "outflow tract arrhythmias" [21]. There is a recent evidence that the pulmonary trunk can also give rise to VT, suggesting a common etiology of these tachycardias [22, 23]. Aortic cusp tachycardia and epicardial LV tachycardia are considered variants of outflow tract arrhythmias [24, 25].

Table 12.1 • Types of idiopathic ventricular tachycardia. Modified from [14]

	Adenosine-sensitive (triggered activity)	Propranolol-sensitive (automatic)	Verapamil-sensitive (intrafascicular re-entry)
Morphology	LBBB, inferior axis	LBBB	RBBB, superior axis
	RBBB, inferior axis	RBBB, polymorphic	RBBB, inferior axis
Clinical characteristics	RMVT; exercise-induced, sustained	Exercise-induced; incessant	May be incessant
Origin	RVOT, LVOT, PA	RV, LV	Intrafascicular, exit site: left posterior fascicle, left anterior fascicle
Drug response			
Adenosine	Terminates	Transient suppression	No effect
Propranol	Terminates	Terminates/transient suppression	Variable
Verapamil	Terminates	No effect	Terminates
Mechanism	cAMP-mediated Triggered activity	Enhanced automaticity	Re-entry
EPS:			
Induction	Programmed stimulation +/− catecholamines	Catecholamines	Programmed stimulation +/− catecholamines
Entrainment	No	No	Yes

EPS, electrophysiological study; *LBBB*, left bundle branch block; *LVOT*, left ventricula outflow tract; *PA*, pulmonary artery; *RBBB*, right bundle branch block; *RMVT*, repetitive monomorphic ventricular tachycardia; *RVOT*, right ventricular outflow tract

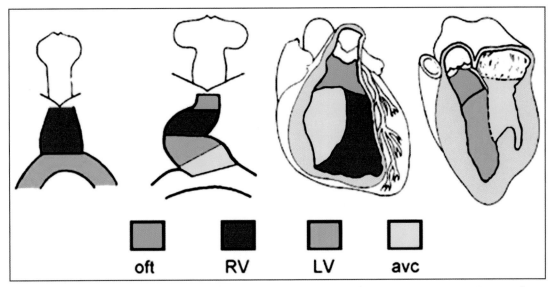

Fig. 12.1 • Embryological origin of the ventricles. In the tubular heart the atrioventricular canal and the outflow tract are separated by ventricular primordial, whereas in the formed heart they are connected. *Left*: embryonic heart tube. *Right*: the formed heart. *oft*, outflow tract (*blue*); *RV*, right ventricle (*red*); *LV*, left ventricle (*green*); *avc*, atrio-ventricular canal (*yellow*). Reproduced from [15]

Idiopathic Right Ventricular Outflow Tract Tachycardia

Definition

The origin of the tachycardia from the RVOT results in a distinctive pattern of QRS complexes with a LBBB and inferior axis morphology (Fig. 12.2). Typically the QRS complex is positive in leads II, III, and aVF. Importantly, it is negative in lead aVL.

The term "right ventricular outflow tract tachycardia" is descriptive and based on the ECG pattern. Occasionally, the arrhythmia source is in the LVOT or in pulmonary trunk [21-25] and ECG features do not always allow differentiation. The term "idiopathic" implies the exclusion of any known cardiac pathology.

Clinical Characteristics and Diagnosis

RVOT tachycardia appears to be more common in women with 2:1 female predominance [26]. Familial occurrence has not been reported. Symptoms develop typically between the ages of 20 and 50 years, but presentation in childhood and infancy has been observed. Patients may present with palpitations, atypical chest pain, or dizziness. About 10% develop syncope during VT [2, 27-31].

The two predominant clinical phenotypes of this tachycardia are nonsustained, repetitive, monomorphic VT (RMVT) and paroxysmal, sustained VT; both are characterized by sensitivity to adenosine. RMVT is more common. Typically, it occurs at rest, has a pattern of a nonsustained salvos, and can be incessant, with frequent premature ventricular beats. In contrast, paroxysmal idiopathic VT is usually exercise-induced or associated with stress, may be sustained and separated by long intervals of sinus rhythm with relatively infrequent premature ventricular beats. There is considerable overlap between these two phenotypes. RVOT monomorphic extrasystoles and sustained RVOT VT appear to be two extremes of the spectrum of the same arrhythmic disorder.

The diagnosis of idiopathic RVOT VT is made after exclusion of other pathologies. ARVC/D in subtle forms may not always be detected even following Task Force criteria [32].

The resting 12-lead electrocardiogram during sinus rhythm is usually normal in RVOT idiopathic VT. Approximately 10% of these patients have complete or incomplete RBBB. The signal-averaged-ECG (SAECG) is typically normal.

Exercise testing reproduces the patient's clinical arrhythmia in 25% to 50% of the cases [2, 27, 30]. Tachycardia can be initiated either during exercise or during recovery. RMVT is often suppressed during exercise but recurs after stopping exercise expressing

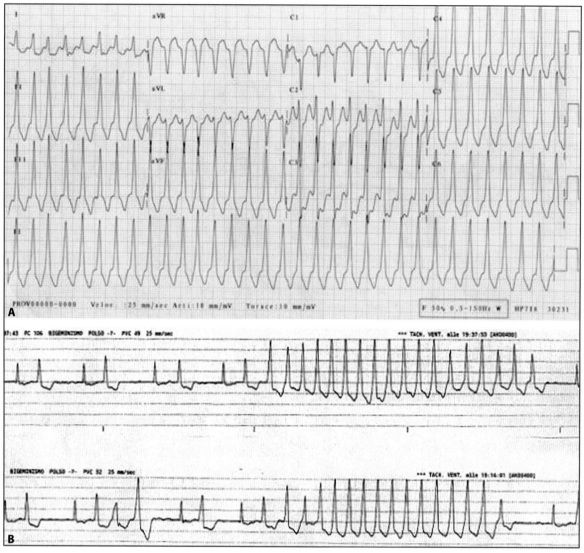

Fig. 12.2 • Idiopathic RVOT tachycardia. **A** The 12 lead ECG shows tachycardia with a left bundle branch block configuration and frontal plane axis directed inferiorly. Note that the QRS in negative in AVL. **B** ECGs of paroxysmal (repetitive) monomorphic RVOT VT

its dependence on a critical heart rate. Relation of the arrhythmia to exercise has not been shown to be of prognostic value [30].

Structural Investigation: Echocardiography and Magnetic Resonance Imaging

The echocardiogram is usually normal. The most frequent abnormality is mitral valve prolapse, not associated with valvular insufficiency or myxomatous thickening of the valve leaflets [27]. This is probably an incidental finding without pathophysiologic significance. Slight enlargement of the right or the left ventricle has been observed.

Several authors have reported a high prevalence of mild abnormalities identified by Magnetic Resonance Imaging (MRI) in hearts of patients with RVOT tachycardia (Table 12.2). MRI studies have reported that as many as two-thirds of patients (up to 95% in early reports) have had right ventricular thinning, fatty infiltration of the myocardium or wall motion abnormalities but the accuracy as well as the clinical and prognostic significance of these findings is uncertain.

Carlson et al. reported MRI abnormalities in the RVOT in 21 of 22 patients (95%) with idiopathic VT [33]. The abnormalities were limited to those observed by cine MRI and consisted of focal wall thinning, excavation, and decreased systolic thickening. No patient had intramyocardial hyperintense signals

Table 12.2 • Diagnostic findings in RVOT tachycardia patients evaluated by MRI

Author	Year	No. patients	ECG	SAECG	ECHO	RV Angiography	MRI abnormalities	MRI abnormalities in controls
Carlson [33]	1994	24	–	–	N 19/21	N 2/5	22/24 (95%)	2/16
Globits [36]	1997	20	N	–	N	–	13/20 (65%)	2/10
Grimm [39]	1997	23	N	N 21/23	N	N 5/5	1/23 (4%)	–
Markowitz [35]	1997	14	N 12/14	N 9/9	N 10/10	–	10/14 (71%)	1/18
White [34]	1998	53	–	–	N 50/53 E 3/53	–	32/53 (60%)	0/15
O'Donnell [42]	2003	33	N 31/33	N	N	N 12/12	18/33 (54%)	–
Tandri [38]	2004	20	N	N	N	–	2/20 (10%)	2/18
Krittayaphong [37]	2006	41	N	N 35/41	N	–	24/41 (58%)	1/15

N, normal; *E*, Equivocal; –, not reported

indicative of fat infiltration. In this cohort of patients with VT, echocardiography showed abnormalities in the RVOT in only 2 of 21 patients. Using a similar MRI protocol and patient selection criteria, White et al. reported MRI abnormalities in 32 of 53 patients (60%). In addition to cine MRI abnormalities, 25% of the patients in this study also had intramyocardial hyperintense signals [34]. Markowitz et al. found abnormalities on MRI scan in 10 of 14 patients (71%) with adenosine-sensitive VT and fatty tissue was present in 4 (29%) [35]. It is of considerable interest that the most common site of abnormal findings was the RV free wall, which did not correspond to the site of origin of the arrhythmia. However, these studies did not exclude patients with 12-lead electrocardiographic abnormalities, and signal-averaged electrocardiogram as well as RV angiography were not performed in most of them. In another study, Globits et al. [36] showed no difference by MRI of RV volumes and systolic function in 20 patients with RVOT VT compared with 10 control subjects. In controls, RV abnormalities were limited to fatty deposits of the right atrioventricular groove extending into the subtricuspid region in 2; MRI demonstrated morphological changes of the RV free wall in 13 of 20 patients (65%) with ventricular tachycardia, including fatty infiltration in 5, wall thinning in 9, and dyskinetic wall segments in 4. Eight of these patients had additional fatty deposits, thinning or a saccular aneurysm in the RV outflow tract, corresponding to the ablation site in 6 patients. In this study signal-averaged electrocardiogram and RV angiography were not performed.

Recently, Krittayaphong et al. reported structural and functional MRI abnormalities in 24 of 41 patients (58%) with RVOT tachycardia. Late potentials

on SAECG were present in only 6 of these patients (11%). MRI abnormalities together with late potentials were associated with unfavorable outcomes of RF ablation [37].

In contrast, the results of the study by Tandri et al. [38], revealed that patients with idiopathic VT who had a normal surface electrocardiogram and signal-averaged electrocardiogram, did not have evidence of structural heart disease on MRI, and were indistinguishable from controls. Quantitative segmental evaluation of the right ventricle demonstrated no differences in the global and regional RV function in idiopathic VT compared with control subjects. These findings are similar to the results of an early study by Grimm et al. who reported normal MRI in 22 of 23 patients with RMVT. However, cine imaging was not performed in this study [39].

Since MRI studies are frequently obtained to distinguish ARVC/D from RVOT tachycardia, it is important to realize that normal RV wall motion may be misinterpreted as abnormal. A recent MRI study by Sievers et al. focused on RV wall motion pattern in 29 normal subjects [40]. Blinded interpretation of the cine MRI studies by experienced radiologists reported wall motion abnormalities in 93%, including areas of apparent dyskinesia in 76% and bulging in 27.6%. The overinterpretation of intramyocardial fat or wall thinning on MRI led to a high frequency of "misdiagnosis" of ARVD/C as reported by Bomma et al. [41].

The study by O'Donnell et al. addressed clinical and electrophysiological differences between patients diagnosed as having ARVC/D or idiopathic RVOT VT. In 18 on 33 of patients (54%) with idiopathic right ventricular tachycardia some structural abnormalities were present on MRI, but no structural abnormalities were found in this group using echocardiography or right ventricular cineangiography [42].

These data indicate that conventional cardiac MRI may not be reliable in most centers to differentiate between idiopathic RVOT tachycardia and ARVC/D. MRI has intrinsic limitations related to technical factors and cardiac anatomy, and a poor agreement among physicians in the interpretation of MRI scans has been observed [43]. Whether recent late enhancement technology may increase cardiac MRI diagnostic accuracy for detection of RV fatty/fibrofatty myocardial replacement remains to be determined. Preliminary data, although promising, indicate limited sensitivity of contrast-enhanced MRI to detect small amounts of fibrosis in early ARVC/D [44].

Mechanisms

Experimental data shows that the electrophysiological mechanism in RVOT tachycardia is triggered activity secondary to cyclic adenosine monophosphate (cAMP)-mediated delayed afterdepolarizations (DADs) [18, 19]. Termination of VT by adenosine is considered to be pathognomonic for VT caused by cAMP-triggered DADs.

Afterdepolarizations are oscillations of membrane potential occurring in phase 3 (early after- depolarization) or after the action potential (phase 4 or late afterdepolarization). If the oscillation is of sufficient amplitude to reach threshold potential, a full action potential is induced, which may result in a sustained arrhythmia. In ventricular myocytes, DADs originate predominantly from M-cells. These cells are localized in the sub- and midmyocardium, and share features of both Purkinje and working myocardial cells. The preponderance of M- cells in the RVOT may explain why idiopathic arrhythmias originate primarily from this area.

Delayed afterdepolarizations responsible for the tachycardia occur under various circumstances that cause an increase in intracellular calcium, including catecholamine release and digitalis. Stimulation of the β adrenergic receptor produces cyclic AMP-mediated phosphorylation and activation of the slow inward calcium channel as well as increased calcium release from the sarcoplasmic reticulum [Fig. 12.3]. The cellular calcium overload leads to activation of a nonspecific transient inward sodium current that induces DADs. Digitalis induces DADs by a different pathway (inhibition of Na^+, K^+-ATPase).

Adenosine terminates VT due to triggered activity through its antiadrenergic effects. By binding to the specific adenosine receptor, it inhibits adenylyl cyclase. This leads to a decrease of the slow inward calcium channel and sarcoplasmic reticulum calcium release with subsequent attenuation of the transient inward current. Adenosine has no effect on digitalis-mediated-DADs.

Vagal maneuvers inhibit triggered activity by decreasing cAMP concentrations via muscarinic-cholinergic receptors. Verapamil exerts its effects directly through inhibition of the slow inward calcium current, whereas β-blockers act earlier in the process by preventing β-receptor activation. The effects of β-blockers and of verapamil on VT are nonspecific, and are also effective in arrhythmias due to re-entry and in abnormal automaticity. In contrast, adenosine's effect is mechanism-specific, terminating only the tachycardia due to cAMP-mediated triggered activity. It has no effect either on arrhythmias triggered by early afterdepolarizations nor on re-entrant VTs. Adenosine's effect on VT caused by automaticity is different from its effect on VT caused by triggered activity. Adenosine transiently (for less than 20 seconds) suppresses catecholamine-induced automaticity, whereas it terminates VT caused by triggered activity.

There is interesting data regarding the etiology of RVOT tachycardia from molecular biology. In a patient with an adenosine-insensitive form of RVOT tachycardia, a point mutation in the inhibitory G-protein has been identified in biopsy samples from the myocardial site of origin of the tachycardia. This mutation, interrupting adenosine signaling, is not present at myocardial sites remote from the arrhythmogenic focus or from peripheral lymphocytes [16].

Electrophysiologic Characteristics

The clinical diagnosis of triggered activity is supported in part by termination of VT with adenosine, by the Valsalva's maneuver, carotid sinus pressure, verapamil and beta-blockade. The tachycardia can also be initiated and terminated with programmed stimulation and cannot be entrained.

The ability to reproducibly initiate an arrhythmia by programmed electrical stimulation is considered a hallmark of re-entrant arrhythmias. Arrhythmias that are the consequence of automaticity, are due to spontaneous depolarization and cannot usually be initiated by programmed stimulation. Tachyarrhythmias that are due to early afterdepolarizations are bradycardia-dependent and are not well suited for study by programmed stimulation. Under certain circumstances, triggered activity due to delayed afterdepolar-

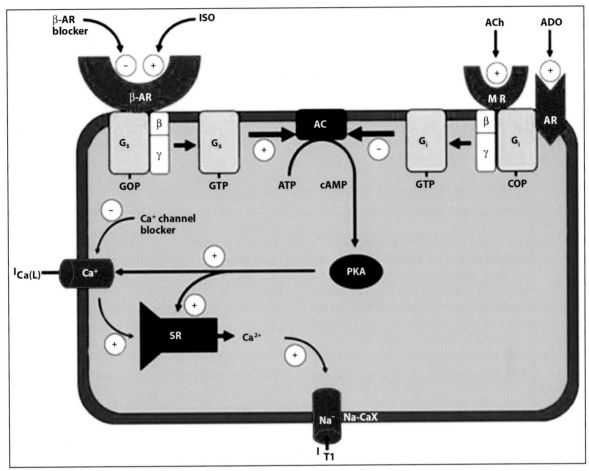

Fig. 12.3 • Receptor schema for activation and inactivation of cAMP-mediated triggered activity caused by delayed after-depolarizations (DADs). A_1, receptor; A_1R, adenosine; *AC*, adenylyl cyclase; *ACH*, acetylcholine; *ADO*, adenosine; *β-AR*, β adrenergic receptor; *cAMP*, cyclic adenosine-monophosphate; G_i, inhibitory G-protein; G_i, stimulatory G-protein; G_s, stimulatory G-protein; $I_{Ca(L)}$, slow inward calcium current; *ISO*, isoproterenol; I_{Ti}, transient inward current; M_2R, muscarinic cholinergic receptor; *Na-CaX*, Na^+-Ca^{2+} exchanger; *PKA*, protein kinase A; *SR*, sarcoplasmic reticulum. Reproduced from [19]

izations can be initiated by programmed stimulation. The response of the triggered activity to programmed stimulation is characteristic: 1) The amplitude and coupling interval of DADs depend on the duration and rate of the preceding pacing stimuli that result in induction; 2) Pacing at progressively shorter cycle lengths is associated with a shortening of the coupling interval for the initial beats of the tachycardia (this phenomenon, termed "overdrive acceleration", is typical for initiation of triggered activity); 3) Rapid burst pacing is more effective than programmed ventricular extrastimuli in inducing tachycardia.

The ability to evoke triggered activity is dependent on the autonomic status of the patient. Reproducibility of induction is unpredictable. A heavily sedated patient is rarely inducible. Frequently, infusion of exogenous catecholamines is necessary for initiation of the arrhyhmia. An isoproterenol infusion is

started at 2 μg/min and the infusion rate is titrated until the heart rate is increased by at least 20% (up to 10 to 14 μg/min as needed). Other agents that directly or indirectly increase cAMP activity can be used to facilitate inducibility: atropine (0.04 mg/kg) and aminophylline (2.8 mg/kg). Atropine attenuates the potential effect of acetylcholine and, at this dose, amino-phylline acts as a competitive adenosine antagonist.

Induction of VT by programmed ventricular stimulation may be consistent with either reentrant excitation or triggered activity. Induction of tachycardia with programmed electrical stimulation in the presence of fragmented electrograms favors re-entry as in ARVC/D. Arrhythmia induction by isoproterenol with cycle length dependence is consistent with a cyclic AMP-mediated triggered activity and favors the diagnosis of idiopathic RVOT tachycardia [45].

Prognosis

The long-term prognosis in patients with idiopathic RVOT tachycardia is excellent despite frequent episodes of VT [2, 27]. Rare cases of sudden death have been reported [28, 30, 46-48], but it is possible that early reports included a heterogeneous patient population. In the series of patients presenting with apparently idiopathic ventricular arrhythmias reported by Deal et al. [28], two of three subjects who died had abnormalities at cardiac catheterization, and in the third right ventricle cardiomyopathy was revealed at postmortem examination.

Long-term follow-up studies indicate a benign course suggesting that this arrhythmia does not represent an early manifestation of a concealed cardiomyopathy. In the European Registry of children from neonatal age to 16 years at time of first manifestation (mean age 5.4 years) with idiopathic VT, patients were followed for a mean of 47 months (12-182 months); no deaths were reported [49]. Several investigators have observed a spontaneous VT remission (5%-20% of patients). This also was observed in patients in whom the arrhythmic disorder was manifest only as premature beats. In a long-term follow-up study by Gaita et al. [50], patients with frequent monomorphic RV ectopy were reassessed 15 years after initial presentation. No patient died of sudden death nor developed ARVC/D and in half of the patients, the arrhythmia disappeared.

The benign nature of RVOT ectopic beats has been recently questioned by data that the RVOT can be the site of origin of ectopic beats triggering polymorphic VT and ventricular fibrillation. It has been reported that, in isolated cases, extrasystoles with short coupling intervals initiated polymorphic RVOT VT; this variant of arrhythmia was called "short-coupled RVOT VT" [51]. Subsequently, the coexistence of monomorphic and polymorphic RVOT VT has been observed. Noda et al. [52] have documented typical monomorphic RVOT VT in 5 of the 16 patients who also had polymorphic VT initiated by ventricular extrasystoles with LBBB morphology and inferior axis configuration. Eleven of the 16 patients with polymorphic tachycardia had prior episodes of syncope, and the remaining 5 patients experienced pre-syncope. Spontaneous episodes of VF were documented in 5 patients. It has been proposed that these two arrhythmias may share the same underlying mechanism (DADs-induced triggered activity) [53].

Tachycardia induced Cardiomyopathy

There is evidence suggesting that frequent RVOT premature ventricular contractions (PVCs) can adversely affect LV function. Several investigators have observed that dilated cardiomyopathy can be induced by VT and can be reversed if the tachycardia is abolished by radiofrequency ablation [54-57].

Kim et al. [54] reported a case of catheter ablation of VT performed in a patient with dilated cardiomyopathy and a long history of repetitive palpitations. VT with LBBB with inferior axis morphology was present for about one third of the daytime hours. During electrophysiological study VT was reproduced by isoproterenol infusion and radiofrequency catheter ablation in the RVOT was performed. Left ventricular ejection fraction improved from 38% to 48% 1 month after ablation, and to 61% 1 year after ablation. In the series of Grimm et al. [55], radiofrequency catheter ablation was performed in four adults with myocardial dysfunction related to RMVT originating in the RVOT. Serial echocardiographic assessment of LV function before and after radiofrequency catheter ablation of RMVT showed complete reversal of LV dysfunction without arrhythmia recurrence during a mean follow-up of 31 months. In the study by Yarlagadda et al. [56], successful ablation of RVOT VT was performed in 23 patients , including 7 of 8 patients with depressed ventricular function. In this latter group, ventricular function improved in all subjects (from 39% to 62%).

Treatment

The decision to treat patients with idiopathic outflow tract tachycardia is based on clinical information. If symptoms are infrequent and relatively mild, treatment may not be necessary and patients may simply be reassured. However, in presence of presyncope/syncope or if frequent ventricular extrasystoles are debilitating, medical therapy or radiofrequency catheter ablation should be indicated. Patients with worsening symptoms and increasing arrhythmia burden during follow-up should be reassessed in order to identify any evolving cardiac functional abnormality.

Antiarrhythmic Drug Therapy

RVOT tachycardia is potentially responsive to all classes of antiarrhythmics [3]. Medical therapy is successful in approximately 25%-50% of patients. Beta blockers are the initial choice for antiarrhythmic therapy. Alternatively, calcium-channel blockers with verapamil or diltiazem, class IA, or class IC agents can be used. Class III antiarrhythmic drugs (sotalol and amiodarone) are effective in approximately 50% of patients.

In the acute setting, termination of the tachycardia can often be achieved by the Valsalva maneuver or carotid sinus pressure. If this is unsuccessful, adenosine can be administered (6-24 mg); other options include verapamil (10 mg given over 1 min), and lidocaine.

Catheter Ablation

Several electrophysiologic characteristics of RVOT tachycardia make this arrhythmia amenable to ablation [3, 54-79]. The focus of origin is well circumscribed and localized in an accessible region. The 12-lead ECG during VT can be helpful in localizing the optimal ablation site [3, 60, 61, 63]. The QRS duration during VT is usually greater than 140 msec and a pattern RR' or Rr' in leads II and III may be observed if VT originates from the free-wall. In contrast, QRS duration less than 140 ms and a monophasic R-wave is seen in VT of septal origin. The relative amplitude of the QS complex in leads aVR versus aVL may differentiate right upper from left upper region of the RVOT. The precordial R-wave transition becomes earlier as the site of origin advances more superiorly along the septum. An R-wave transition in lead V2 suggests a site of origin immediately inferior to the pulmonic wave or a left septal origin of VT. R-wave amplitudes in the inferior leads, aVL/aVR ratio of Q-wave amplitude, and R/S ratio on lead V_2 were significantly greater in VTs originating above the pulmonary valve compared to the RVOT VT group [23]. Useful algorithms for determination of the site of origin of the tachycardia have been proposed [63, 76].

The arrhythmogenic focus is located by means of activation sequence mapping (earliest site of activation during tachycardia) or by pacemapping (the site where pacing reproduces the QRS morphology of the tachycardia). Techniques to identify the earliest site of activation rely primarily on bipolar activation mapping. In general, successful ablation sites are associated with activation times 10-60 ms before the onset of the earliest surface QRS. Normal bipolar endocardial electrograms have high amplitudes and rapid slew rates. Recording of fractionated complex electrograms and diastolic potentials should raise the suspicion of un-

derlying structural disease. In a recent series of patients undergoing 3D electroanatomic mapping during RVOT VT, the mean area of myocardium activated within the first 10 ms was 3.0 ± 1.6 cm^2 (range 1.3 to 6.4 cm^2) [78]. Therefore, ablation guided by activation mapping alone may have limited utility. Addition of high-density electroanatomical mapping allows better identification of the early activation area.

Pace mapping is performed during sinus rhythm at a cycle length identical to that of spontaneous or induced tachycardia. The QRS morphology, R:S ratio and notching in the QRS complex is evaluated. An identical match is necessary in at least 11 of 12 or more (typically 12 of 12 leads). Pace mapping was initially considered to be more useful in identifying the successful ablation site than activation mapping, but this approach has important limitations. Exact matches can be observed up to 2 cm from a tachycardia focus [78].

The distance between the VT exit site (determined by activation mapping) and the VT site of origin (determined by pace mapping) is usually relatively small (6 ± 5 mm). Pace mapping seems to add little information to sites selected on the basis of 3D activation mapping alone.

Most successful ablation sites are located within the septal region of the RVOT, usually inferior to the pulmonary valve.

Published studies of catheter ablation for RVOT VT including about seven hundred patients reported that it was successful in >90% with a recurrence rate of approximately 5% (Table 12.3). Failures are caused either by an inability to induce the arrhythmia during the procedure, preventing adequate mapping, or by the location of the focus deep within the septum or in the epicardium over the septum. Occasionally, ablation from the left side of the interventricular septum or from the epicardium is required. Complications are infrequent and serious complications occur in less than 1% of cases (cardiac perforation with tamponade, injury to the left main coronary artery, and heart block due to inadvertent movement of the catheter toward the His bundle during ablation) [3, 79]. Death is extremely rare. A new right bundle branch block (RBBB) develops in about 1% of patients.

There are some high-risk characteristics that should induce the physician to recommend radiofrequency ablation without delay: 1) a history of unexplained syncope [52]; 2) very fast VT (rates >230 beats/min) [52]; 3) extremely frequent ectopy (>20,000 PVCs/day) [57]; 4) ventricular ectopy with short coupling interval [51].

Over the last 10 years new techniques in arrhythmia mapping have been developed. These include

Table 12.3 • Outcome of radiofrequency catheter ablation in RVOT-V. Modified from [3]

Author	Year	Patients (N)	Acute success (%)	Mean follow-up (months)	Recurrence
Calkins [60]	1993	10	100	8	0/10
Coggins [61]	1994	20	85	10	1/17
Mandrola [62]	1995	35	100	24	0/35
Movsowitz [64]	1996	18	89	12	5/16
Gumbrielle [65]	1997	10	100	16	0/10
Chinushi [66]	1997	13	100	28	1/13
Rodriguez [67]	1997	35	83	30	4/28
Almendral [68]	1998	15	87	21	1/13
Wen [69]	1998	44	87	41	4/39
Aiba [71]	2001	50	94	NA	NA
Lee [72]	2002	35	86	NA	NA
Freidman [73]	2002	10	90	11	2/9
O'Donnell [42]	2003	33	97	56	1/32
Ribbing [74]	2003	33	82	54	1/27
Ito [76]	2003	109	97	21	0/106
Joshi [3]	2005	72	99	51	2/71
Azegami [78]	2005	15	100	15	0/15
Krittayaphong [75]	2006	144	92	72	16/133
Total		701	93%		38/574 (6.6%)
Range			82-100%		0-12%
NA, not available					

multielectrode baskets, electroanatomic mapping, and non-contact mapping. These new techniques overcome the limitation of traditional electrophysiological methods and offer new therapeutic opportunities [71, 73, 78, 79].

ARVC/D vs. Idiopathic RVOT Ventricular Tachycardia: Differential Diagnosis

VT associated with ARVC/D may be localized in the outflow tract mimicking idiopathic RVOT tachycardia. Discrimination between the two entities is mandatory for prognostic and therapeutic reasons as well as for genetic implication [80, 81].

Standardized diagnostic criteria for the diagnosis of ARVC/D have been proposed and are known as the Task Force criteria [32]. According to these Task Force guidelines, the diagnosis of ARVC/D is based on the presence of major and minor criteria including ECG, arrhythmic, morphofunctional, and histopathological findings as well as a family history of this disease. The diagnosis of ARVC/D is made by the presence of 2 major criteria or 1 major plus 2 minor or 4 minor criteria from different groups. Recently, revisions have been proposed to

increase diagnostic sensitivity, particularly in the context of family screening. First degree family members having a single feature including T wave inversion in right precordial leads (V1, V2, and V3), late potentials on SAECG, VT with left bundle branch morphology, more than 200 extrasystoles over a 24-h period, mild structural or functional abnormalities of the RV, should be considered affected with ARVC/D [82].

Another proposed new ECG criterion is a prolonged S-wave upstroke ($\geq$55 ms) in leads V1-V3. This criterion was found in all patients with diffuse ARVC/D and in 90% of patients in localized ARVC/D [83].

Although RVOT tachycardia is considered a benign and not progressive entity, it may cause syncope and, sometimes, sudden cardiac death [46-48]. These malignant events, although occasionally correlated with polymorphic or very fast VT [51-53], are most likely explained by the clinical overlap between idiopathic RVOT tachycardia and early and/or segmental ARVC/D.

In order to exclude ARVC/D in patients with RVOT tachycardia, careful personal and family history is recommended, and a broad spectrum of non-invasive and invasive tests are performed including

12-lead ECG, signal-averaged ECG, exercise stress testing, echocardiography, magnetic resonance imaging, cardiac catheterization, ventriculography, electrophysiological study, and endomyocardial biopsy.

There are several findings which can help in the differentiation between the two conditions (Table 12.4). First, ARVC/D is a genetically determined disease, so family history for ARVC/D or sudden death should induce a high degree of suspicion. A negative family history does not exclude ARVC/D, because of sporadic variants and incomplete disease penetrance. Usually the ECG during sinus rhythm in RVOT VT patients is normal and abnormal late potentials are absent. In contrast, ECG abnormalities are detected in up to 95% of ARVC/D patients [42, 83-86]. The most common abnormality consists of T-waves inversion in the precordial leads V1-V3, complete or incomplete RBBB, prolongation of right precordial QRS duration more than 110 ms in V1-V3 in the absence of right bundle branch block, prolonged S-wave upstroke,

and postexcitation epsilon waves. These electrical markers reflect the distinctive pathologic substrate of ARVC/D, i.e., a fibrofatty scar, which accounts for the right intraventricular conduction defect. However, in patients with early/minor ARVC/D, 12-lead ECG and SAECG may be unremarkable, thus limiting their diagnostic role. Conventional imaging modalities including echocardiography and contrast angiography demonstrate RV structural and functional abnormalities in overt forms of ARVC/D. Two-dimensional echocardiography has significant limitations in the visualization and definition of morphofunctional abnormalities of the anterior wall and RVOT. It has been reported that some forms of localized ARVC/D, particularly in the infundibulum, may exhibit normal RV volumes and preserved RV ejection fraction by RV angiography. A recent angiographic study of computer-based quantitative segmental contraction analysis of the RV free wall demonstrated that wall motion is nonuniform in different RV regions: the tricuspid

Table 12.4 • Differential diagnosis of ventricular tachycardia with LBBB and inferior axis configuration (idiopathic RVOT VT vs. ARVC/D)

	Idiopathic RVOT VT*	ARVC/D*
Baseline ECG (83-85)	Usually normal	Frequent depolarization/repolarization abnormalities
RBBB	RBBB/rr' possible	RBBB varying degree (11-22%)
T-wave inversion in V2-V3 in the absence of RBBB	0-20%	50-85%
Epsilon waves	0%	22-33%
QRS duration ≥110 ms in V1-V3	0-20%	50-77%
QRSd duration V1+V2+V3/V4+V5+V6≥1.2	3.5-7%	77%
Prolonged S-wave upstroke in V1-V3 ≥55 ms	7%	95%
QRS dispersion ≥40 ms	4%	44%
QT dispersion ≥65 ms	10%	69%
Morphology during VT tachycardia	Usually monomorphic; QRS axis inferior	Multiple morphologies common; QRS axis variable (inferior, superior, intermediate)
Adenosine sensitivity	Yes	No
Programmed stimulation	Induciblity +–	Inducible
Entrainment	No	Yes
(Mechanism)	(Triggered activity)	(Re-entry)
SAECG [42, 83-85]	Usually normal (0-25%)	Abnormal late potentials in 56%-78%
RV (imaging studies)	Normal or mild abormalities	Dilation, dysfunction ("triangle of dysplasia"); Normal or mild abnormalities in early stage
Endocardial mapping	Normal	Low-voltage, fragmented electrograms ("scars")
History	Nonfamilial	Family history in 50%
* % of patients with positive findings		

valve zones show the greatest movement during contraction, whereas anterior and infundibular regions the least movement [84]. MRI findings should be interpreted with caution and confirmed by other imaging morphologies in order to avoid over diagnosis [40, 41, 43]. MRI should be performed only in a few centers with extensive experience with MR imaging in the interpretation of ARVC/D.

Unlike RVOT VT, the VT in ARVC/D does not respond to adenosine. This may be explained by different pathophysiologic mechanisms proposed for the two tachycardias. Usually, VT associated with ARVC/D can be induced by programmed ventricular stimulation and can be entrained. However, the response to programmed ventricular stimulation may be of limited value because a proportion of patients with spontaneous ventricular arrhythmia are not inducible regardless of the underlying substrate predisposing to reentrant arrhythmias [11]. Induction of tachycardia by programmed ventricular stimulation is also compatible with the mechanism of triggered activity. Idiopathic RVOT VT, which is due to cAMP-mediated-triggered activity, can be initiated and terminated with programmed stimulation although it cannot be entrained [45].

More than one VT morphology is characteristic for ARVC/D rather than for idiopathic RVOT VT, suggesting multiple right ventricular arrhythmogenic foci.

It has been noted that QRS duration during VT may be indicative of the septal or free-wall origin of the tachycardia. Because ARVC/D typically involves the free wall sparing the septum, this would be expected to result in a longer QRS duration through slowly conducting tissue. RVOT VT occurs in the absence of slowly conducting tissue, resulting in less conduction delay. Ainsworth et al. [87] analyzed the QRS morphology in ARVC/D patients diagnosed according to standardized criteria and in idiopathic RVOT VT. QRS prolongation during VT was consistent with ARVC/D. QRS duration in lead I ≥120 ms had a sensitivity of 100%, specificity of 46%, positive predictive value 61%, and negative predictive value 100% for ARVC/D. A mean QRS axis less than 30° (R<S in lead III) increased specificity for ARVC/D to 100%. In the subgroup of VT axis compatible with RVOT origin, QRS duration remained a strong discriminating factor for ARVC/D.

Niroomand et al. [80] analyzed clinical and electrophysiological data of patients referred for arrhythmias originating from the right ventricle. Fifteen of them were classified as having ARVC/D and 41 affected with idiopathic RV arrhythmias (IRVA).

Seven (48%) of ARVC/D subjects and 37 (90%) of IRVA patients had inferior axis configuration during arrhythmia. The ARVC/D patients were clearly distinguished by inducibility of VT by programmed electrical stimulation (93% vs. 3% IRVA), presence of multiple morphologies during tachycardia (73% vs. 0% IRVA), and abnormal fragmented diastolic potentials during ventricular arrhythmia (93% vs. 0% IRVA). A similar comparison was made by O'Donnell et al. [42]. This series included only patients with RVOT VT morphology. Seventeen patients who fulfilled standard criteria for ARVC/D and 33 with idiopathic RVOT VT had an electrophysiological study. In 82% of patients with ARVC/D VT was inducible by programmed ventricular stimulation vs. 3% in RVOT VT group. In RVOT VT patients tachycardia was inducible with isoproterenol and was cycle length dependent. Moreover, 70% of patients in the ARVC/D group had more than one morphology, while all RVOT VT patients showed a single VT morphology. Significant areas of fragmented electrograms were present in ARVC/D and only rarely seen in RVOT VT group. These results are consistent with the character of the pathologic substrate underlying ARVC/D and with different arrhythmia mechanisms in two conditions.

The most important pathologic lesion of ARVC/D is replacement of the myocardium of the RV free wall with fibrofatty tissue. The significant loss of myocardium results in the recording of low-amplitude, fractionated endocardial electrograms. This was first noted in patients with ischemic ventricular scar by traditional electrophysiological methods. Subsequently, a new technique allowing three-dimensional electroanatomic color-coded voltage mapping (3-D CARTO system) has been introduced. Boulos et al. reported the utility of electroanatomical voltage mapping in detection of pathological substrate in patients with ARVC/D and documented the presence of low-amplitude local electrograms in the right ventricle in ARVC/D patients [88]. Later, Corrado et al. [89] demonstrated that the electroanatomic low-amplitude areas were associated with the histopathological finding of myocyte loss and fibrofatty replacement at endomyocardial biopsy confirming that RV loss of voltage reflects the replacement of action potential-generating myocardial tissue with electrically silent fibrofatty tissue. Recently, Boulos et al. compared electroanatomic findings in patients with a diagnosis of idiopathic RVOT tachycardia with those in patients who had ARVC/D [90]. They found that mapping results were concordant with the previous clinical diagnosis, by showing normal voltages in the idiopathic RVOT tachycardia group and abnormal low-amplitude areas in ARVC/D patients. Another study by Corrado et al. indicated that 3D electroanatomic voltage mapping of the RV may differentiate patients with idiopathic RVOT tachycardia and those with underlying subtle ARVC/D. This technique provided evidence of electroanatomic RV scar(s) in approximately one third (7/24) of patients with RVOT tachycardia, in whom a normal RV size and function were diagnosed by traditional imaging studies. Thus, electroanatomic voltage mapping by assessing the electrical consequences of loss of RV myocardium obviated limitations in RVOT wall motion analysis and increased sensitivity for detecting otherwise concealed ARVC/D myocardial substrate. From these preliminary data it would appear that a carefully performed, high density voltage map may be able to differentiate normal from abnormal myocardial substrate. Confirmation of these data in a larger series of patients is needed.

Acknowledgements

The study was supported by grants from the Ministry of Health, Rome, Italy, European Comunity research contract #QLG1-CT-2000-01091 and the Veneto Region, Venice, Italy.

References

1. Nava A, Thiene G, Canciani B et al (1992) Clinical profile of concealed form of arrhythmogenic right ventricular cardiomyopathy presenting with apparently idiopathic ventricular arrhythmias. Int J Cardiol 35:195-206
2. Buxton A, Waxman H, Marchlinski F et al (1983) Right ventricular tachycardia: Clinical and electrophysiologic characteristics. Circulation 68:917-927
3. Joshi S, Wilber DJ (2005) Ablation of idiopathic right ventricular outflow tract tachycardia: current perspectives. J Cardiovasc Electrophysiol 16:52-58
4. Marcus FI, Fontaine GH, Guiraudon G et al (1982) Right ventricular dysplasia: a report of 24 adult cases. Circulation 65:384-398
5. Thiene G, Nava A, Corrado D et al (1988) Right ventricular cardiomyopathy and sudden death in young people. N Engl J Med 318:129-133
6. Corrado D, Basso C, Thiene G (2000) Arrhythmogenic right ventricular cardiomyopathy: diagnosis, prognosis, and treatment. Heart 83:588-595
7. Hulot JS, Jouven X, Empana JP et al (2004) Natural history and risk stratification of arrhythmogenic right ventricular dysplasia/cardiomyopathy. Circulation 110:1879-1884
8. Lemola K, Brunckhorst C, Helfenstein U et al (2005) Predictors of adverse outcome in patients with arrhythmogenic right ventricular dysplasia/cardiomyopathy: long-term experience of a tertiary care center. Heart 91:1167-1172
9. Verma A, Kilicaslan F, Schweikert RA et al (2005) Short- and long-term success of substrate-based mapping and ablation of ventricular tachycardia in arrhythmogenic right ventricular dysplasia. Circulation 111:3209-3216
10. Marchlinski FE, Zado E, Dixit S et al (2004) Electroanatomic substrate and outcome of catheter ablative therapy for ventricular tachycardia in setting of right ventricular cardiomyopathy. Circulation 110:2293-2298
11. Corrado D, Leoni L, Link MS et al (2003) Implantable cardioverter-defibrillator therapy for prevention of sudden death in patients with arrhythmogenic right ventricular cardiomyopathy/dysplasia. Circulation 108:3084-3091
12. Wichter T, Paul M, Wollmann C et al (2004) Implantable cardioverter/defibrillator therapy in arrhythmogenic right ventricular cardiomyopathy. Single-center experience of long-term follow-up and complications in 60 patients. Circulation 19:1503-1508
13. Maron BJ, Towbin JA, Thiene G et al (2006) Contemporary definitions and classification of the cardiomyopathies: An American Heart Association Scientific Statement from the Council on Clinical Cardiology, Heart Failure and Transplantation Committee; Quality of Care and Outcomes Research and Functional Genomics and Translational Biology Interdisciplinary Working Groups; and Council on Epidemiology and Prevention. Circulation 113:1807-1816
14. Lerman BB, Stein KM, Markowitz SM et al (2000) Ventricular arrhythmias in normal hearts. Cardiology Clin 18:265-291
15. Moorman AFM, Christoffels VM (2003) Cardiac chamber formation: development, genes, and evolution. Physiol Rev 83:1223-1267
16. Schafers M, Lerch H, Wichter T et al (1998) Cardiac sympathetic innervation in patients with idiopathic right ventricular outflow tract tachycardia. J Am Coll Cardiology 32:181-186
17. Lerman BB, Dong B (1998) Right ventricular outflow tract tachycardia due to a somatic cell mutation in G protein subunit alpha i2. J Clin Invest 101:2862-2868
18. Lerman BB, Belardinelli L, West A et al (1986) Adenosine-sensitive ventricular tachycardia evidence suggesting cyclic AMP-medicated triggered activity. Circulation 74:270-280
19. Farzaneh-Far A, Lerman BB (2005) Idiopathic ventricular ventricular outflow tract tachycardia. Heart 91:136-138
20. Sugishita Y, Watanabe M, Fisher S (2004) The development of the embryonic outflow tract provides novel insights into cardiac differentiation and remodeling. Trends Cardiovasc Med 14:235-241
21. Iwai S, Cantillon DJ, Kim RJ et al (2006) Right and left ventricular outflow tract tachycardias: Evidence for a

common electrophysiologic mechanism. J Cardiovasc Electrophysiol; 17:1052-1058

22. Timmermans C, Rodriguez LM, Medeiros A et al (2002) Radiofrequency catheter ablation of idiopathic ventricular tachycardia originating in the main stem of the pulmonary artery J Cardiovasc Electrophysiol 13:281-284

23. Sekiguchi Y, Aonuma K, Takahashi A et al (2005) Electrocardiographic and electrophysiologic characteristics of ventricular tachycardia originating within the pulmonary artery. J Am Coll Cardiol 45:887-895

24. Ouyang F, Fotuhi P, Ho SY et al (2002) Repetitive monomorphic ventricular tachycardia originating from the aortic sinus cusp: electrocardiographic characterization for guiding catheter ablation. J Am Coll Cardiol 39:500-508

25. Tada H, Nogami A, Naito S et al (2001) Left ventricular epicardial outflow tract tachycardia: A new distinct subgroup of outflow tract tachycardia. Jpn Circ J 65:723-730

26. Nakagawa M, Takahashi N, Nobe S et al (2002) Gender differences in various types of idiopathic ventricular tachycardia. J Cardiovasc Electrophysiol 13:633-638

27. Lemery R, Brugada P, Della Bella P et al (1989) Nonischemic ventricular tachycardia. Clinical course and long-term follow-up in patients without clinically overt heart disease. Circulation 79:990-999

28. Deal BJ, Miller SM, Scagliotti D et al (1986) Ventricular tachycardia in a young population without overt heart disease. Circulation 73:1111-1118

29. Goy JJ, Tauxe F, Fromer M et al (1990) Ten-years follow-up of 20 patients with idiopathic ventricular tachycardia. PACE 13:1142-1147

30. Mont L, Seixas T, Brugada P et al (1991) Clinical and electrophysiologic characteristics of exercise-related idiopathic ventricular tachycardia. Am J Cardiol 68:897-900

31. Harris KC, Potts JE, Fournier A et al (2006) Right ventricular outflow tract tachycardia in children. J Pediatr 149:822-826

32. McKenna WJ, Thiene G, Nava A et al (1994) Diagnosis of arrhythmogenic right ventricular dysplasia/cardiomyopathy. Br Heart J 71:215-221

33. Carlson MD, White RD, Trohman RG et al (1994) Right ventricular outflow tract tachycardia: detection of previously unrecognized anatomic abnormalities using cine magnetic resonance imaging. J Am Coll Cardiol 24:720-727

34. White RD, Trohman RG, Flam SD et al (1998) Right ventricular arrhythmia in the absence of arrhythmogenic dysplasia: MR imaging of myocardial abnormalities. Radiology 207:743-751

35. Markowitz SM, Litvak BL, Ramirez de Arellano EA et al (1997) Adenosine sensitive ventricular tachycardia: Right ventricular abnormalities delineated by magnetic resonance imaging. Circulation 96:1192-2000

36. Globits S, Kreiner G, Frank H et al (1997) Significance of morphological abnormalities detected by MRI in patients undergoing successful ablation of right ventricular outflow tract tachycardia. Circulation 96:2633-2640

37. Krittayaphong R, Saiviroonporn P, Boonyasirinant T et al (2006) Magnetic resonance imaging abnormalities in right ventricular outflow tract tachycardia and the prediction of radiofrequency ablation outcome. PACE 29:837-845

38. Tandri H, Bluemke DA, Ferrari VA et al (2004) Findings on magnetic resonance imaging of idiopathic right ventricular outflow tachycardia. Am J Cardiol 94:1441-1445

39. Grimm W, List-Hellwig E, Hoffman J et al (1997) Magnetic resonance imaging and signal-averaged electrocardiography in patients with repetitive monomorphic ventricular tachycardia and otherwise normal electrocardiogram. Pacing Clin Electrophysiol 17:1826-1833

40. Sievers B, Addo M, Franken U et al (2004) Right ventricular wall motion abnormalities found in healthy subjects by cardiovascular magnetic resonance imaging and characterized with a new segmental model. J Cardiovasc Magn Reson 6:601-608

41. Bomma C, Rutberg J, Tandri H et al (2004) Misdiagnosis of arrhythmogenic right ventricular dysplasia/cardiomyopathy. J Cardiovasc Electrophysiol 15:300-306

42. O'Donnell D, Cox D, Bourke J et al (2003) Clinical and electrophysiological differences between patients with arrhythmogenic right ventricular dysplasia and right ventricular outflow tract tachycardia. Eur Heart J 24:801-810

43. Bluemke DA, Krupinski EA, Ovitt T et al (2003) MR Imaging of arrhythmogenic right ventricular cardiomyopathy: morphologic findings and interobserver reliability. Cardiology 99:153-162

44. Tandri H, Saranathan M, Rodriguez ER et al (2005) Non-invasive detection of myocardial fibrosis in arrhythmogenic right ventricular cardiomyopathy using delayed-enhancement magnetic resonance imaging. J Am Coll Cardiol 45:98-103

45. Josephson M (2002) Recurrent ventricular tachycardia. In: Clinical cardiac electrophysiology. Lippincott Wiliams and Wilkins, Philadelphia

46. Pederson DH, Zipes DP, Foster PR et al (1979) Ventricular tachycardia and ventricular fibrillation in a young population. Circulation 60:988-992

47. Maddox K (1947) Intermittent ventricular tachycardia in youth: report of case with fatal termination. Am Heart J 33:739-740

48. Lesch M, Lewis E, Humphries JO et al (1967) Paroxysmal ventricular tachycardia in the absence of organic heart disease. Ann Intern Med 66:950-960

49. Pfammatter JP, Paul T (1999) Idiopathic ventricular tachycardia in infancy and childhood: a multicenter study on clinical profile and outcome. Working Group on Dysrhythmias and Electrophysiology of the Association for European Pediatric Cardiology. J Am Coll Cardiol 3:2067-2072

50. Gaita F, Giustetto C, Di Donna P et al (2001) Long-term follow-up of right ventricular monomorphic extrasystoles. J Am Coll Cardiol 38:364-370

51. Viskin S, Rosso R, Rogowski O et al (2005) The short-coupled variant of right ventricular outflow ventricu-

lar tachycardia. A not so benign form of benign ventricular tachycardia. J Cardiovasc Electrophysiol 16:912-916

52. Noda T, Shimizu W, Taguchi A et al (2005) Malignant entity of idiopathic ventricular fibrillation and polymorphic ventricular tachycardia initiated by premature extrasystoles originating from right ventricular outflow tract. J Am Coll Cardiol 46:1288-1294

53. Viskin S, Antzelevitch C (2005) The cardiologists' worst nightmare: Sudden death from "benign" ventricular arrhythmias. J Am Coll Cardiol 46:1295-1297

54. Kim YH, Goldberger J, Kadish A (1996) Treatment of ventricular tachycardia-induced cardiomyopathy by transcatheter radiofrequency ablation. Heart 76:550-552

55. Grimm W, Menz V, Hoffman J et al (2001) Reversal of tachycardia induced cardiomyopathy following ablation of repetitive monomorphic right ventricular outflow tract tachycardia. Pacing Clin Electrophysiol 24:166-71

56. Yarlagadda RK, Iwai S, Stein KM et al (2005) Reversal of cardiomyopathy in patients with repetitive monomorphic ventricular ectopy originating from the right ventricular outflow tract. Circulation 112:1092-1097

57. Takemoto M, Yoshimura H, Ohba Y et al (2005) Radiofrequency catheter ablation of premature ventricular complexes from right ventricular outflow tract improves left ventricular dilation and clinical status in patients without structural heart disease. J Am Coll Cardiol 45:1259-1265

58. Breithardt G, Borggrefe M, Wichter T (1990) Catheter ablation of idiopathic right ventricular tachycardia. Circulation 82:2273-2276

59. Wilber DJ, Baerman J, Olshansky B et al (1993) Adenosine-sensitive ventricular tachycardia. Clincial characteristics and response to catheter ablation. Circulation 87:126-134

60. Calkins H, Kalbfleisch SJ, El-Atassi R et al (1993) Relation between efficacy of radiofrequency catheter ablation and site of origin of idiopathic ventricular tachycardia. Am J Cardiol 71:827-833

61. Coggins DL, Lee RJ, Sweeney J et al (1994) Radiofrequency catheter ablation as a cure for idiopathic ventricular tachycardia of both right and left ventricular origin. J Am Coll Cardiol 23:1333-1341

62. Mandrola JM, Klein LS, Miles WM et al (1995) Radiofrequency catheter ablation of idiopathic ventricular tachycardia in 57 patients: Acute success and long term follow-up. J Am Coll Cardiol 19A (abstract)

63. Jadonath RL, Schwartzman DS, Preminger MW et al (1995) Utility of the 12-lead electrocardiogram in localizing the origin of right ventricular outflow tract tachycardia. Am Heart J 130:1107-1113

64. Movsowitz C, Schwartzman D, Callans DJ et al (1996) Idiopathic right ventricular outflow tract tachycardia. Narrowing the anatomic location for successful ablation. Am Heart J 131:930-936

65. Gumbrielle TP, Bourke JP, Doig JC et al (1997) Electrocardiographic features of septal location of right ventricular outflow tract tachycardia. Am J Cardiol 79:213-216

66. Chinushi M, Aizawa Y, Takahashi K et al (1997) Radiofrequency catheter ablation for idiopathic right ventricular tachycardia with special reference to morphological variation and long term outcome. Heart 78:255-261

67. Rodriguez LM, Smeets JL, Timmermans C et al (1997) Predictors for successful ablation of right- and left-sided idiopathic ventricular tachycardia. Am J Cardiol 79:309-314

68. Almendral J, Peinado R (1998) Radiofrequency catheter ablation of idiopathic right ventricular outflow tract tachycardia. In: Farre J, Concepcion M (eds) Ten years of radiofrequency catheter ablation. Futura, pp 249-262

69. Wen MS, Taniguchi Y, Yeh SJ et al (1998) Determinants of tachycardia recurrences after radiofrequency ablation of idiopathic ventricular tachycardia. Am J Cardiol 81:500-503

70. Merino JL, Jimenez-Borreguero J, Peinado R et al (1998) Unipolar mapping and magnetic resonance imaging of "idiopathic" right ventricular outflow tract ectopy. J Cardiovasc Electrophysiol 9:84-87

71. Aiba T, Shimizu W, Taguchi A et al (2001) Clinical usefulness of a multielectrode basket catheter for idiopathic ventricular tachycardia originating from right ventricular outflow tract. J Cardiovasc Electrophysiol 12:518-520

72. Lee SH, Tai CT, Chiang CE et al (2002) Determinants of successful ablation of idiopathic ventricular tachycardias with left bundle branch block morphology from the right ventricular outflow tract. Pacing Clin Electrophysiol 25:1346-1351

73. Friedman PA, Asirvatham SJ, Grice S et al (2002) Noncontact mapping to guide ablation of right ventricular outflow tract tachycardia. J Am Coll Cardiol 39:1808-1812

74. Ribbing M, Wasmer K, Monnig G et al (2003) Endocardial mapping of right ventricular outflow tract tachycardia using noncontact activation mapping. J Cardiovasc Electrophysiol 14:602-608

75. Krittayaphong R, Sriratanasathavorn C, Dumavibhat C et al (2006) Electrocardiographic predictors of long-term outcomes after radiofrequency ablation in patients with right-ventricular outflow tract tachycardia. Euopace 8:601-606

76. Ito S, Tada H, Naito S et al (2003) Development and validation of an ECG algorithm for identifying the optimal ablation site for idiopathic ventricular outflow tract tachycardia. J Cardiovasc Electrophysiol 14:1280-1286

77. Yarlagadda RK, Iwai S, Stein KM et al (2005) Reversal of cardiomyopathy in patients with repetitive monomorphic ventricular ectopy originating from the right ventricular outflow tract. Circulation 112:1092-1097

78. Azegami K, Wilber DJ, Arruda M et al (2005) Spatial resolution of pace mapping and activation mapping in patients with idiopathic right ventricular outflow tract tachycardia. J Cardiovasc Electrophysiol 16:823-829

79. Miller JM, Pezeshkian NG, Yadav AV (2006) Catheter mapping and ablation of right ventricular outflow tract ventricular tachycardia. Journal of Cardiovascular Electrophysiology 17:800-802

80. Niroomand F, Carbucicchio C, Tondo C et al (2002) Electrophysiological characteristics and outcome in patients with idiopathic right ventricular arrhythmia compared with arrhythmogenic right ventricular dysplasia. Heart 87:41-47

81. Cassidy DM, Vassallo JA, Miller JM et al (1986) Endocardial catheter mapping in patients in sinus rhythm: relationship to underlying heart disease and ventricular arrhythmias. Circulation 73:645-652

82. Hamid MS, Norman M, Quraishi A et al (2002) Prospective evaluation of relatives for familial arrhythmogenic right ventricular cardiomyopathy/dysplasia reveals a need to broaden diagnostic criteria. J Am Coll Cardiol 40:1445-1450

83. Nasir K, Bomma C, Tandri H et al (2004) Electrocardiographic features of arrhythmogenic right ventricular dysplasia/cardiomyopathy according to disease severity: a need to broaden diagnostic criteria. Circulation 110:1527-1534

84. Kazmierczak J, De Sutter J, Tavernier R et al (1998) Electrocardiographic and morphometric features in patients with ventricular tachycardia of right ventricular origin. Heart 79:388-393

85. Arana E, Pedrote A, Romero N et al (2006) Electrocardiogram analysis in right ventricular tachycardias in patients without apparent structural heart disease. Pacing Clin Electrophysiol 29:56 (abstract)

86. Indik JH, Dallas WJ, Ovitt T et al (2005) Do patients with right ventricular outflow tract ventricular arrhythmias have a normal right ventricular wall motion? A quantitative analysis compared to normal subjects. Cardiology 104:10-15

87. Ainsworth CD, Skanes AC, Klein GJ et al (2006) Differentiating arrhythmogenic right ventricular cardiomyopathy from right ventricular outflow tract ventricular tachcardia using multilead QRS duration and axis. Heart Rhythm 3:416-423

88. Boulos M, Lashevsky I, Reisner S et al (2001) Electroanatomical mapping of arrhythmogenic right renticular dysplasia. J Am Coll Cardiol 38:2020-2027

89. Corrado D, Basso C, Leoni L et al (2005) Three-dimensional electroanatomic voltage mapping increases accuracy of diagnosing arrhythmogenic right ventricular cardiomyopathy/dysplasia. Circulation 111:3042-3050

90. Boulos M, Lashevsky I, Gepstein L (2005) Usefulness of electroanatomical mapping to differentiate between right ventricular outflow tract tachycardia and arrhythmogenic right ventricular dysplasia. Am J Cardiol 95:935-940

91. Corrado D, Tokaiuk B, Leoni L et al (2005) Differential diagnosis between right ventricular outflow tract tachycardia and arrhythmogenic right ventricular cardiomyopathy/dysplasia by 3-D electroanatomic voltage mapping. Eur Heart J 26:373 (abstract)

ELECTROCARDIOGRAPHIC MANIFESTATIONS

Wojciech Zareba, Katarzyna Piotrowicz, Pietro Turrini

Electrocardiographic Findings in the ARVC/D Task Force Criteria

Electrocardiographic (ECG) findings usually are the first clinical abnormalities recognized in patients suspected of arrhythmogenic right ventricular cardiomyopathy/dysplasia (ARVC/D) [1-5]. Typically, ARVC/D is considered in a young or middle-aged individual with a history of ventricular arrhythmias who does not have evidence of ischemic heart disease. The suspicion of ARVC/D is increased if the standard 12-lead ECG shows features suggestive of ARVC/D such as negative T waves in the precordial leads beyond V2 [1-3]. The standard ECG may also show abnormalities of the QRS complex, consisting of localized QRS prolongation in V1-V3 and epsilon waves indicating delayed activation of the right ventricle. Complete and incomplete right bundle branch block (RBBB) may also be observed. If the signal-averaged ECG shows late potentials, it further confirms that there is delayed ventricular activation due to myocardial fibrosis. Holter recordings assist with the diagnosis when there are frequent ventricular premature beats, (>1,000 per 24 h) usually of left bundle branch block (LBBB) morphology. As seen in Table 13.1, there is a great emphasis on ECG findings

in the Task Force criteria for the diagnosis of ARVC/D [4]. This chapter provides an overview regarding the clinical significance and utility of ECG findings in patients suspected of ARVC/D.

Ventricular Arrhythmias

Ventricular arrhythmias manifest clinically with palpitations, or episodes of ventricular tachycardia (VT) associated with syncope, and are frequently the first manifestations of the disorder. There is evidence that ARVC/D is a common cause of sudden cardiac death in young people [6]. Patients with VT who have associated hemodynamics impairment or those who had ventricular fibrillation have a worse prognosis than patients with hemodynamically stable VT [7]. They usually also have more advanced right ventricular disease, as described by Turrini et al. [7] who demonstrated the association between sustained VT and reduced RV ejection fraction.

Dalal et al. [8] compared the incidence of induced or spontaneous ventricular arrhythmias in patients with plakophilin-2 (PKP2) gene mutation with those who did not have an identified form of the disease. There was no significant difference between the two groups, suggesting that the PKP2 mutation is not as-

Table 13.1 • ECG-Based Task Force criteria for Diagnosing ARVC/D [4]

	Minor	Major
III. Repolarization Abnormalities	Inverted T waves in precordial leads (V2 and V3) in absence of right bundle block	
IV. Depolarization/Conduction Abnormalities	Late potentials in signal-averaged ECG	Epsilon waves/Localized prolongation (>110 ms) of QRS in right precordial leads (V1-V3)
V. Arrhythmias	Left bundle branch block type ventricular tachycardia (sustained & nonsustained) by ECG, Holter, or exercise testing	
	Frequent ventricular extrasystoles in Holter (>1000/24 h)	

tion between right and left precordial leads >25 ms are characteristic of ARVC/D. This localized prolongation of the QRS complex is a major criterion for the diagnosis of ARVC/D. Wichter et al. [17] found that QRS duration prolongation in the right precordial leads was present in 52% of 151 patients. Nasir et al. [15] observed this finding in 64% of 39 patients. They also [15] reported that the ratio of the sum of QRS in V1-V3/V4-V6 >1.2 was observed in 77% of these patients. Peters et al. [21] reported localized right precordial QRS prolongation (V1 + V2 + V3)/(V4 + V5 + V6) ≥1.2 in 261 of 265 patients (98% with ARVC/D). Localized prolongation of inferior QRS complexes was found in 58 cases (22%). These authors indicate that localized right precordial QRS prolongation is the most typical ECG finding for ARVC/D.

Another way of presenting these interlead differences in QRS duration is by measuring QRS dispersion, i.e., the differences in QRS duration between precordial leads, which could represent regional inhomogeneity of depolarization. Peters et al. [22] reported that QRS dispersion ≥50 ms is a noninvasive predictor of recurrent arrhythmic events. In 20 patients who died suddenly with ARVC/D proven at autopsy, Turrini et al. [18] found that QRS dispersion ≥40 ms was the strongest independent predictor of sudden death, with a sensitivity of 90% and a specificity of 77%. Hulot et al. [23] confirmed the value of QRS dispersion ≥40 ms as a risk factor for cardiovascular death during the natural history of the disease. Nasir et al. [15] identified QRS dispersion ≥40 ms as one of the most significant ECG predictor of inducibility of VT at EPS. Localized depolarization abnormalities are more commonly associated with cardiac arrest and may be predictive of sustained ventricular arrhythmias.

Localized delay of depolarization may also be manifest by a widened QRS wave frequently with notches on the upstroke of this wave. Nasir et al. [15] reported that 95% of 39 patients with ARVC/D had an S wave in V1-V3 ≥55 ms. This ECG abnormality might be the most specific indicator of the selective increase of QRS duration in the precordial leads in ARVC/D. It is the terminal part of the QRS represented by the S wave in V1-V3 that reflects preferential repolarization of the last part of the heart to be depolarized, the right ventricle. These abnormalities seem to correlate with the inducibility of ventricular arrhythmias [15].

The above abnormalities are not valid in patients with RBBB, which is a frequent finding in patients who present more advanced stages of the disease. Complete RBBB was reported in 15% of ARVC/D patients described by Turrini et al. [18]. More frequently, features of incomplete RBBB or parietal block reflecting intraventricular myocardial conduction defect (not conduction system defect) is observed. The term parietal block seems to reflect localized right precordial QRS prolongation with features resembling RBBB but not fulfilling RBBB criteria [19, 20]. Nasir et al. [15] found parietal block in 52% of patients without RBBB. Peters et al. [21] reported complete RBBB with T inversions beyond V2 in 17 patients (6%) and incomplete RBBB in 38 cases (14%) of studied 265 ARVC/D patients. More advanced forms of the disease, especially with decompensation of the right ventricle function, are associated with complete RBBB [22, 23].

Epsilon Waves

The epsilon wave consists of high-frequency notches located on the ST segment immediately after the QRS complex, usually recorded in the right precordial leads on the standard ECG (Fig. 13.3). This ECG wave was first described in patients with ARVC/D [2, 20]. It is believed that epsilon waves represent delayed activation of affected areas of right ventricle. Late potentials in the signal average ECG (SAECG) are another manifestation of the same phenomenon. It is recommended that the ECG should be recorded at double speed (50 mm/s) and double amplitude (20 mm/mv) to increase the sensitivity to detect epsilon waves. Improvement in detecting epsilon waves can also be obtained by using the limb leads placed on the chest with the left arm lead over the xyphoid process, the right arm lead on the manubrium sternum, and the left leg lead over a rib at the V4 or V5 position [24]. Further

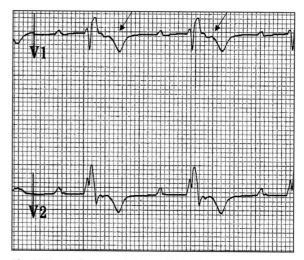

Fig. 13.3 • Epsilon wave in V1 and V2 in the presence of right bundle branch block

enhancement can be obtained by resetting the filter of the ECG machine from the usual 150 Hz to 40 Hz.

Wichter et al. [17] found epsilon waves in 22.5% of 151 ARVC/D patients and late potentials in 41% of the 151 patients. Turrini et al. [18] reported epsilon waves in 25%-35% of patients with different arrhythmogenic potential. These data suggest that the epsilon wave is not predictive of arrhythmic events. In a series of 265 patients, Peters et al. [21] recorded precordial epsilon waves using the standard ECG setting in 23% and using highly amplified and modified recording technique in 75% of the patients.

Abnormal SAECG

The presence of late potentials and delayed activation of ventricular myocardium detected in the SAECG is considered to represent slowed ventricular conduction, which is a substrate for reentrant tachyarrhythmias (Fig. 13.4). In the first reported series of patients with this disease, late potentials were recorded in 81% of patients by Marcus, Fontaine et al. [1]. In the 151 patients described by Wichter et al. [17], late potentials were found in 41%. Kinoshita et al. [25] analyzed the SAECG in 28 patients with ARVC/D and 35 age-matched normal subjects at two different high-pass filter settings, 25 Hz and 40 Hz. Positive SAECG criteria were found in 20 (71%) and 18 (64%) patients at filter settings of 25 Hz and 40 Hz, respectively. Nazir et al. [26] also indicated that detection of late potentials in ARVC/D can be improved by employing a high-pass filter of 25 Hz and specifically looking for changes in the Z leads.

As with other ECG markers, there is a correlation between abnormal SAECG values and the extent of right ventricular disease. Nasir et al. [26] reported that a positive SAECG predicted inducibility of sustained VT during programmed electrical stimulation testing. They performed electrophysiological studies in 40 pa-

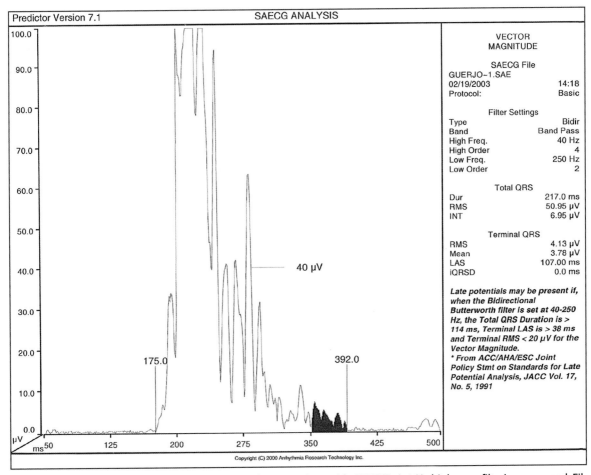

Fig. 13.4 • Signal-averaged ECG with late potentials in a patient with ARVC/D. A 4-Hz high-pass filtering was used; Filtered QRS duration (QRSD) = 217 ms; Low Amplitude Signal (LAS) = 107 ms, and Root-Mean Square voltage of terminal 40 ms (RMS) = 4 μV

tients (37±12 years) with ARVC/D. Of the 31 without bundle branch blocks, 21 (76%) had inducible monomorphic VT. At an fQRS ≥110 msec the sensitivity of an fQRS >110 msec was 91% to predict inducibility of VT; the specificity was 90%, and the predictive value was 90%. In general, the larger the right ventricular size, the greater the possibility of inducing VT/VF at electrophysiological study and of having sustained ventricular arrhythmias. However, data on arrhythmic risk stratification using signal averaged ECG in ARVC/D are limited [27]. Recently, Pezawas et al. [28] reported that an abnormal SAECG and decreased left ventricular ejection fraction were statistically significant predictors for VT recurrence by multivariate analysis. Folino et al. [29] found that patients with ARVC/D who have sustained VT tend to have longer fQRS. Therefore, the presence of an abnormal SAECG might be considered as risk factor, although larger studies with long-term follow-up are needed to determine the predictive value of SAECG in ARVC/D.

It is important to realize that the definitions of abnormal values of SAECG parameters were derived for the purpose of risk stratification of sudden death and ventricular arrhythmias in postinfarction patients. These values may not apply to identification of abnormal SAECG when evaluating young subjects suspected of ARVC/D. Recently, Marcus et al. [30] investigated this topic and based on published literature of the SAECG of normal subjects, gender- and recording device-specific criteria for SAECG parameters were proposed. These proposed SAECG criteria require evaluation and validation in future studies.

QT Dispersion

In ARVC/D there is increased electrical heterogeneity that is likely to be responsible for ventricular instability. Fontaine et al. [31] suggested the coexistence of two different mechanisms for the occurrence of ventricular arrhythmias leading to SCD, i.e., depolarization abnormalities mediated by a sympathetic mechanism and repolarization abnormalities facilitated by parasympathetic drive. The interlead variability in QT interval duration on the standard 12-lead ECG, the so-called QT dispersion, has been suggested to reflect regional variations in ventricular repolarization and to provide an indirect measure of the extent of nonuniformity of myocardial repolarization. The concept of QT dispersion is controversial. There are studies that raise concern about methodological and conceptual aspects of this approach. In addition, there is a lack of consistency on findings regarding the prognostic significance of QT

dispersion for risk stratification. The value of QT dispersion as an arrhythmic marker in ARVC/D is controversial. Benn et al. [32] found increased QT dispersion in ARVC/D patients, without significant differences between patients considered at low and high risk for life-threatening arrhythmias. Peters et al. [33], analyzing ARVC/D patients with sustained VT who had the overt form of disease, did not find an increased QT dispersion. However, they demonstrated that repolarization abnormalities were present at body surface mapping and might be related to the occurrence of ventricular arrhythmias. In the series of Turrini et al. [18], QT dispersion was significantly greater in the patients who died suddenly as compared to those presenting different arrhythmic profiles. A cut-off value for QT dispersion >65 ms was associated with a high risk of sudden death with a sensitivity of 85% and a specificity of 75%. However, in this report, QT dispersion was not an independent predictor of high arrhythmic risk at multivariate analysis. In the series of Nasir et al. [15], QT dispersion ≥65 ms did not discriminate patients with spontaneous and/or induced sustained ventricular arrhythmias from those without. Notably, the localized form of ARVC/D showed a similar frequency of QT dispersion as compared with the diffuse form of the disease. Interestingly, in ARVC/D, an increased QT dispersion showed a similar frequency of negative T waves in V1-V3, which is a marker of repolarization abnormalities [15, 18]. It is important to stress that QRS dispersion is considered as the major determinate of QT dispersion.

Serial Electrocardiographic Evaluation in ARVC/D

The ARVC/D is a progressive disorder and ECG testing should be considered as the most useful tool for detecting progression of this disorder. Jaoude et al. [34] performed long-term electrocardiographic follow-up in 36 patients presenting with ARVC/D-related VT and showed that after a maximum of 6 years all patients had developed ECG abnormalities. The authors concluded that long-term electrocardiographic follow-up is necessary to confirm or exclude ARVC/D in patients presenting with a VT originating from the RV. In a study by Kies et al. [35], 60 patients suspected of having ARVC/D were evaluated. Initially, 22 (37%) of these patients were diagnosed as having ARVC/D. After a mean 4-year follow-up, 23 initially ARVC/D-negative patients were re-evaluated because of recurrent symptoms. Of those, 12 (52%) met the ARVC/D Task Force criteria. Eleven of the 12 (92%) patients first presented with ECG abnormalities only, but developed structural abnormalities on imaging at follow-up. The authors concluded that ECG abnormalities may precede structural abnormalities, warranting serial re-evaluation for ARVC/D in initially Task Force criteria-negative patients presenting with LBBB VT with only ECG abnormalities.

Conclusions

The electrocardiographic manifestations of ARVC/D are highly variable depending upon the stage of the disease. In the concealed form, the ECG may be normal. When there is overt disease including congestive heart failure, there is an increasing incidence of ECG abnormalities. Both myocardial conduction abnormalities and repolarization abnormalities are important clinical findings which raise the suspicion of the presence of ARVC/D. There is a need for more studies to evaluate the progression of the disease and its ECG manifestations over a long period of time. At present there is no clear evidence for a specific association between known ARVC/D genes and ECG abnormalities. ECG abnormalities are generally related to the extent of myocardial changes, but clinical experience indicates that ECG changes may precede morphological and functional abnormalities of right ventricle.

References

1. Marcus FI, Fontaine GH, Guiraudon G et al (1982) Right ventricular dysplasia: A report of 24 adult cases. Circulation 65:384-389
2. Fontaine G, Frank R, Guiraudon C et al (1984) Signification des troubles de conduction intraventriculaire observés dans la dysplasie ventriculaire droite arhytmogène. Arch Mal Cœur 77:872-879
3. Nava A, Canciani B, Buja G et al (1988) Electrovector-cardiographic study of negative T waves on precordial leads in arrhythmogenic right ventricular dysplasia: Relationship with right ventricular volumes. J Electrocardiol 21:239-245
4. McKenna WJ, Thiene G, Nava A et al (1994) Diagnosis of arrhythmogenic right ventricular dysplasia/cardiomyopathy. Task Force of the Working Group Myocardial and Pericardial Disease of the European Society of Cardiology and of the Scientific Council on Cardiomyopathies of the International Society and Federation of Cardiology. Br Heart J 71:215-218
5. Turrini P, Corrado D, Basso C et al (2003) Noninvasive risk stratification in arrhythmogenic right ventricular cardiomyopathy. ANE 8:161-169
6. Thiene G, Nava A, Corrado D et al (1988) Right ventricular cardiomyopathy and sudden death in young people. N Engl J Med 318:129-133
7. Turrini P, Angelini A, Thiene G et al (1999) Late potentials and ventricular arrhythmias in arrhythmogenic right ventricular cardiomyopathy. Am J Cardiol 83:1214-1219
8. Dalal D, Molin LH, Piccini J et al (2006) Clinical features of arrhythmogenic right ventricular dysplasia/cardiomyopathy associated with mutation in plakophilin-2. Circulation 113:1641-1649
9. Ainsworth CD, Skanes AC, Klein GJ et al (2006) Differentiating arrhythmogenic right ventricular cardiomyopathy from right ventricular outflow tract ventricular tachycardia using multilead QRS duration and axis. Heart Rhythm 3:416-423
10. Hamid MS, Norman M, Quraishi A et al (2002) Prospective evaluation of relatives for familial arrhythmogenic right ventricular cardiomyopathy/dysplasia reveals a need to broaden diagnostic criteria. J Am Coll Cardiol 40:1445-1450
11. Marcus FI (2005) Prevalence of T-wave inversion beyond V1 in young normal individuals and usefulness for the diagnosis of arrhythmogenic right ventricular cardiomyopathy/dysplasia. Am J Cardiol 95:1070-1071
12. Suarez RM, Suarez RM Jr. (1946) The T wave of the precordial electrocardiogram at different age levels. Am Heart J 32:480-493
13. Nava A, Bauce B, Basso C et al (2000) Clinical profile and long-term follow-up of 37 families with arrhythmogenic right ventricular cardiomyopathy. J Am Coll Cardiol 36:2226-2233
14. Dalal D, Nasir K, Bomma C et al (2005) Arrhythmogenic right ventricular dysplasia. A United States experience. Circulation 112:3823-3832
15. Nasir K, Bomma C, Tandri H et al (2004) Electrocardiographic features of arrhythmogenic right ventricular dysplasia/cardiomyopathy according to disease severity. Circulation 110:1527-1534
16. Lemola K, Brunckhorst C, Helfenstein U et al (2005) Predictors of adverse outcome in patients with arrhythmogenic right ventricular dysplasia/cardiomyopathy: Long term experience of a tertiary care centre. Heart 91:1167-1172
17. Wichter T, Wilke K, Haverkamp W et al (1999) Identification of arrhythmogenic right ventricular cardiomyopathy from the surface ECG: Parameters for discrimination from idiopathic right ventricular tachycardia. Eur Heart J 20:485 (abstract)
18. Turrini P, Corrado D, Basso C et al (2001) Dispersion of ventricular depolarization-repolarization: A non invasive marker for risk stratification in arrhythmogenic right ventricular cardiomyopathy. Circulation 103:3075-3080
19. Fontaine G, Umemura J, Di Donna P et al (1993) Duration of QRS complexes in arrhythmogenic right ventricular dysplasia. A new non-invasive diagnostic marker. Ann Cardiol Angeiol 42:399-405
20. Fontaine G, Fontaliran F, Hebert JL et al (1999) Arrhythmogenic right ventricular dysplasia. Annu Rev Med 50:17-35

21. Peters S, Trummel M (2003) Diagnosis of arrhythmogenic right ventricular dysplasia-cardiomyopathy: Value of standard ECG revisited. Ann Noninvasive Electrocardiol 8:238-245
22. Peters S, Peters H, Thierfelder L (1999) Risk stratification of sudden cardiac death and malignant ventricular arrhythmias in right ventricular dysplasia-cardiomyopathy. Int J Cardiol 71:243-250
23. Hulot JS, Jouven X, Empana JF et al (2004) Natural history and risk stratification of arrhythmogenic right ventricular dysplasia/cardiomyopathy. Circulation 110:1879-1884
24. Marcus FI, Fontaine G (1995) Arrhythmogenic right ventricular dysplasia/cardiomyopathy: A review. Pacing Clin Electrophysiol 18:1298-1314
25. Kinoshita O, Fontaine G, Rosas F et al (1995) Time- and frequency-domain analyses of the signal-averaged ECG in patients with arrhythmogenic right ventricular dysplasia. Circulation 91:715-721
26. Nasir K, Rutberg J, Tandri H et al (2003) Utility of SAECG in Arrhythmogenic Right Ventricle Dysplasia. ANE 8:112-118
27. Oselladore L, Nava A, Buja G et al (1995) Signal-averaged electrocardiographic in familial form of arrhythmogenic right ventricular cardiomyopathy. Am J Cardiol 75:1038-1041
28. Pezawas T, Stix G, Kastner J et al (2006) Ventricular tachycardia in arrhythmogenic right ventricular dysplasia/cardiomyopathy: Clinical presentation, risk stratification and results of long-term follow-up. Intl J Cardiol 110:279-287
29. Folino AF, Bauce B, Frigo G et al (2006) Long term follow up of the signal averaged ECG in arrhythmogenic right ventricular cardiomyopathy: Echocardiographic findings. Europace 8:423-429
30. Marcus FI, Zareba W, Sherrill D (2007) Evaluation of the normal values for signal averaged electrocardiogram. J Cardiovasc Electrophysiol 18:231-233
31. Fontaine G, Aouate P, Fontaliran F (1997) Repolarization and the genesis of cardiac arrhythmias. Circulation 95:2600-2602
32. Benn M, Hansen PS, Pedersen AK (1999) QT dispersion in patients with arrhythmogenic right ventricular dysplasia. Eur Heart J 20:764-770
33. Peeters HAP, SippensGroenewegen A, Schoonderwoerd BA et al (1997) Body-surface QRST integral mapping: Arrhythmogenic right ventricular dysplasia versus idiopathic right ventricular tachycardia. Circulation 95:2668-2676
34. Jaoude SA, Leclercq JF, Coumel P (1996) Progressive ECG changes in arrhythmogenic right ventricular disease. Evidence for an evolving disease. Eur Heart J 17:1717-1722
35. Kies P, Boostma M, Bax JJ et al (2006) Serial reevaluation for ARVD/C is indicated in patients presenting with left bundle branch block ventricular tachycardia and minor ECG abnormalities. J Cardiovasc Electrophysiol 17:586-593

CHAPTER 14

ECHOCARDIOGRAPHY

Danita Yoerger-Sanborn, Michael H. Picard, Barbara Bauce

Introduction

Cardiac imaging plays a key role in the evaluation of a patient suspected of having arrhythmogenic right ventricular cardiomyopathy/dysplasia (ARVC/D). Global or regional abnormalities of right ventricular (RV) structure and function are an important component of the Task Force of the Working Group on Cardiomyopathies diagnostic criteria [1]. The criterion for RV structure and function currently lacks quantitative cut points for clinicians to use when facing the study of an individual suspected of ARVC/D. Moreover, the ability to correctly categorize individuals at risk for ARVC/D, such as family members of affected individuals or those who may have a subclinical form of the disease, is limited by the lack of a gold standard for the diagnosis of ARVC/D. Additionally, the echocardiographic natural history of the disease has not yet been defined.

Echocardiography is an ideal tool to assess RV size and function, due to its widespread availability, portability, and ease of performance and interpretation, even in the setting of implantable cardioverter/defibrillators (ICDs).

Qualitative Echocardiographic Features of ARVC/D

There are several structural abnormalities that have been noted with increased frequency in individuals with ARVC/D. Morphologic abnormalities on echocardiography including a hyperreflective moderator band, trabecular prominence and derangement, and focal aneurysms or sacculations have been described [2, 3]. In a study comparing ARVC/D probands from the North American Registry to matched controls, trabecular derangement was the most frequently noted abnormality, occurring in 54% of affected individuals and not in any matched controls [3]. Figure 14.1 shows representative echocardiograms from subjects in the North American

Registry demonstrating these morphologic abnormalities. Additionally, qualitative abnormalities in RV function are frequently noted in individuals with ARVC/D. In the North American Registry echo study, 79% of probands demonstrated abnormal regional wall motion [3] by echocardiography. The frequency of abnormal wall motion by region is shown in Table 14.1. The anterior wall and apex were the most common regions affected in the ARVC/D probands.

Quantitative Echocardiographic Features of ARVC/D

RV dilatation is a common finding in individuals with ARVC/D [2, 4, 5]. The echocardiographic study from the North American ARVC/D Registry provided potential quantitative parameters to differentiate probands from matched controls [3]. Table 14.2 shows the mean RV dimensions at end-systole and end-diastole in probands and matched controls. An enlarged right ventricular outflow tract (RVOT) was found in 100% of probands. RVOT long axis dimension of >30mm had a sensitivity of 89% and specificity of 84% for ARVC/D. Since there have been no large population studies on normal RV dimensions with normalization for gender or body size, determining appropriate cut off values for mild or moderate enlargement in order to apply the Task Force criteria remains challenging. Based on the preliminary data available from the North American ARVC/D registry patients, an RVOT dimension greater than 2 and less than 3 standard deviations above the mean value in the control subjects should be considered mildly enlarged.

Highly trained athletes can present an important diagnostic challenge when considering the diagnosis of ARVC/D. RV enlargement has been described as an adaptation to endurance sports [6]. However, ARVC/D with RV enlargement has been associated with ventricular arrhythmias and sudden death in athletes, particularly from the Veneto region of Italy

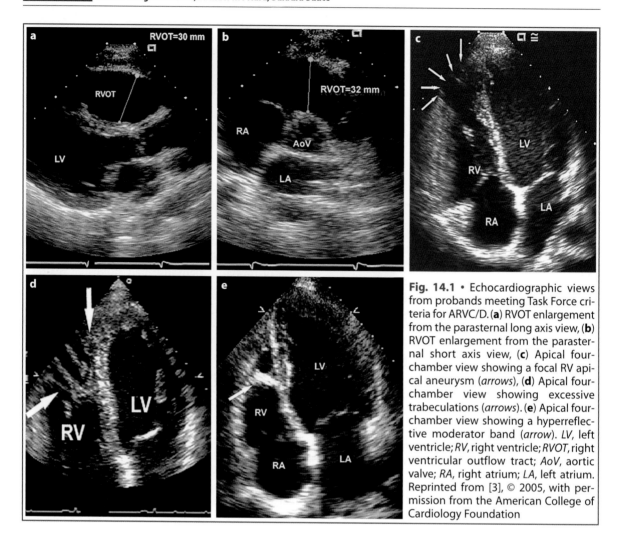

Fig. 14.1 • Echocardiographic views from probands meeting Task Force criteria for ARVC/D. (**a**) RVOT enlargement from the parasternal long axis view, (**b**) RVOT enlargement from the parasternal short axis view, (**c**) Apical four-chamber view showing a focal RV apical aneurysm (*arrows*), (**d**) Apical four-chamber view showing excessive trabeculations (*arrows*). (**e**) Apical four-chamber view showing a hyperreflective moderator band (*arrow*). *LV*, left ventricle; *RV*, right ventricle; *RVOT*, right ventricular outflow tract; *AoV*, aortic valve; *RA*, right atrium; *LA*, left atrium. Reprinted from [3], © 2005, with permission from the American College of Cardiology Foundation

Table 14.1 • Frequency of qualitative echocardiographic abnormalities in individuals with ARVD (n=29)

	Number	Percent
RV global function:		
Normal	11	38
Mildly reduced	8	28
Severely reduced	10	34
RV Regional WMA	23	79
RVOT	13	45
Anteroseptal	16	55
Anterior	20	70
Apex	21	72
Septal	16	55
Inferior Basal	17	59
Inferior Apical	15	52
Hyperreflective moderator band	9	31
Excessive/abnormal trabeculations	15	54
Sacculations	5	17

RV, right ventricular; *RVOT*, right ventricular outflow tract; *WMA*, wall motion abnormality. Reprinted from [3], © 2005, with permission from the American College of Cardiology Foundation

[7, 8]. A careful medical and family history, as well as application of the Task Force diagnostic criteria exclusive of RV structure and function, may help distinguish normal adaptation from disease. In the future, novel echocardiographic parameters such as tissue Doppler and strain imaging may help better refine diagnostic utility of echocardiography in this situation.

Global RV dysfunction is also often noted in individuals with ARVC/D. Because of the geometry of the RV and problems with complete RV visualization in some individuals, estimation of RV volume by echo is challenging, thus making accurate estimation of an RV ejection fraction difficult. The RV fractional area change (FAC) from the parasternal long axis view has been shown to be a useful correlate of RV function [9], and is increased in individuals with ARVC/D compared with controls [3]. Table 14.3 shows the mean values for RV FAC in probands compared with controls from the North

Table 14.2 • Quantitative echocardiographic abnormalities

Right heart dimensions	ARVC/D probands (mean±SD)	Matched controls (mean±SD)	P-value	Reference values (mean±SD)	% of probands enlarged
RA medial-lateral (mm)	44.8±11.4	36.6±6.9	0.0035	37±4	41%
RA superior-inferior (mm)	51.3±10.6	45.7±5.8	0.023	42±4	45%
RVOT-PLAX diastole (mm)	37.9±6.6	26.2±4.9	0.00001	22±1.5	100%
RVOT-PLAX systole (mm)	32.8±7.2	20.1±4.0	0.00001	NA	
RVOT-PSAX diastole (mm)	38.9±4.7	31.1±4.7	0.00001	27±1	96%
RVOT-PSAX systole (mm)	28.3±6.1	19.0±5.1	0.00001	NA	
RVOT/aortic valve	1.28±0.2	1.04±0.2	0.0001	NA	
RVIT PLAX diastole (mm)	57.0±12.2	49.2±8.8	0.0065	45±2.5	73%
RVIT PLAX systole (mm)	46.5±12.6	34.2±6.8	0.0001	NA	
RVIT PSAX diastole (mm)	37.3±8.5	28.1±5.2	0.0004	30±1.5	60%
RVIT PSAX systole (mm)	32.3±8.5	21.6±5.6	0.0004	NA	
RV medial-lateral - Apical 4 Chamber diastole (mm)	34.0±8.9	25.1±4.0	0.00001	30±5	18%
RV medial-lateral - Apical 4 Chamber systole (mm)	27.26± 9.8	17.6±3.9	0.00001	24±3	36%
RV LAX length - Apical 4 chamber diastole (mm)	79.2± 15.6	76.1 ±7.6	0.2281	71±8	24%
RV LAX length - Apical 4 chamber systole (mm)	66.7±15.8	61.2±6.0	0.0802	55±8	38%

LAX, long axis; *NA*, not available; *PLAX*, parasternal long axis; *PSAX*, parasternal short axis; *RA*, right atrial; *RV*, right ventricular; *RVIT*, right ventricular inflow tract; *RVOT*, right ventricular outflow tract; *SD*, standard deviation. Reprinted from [3], © 2005, with permission from the American College of Cardiology Foundation

Table 14.3 • RV function

	ARVC/D probands (mean±SD)	Matched controls (mean±SD)	P-value	Reference value
RV end diastolic area (cm^2)	25.2±7.7	17.9±3.5	0.00001	19.5±4.3
RV end systolic area cm^2)	18.9±8.4	10.5±2.3	0.00001	10.5±3.0
RV FAC (%)	27.2±16	41.0±7.1	0.0003	46.5±7.1
Percent with FAC ≥32	35%	97%		
Percent with FAC 26%-32% (mildly impaired)	24%	3%		
Percent with FAC <26 (severely impaired)	41%	0%		

FAC, fractional area change; *RV*, right ventricular; *SD*, standard deviation. Reprinted from [3], © 2005, with permission from the American College of Cardiology Foundation

American ARVC/D Registry. In this study, RV FAC was measured from the apical four-chamber view. An RV FAC <32% was present in 65% of probands and only 3% of matched controls. As mentioned previously for RV enlargement, there have been no large population studies on normal values for RV FAC with normalization for gender or body size. Thus, determining appropriate cut off values for mild or moderate RV dysfunction in order to apply the Task Force criteria remains challenging.

Novel Echocardiographic Tools to Assess ARVC/D

Tissue Doppler echocardiography is another tool which may help aid in the diagnosis of ARVC/D. Lindstrom and colleagues studied 15 patients who met Task Force diagnostic criteria and 25 unmatched controls, and noted reduced systolic (S) and early diastolic (E$_A$) RV annular velocity compared to unmatched control subjects [5]. The ratio of E$_A$ to the late diastolic (A_A) velocity was also significantly reduced in those with ARVC/D. While this is a promising tool which may help in the diagnosis of ARVC/D, normal reference values for the RV annular velocities are still being defined.

The RV myocardial performance index (MPI) has been proposed as a simple Doppler index of RV function which is independent of geometric assumptions [10] and has been applied in diseases affecting the RV such as Ebstein's anomaly [11] and pulmonary hypertension [12]. Yoerger et al. reported preliminary data regarding the utility of this index [13], demonstrating reduced RV MPI in ARVC/D probands, even when global RV function assessed by FAC was normal. This index needs to be tested in larger populations in order to determine its diagnostic utility in ARVC/D.

Because visualization of the RV can be challenging, echocardiographic contrast has been used for RV opacification. Case reports have suggested that use of intravenous echocardiographic contrast can improve detection of subtle areas of regional dysfunction [14], and have even suggested that abnormalities of RV perfusion can be detected in areas affected by fatty infiltration [15]. The utility of intravenous echo contrast for these indications has yet to be studied in larger populations suspected of ARVC/D.

Echocardiographic Diagnosis in "Concealed Forms" of the Disease

The majority of echocardiographic studies in patients with ARVC/D refer to subjects who had symptoms and who usually presented a moderate or severe form of the disease [3, 4]. However, clinical screening of families affected by ARVC/D have demonstrated that in addition to family members with extensive involvement from the disease there are others with minor or "concealed" forms [16].

The identification of these concealed forms relies on recognition of "minor" echocardiographic signs. These signs may suggest the presence of the disease, particularly in subjects who are preselected on the basis of family history of ARVC/D and/or juvenile sudden death or electrocardiographic findings (12-lead ECG abnormalities, presence of late potentials at signal-averaged ECG, ventricular arrhythmias with left bundle branch block morphology).

The relationship of qualitative echocardiographic signs and concealed forms of ARVC/D was initially studied by Scognamiglio et al. [2] who analyzed a series of family members of affected individuals and compared them to subjects with ventricular arrhythmias with left bundle branch block morphology. The following echocardiographic findings were reported as "suggestive" of a concealed form of the disease:

1. A diastolic localized bulge and/or systolic dyskinesia of postero-inferior wall just below the tricuspid valve (Fig. 14.2);
2. A highly reflective moderator band as well as the presence of a trabecular disarrangement (Figs. 14.1d, 14.1e, and 14.3);
3. An isolated dilatation of RVOT;
4. Presence of sacculations of the RVOT;
5. Isolated wall motion abnormalities (hypokinesia, dyskinesia) of apical, subtricuspid, or RVOT (Fig. 14.1c).

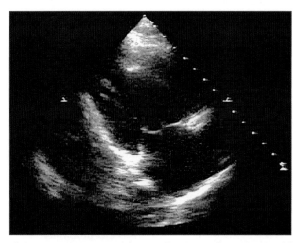

Fig. 14.2 • Parasternal long axis view of a 34-year-old woman who was found to be affected by ARVC/D during familial screening. Note the presence of a diastolic localized bulge of the postero-inferior wall below the tricuspid valve

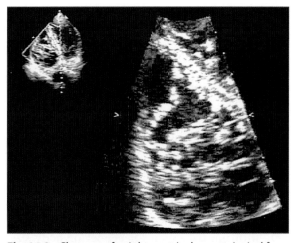

Fig. 14.3 • Close-up of a right ventricular apex (apical four-chamber view) of a 50-year-old man diagnosed with ARVC/D during evaluation for sport eligibility: note the presence of trabecular derangement

The prevalence of each of these findings has yet to be determined in a large population study, which will be challenging given the fact that the prevalence may vary as a function of duration of the disease. Correlating these echocardiographic findings with genotype will also be possible in the near future.

Usefulness of Echocardiography in Familial Screening

In patients affected by ARVC/D, a family history of the disease has been found in 30%-50% of cases, with autosomal dominant transmission in the majority of cases [16].

Nava et al. [16] studied 132 subjects belonging to 37 families affected by ARVC/D and classified subjects into three groups according to the RV size and/or wall motion abnormalities observed on echocardiogram:

1. Mild form: a slightly increased (<75 ml/m^2) or normal right ventricular end-diastolic volume (RVEDV) with localized hypokinetic or akinetic areas of the RV, in the presence or absence of trabecular derangements and thickened, hyperreflective or dense moderator band;
2. Moderate form: RVEDV ranging from 75 to 120 ml/m^2 with localized hypokinetic or akinetic and/or dyskinetic areas of the RV in the presence of trabecular derangement and thickened, hyperreflective or dense moderator band;
3. Severe form: RVEDV greater than 120 ml/m^2 with widespread akinetic and/or dyskinetic areas of the RV with parietal diastolic bulging.

In this series 64% of family members were found to have a mild form of the disease, 30% a moderate form, and 6% a severe form. Moreover, evaluation of RV wall motion abnormalities demonstrated that the regional dysfunction was more frequent in the inferoposterior wall regardless of the extent of disease. Akinesia or hypokinesia of the RV apical region were more common in mild or moderate forms, while in patients with the severe forms, RV wall motion abnormalities of the apical and anterior regions were present in a similar proportion.

Finally, echocardiography in these family members demonstrated that RVOT dilation was related to the disease extent, being present in 100% of severe forms, 50% of moderate, and 29% of mild forms.

The recent identification of several genes whose mutations have been associated with the disease [17-23] offers for the first time the opportunity to study families carrying ARVC/D gene mutations. This allows evaluation of the entire clinical spectrum from concealed to overt forms of the disease. In a study of four families with desmoplakin mutation, echocardiographic abnormalities were found in 14 of 26 mutation carriers (54%), with left ventricular involvement in half of them [24]. Interestingly, subjects with the same mutations could have different clinical presentations, with disease extent ranging from mild to severe forms. Similarly, a recent paper analyzing nine families with plakophilin-2 mutations found that of 32 subjects mutation carriers who underwent clinical evaluation, right ventricular abnormalities on imaging techniques were present in 22 (68%) [25].

Echocardiographic Natural History of ARVC/D

Although changes in RV structure and function over time would be expected to be seen in affected ARVC/D probands, there are no published data reporting on serial changes. Prior echocardiographic studies have included individuals at varying time points in the disease process, and it is unclear what happens to RV structure and function in an affected individual over years. Nava et al. reported on mild, moderate and severe forms of the disease in families with ARVC/D [16] and observed that a subset of patients that were unaffected at initial screening later developed structural changes. The rate of such progression remains unknown, as well as whether those with mild forms progress to have more severe forms of the disease over time.

Conclusions

Echocardiography is a useful tool in individuals suspected of ARVC/D. Dilatation of the RV and, in particular, of RVOT are common, with an RVOT diameter greater than 30 mm being a sensitive and reasonably specific marker for the disease. Moreover, RV dysfunction, both global and regional, is frequently noted. Quantitative cut points for diseased versus normal conditions [26, 27] need to be established in order to help diagnose borderline cases or family members who may have subclinical forms of the disease. Additionally, studies defining the echocardiographic natural history of the disease need to be performed to better aid clinicians in the diagnosis and management of this disease.

References

1. McKenna WJ, Thiene G, Nava A et al (1994) Diagnosis of arrhythmogenic right ventricular dysplasia/cardiomyopathy. Task Force of the Working Group Myocardial and Pericardial Disease of the European Soci-

ety of Cardiology and of the Scientific Council on Cardiomyopathies of the International Society and Federation of Cardiology. Br Heart J 71:215-218

2. Scognamiglio R, Fasoli G, Nava A et al (1989) Contribution of cross-sectional echocardiography to the diagnosis of right ventricular dysplasia at the asymptomatic stage. Eur Heart J 10:538-542

3. Yoerger DM, Marcus F, Sherrill D et al (2005) Echocardiographic findings in patients meeting task force criteria for arrhythmogenic right ventricular dysplasia: New insights from the multidisciplinary study of right ventricular dysplasia. J Am Coll Cardiol 45:860-865

4. Blomstrom-Lundqvist C, Beckman-Suurkula M, Wallentin I et al (1988) Ventricular dimensions and wall motion assessed by echocardiography in patients with arrhythmogenic right ventricular dysplasia. Eur Heart J 9:1291-1302

5. Lindstrom L, Wilkenshoff UM, Larsson H, Wranne B et al (2001) Echocardiographic assessment of arrhythmogenic right ventricular cardiomyopathy. Heart 86:31-38

6. Henriksen E, Kangro T, Jonason T et al (1998) An echocardiographic study of right ventricular adaptation to physical exercise in elite male orienteers. Clin Physiol 18:498-503

7. Thiene G, Nava A, Corrado D et al (1988) Right ventricular cardiomyopathy and sudden death in young people. N Engl J Med 318:129-133

8. Basso C, Thiene G, Corrado D et al (1996) Arrhythmogenic right ventricular cardiomyopathy. Dysplasia, dystrophy, or myocarditis? Circulation 94:983-991

9. Lang RM, Bierig M, Devereux RB et al (2005) Recommendations for chamber quantification: A report from the American Society of Echocardiography's Guidelines and Standards Committee and the Chamber Quantification Writing Group, developed in conjunction with the European Association of Echocardiography, a branch of the European Society of Cardiology. J Am Soc Echocardiogr 18:1440-1463

10. Tei C, Dujardin KS, Hodge DO et al (1996) Doppler echocardiographic index for assessment of global right ventricular function. J Am Soc Echocardiogr 9:838-847

11. Eidem BW, Tei C, O'Leary PW et al (1998) Nongeometric quantitative assessment of right and left ventricular function: Myocardial performance index in normal children and patients with Ebstein anomaly. J Am Soc Echocardiogr 11:849-856

12. Sebbag I, Rudski LG, Therrien J et al (2001) Effect of chronic infusion of epoprostenol on echocardiographic right ventricular myocardial performance index and its relation to clinical outcome in patients with primary pulmonary hypertension. Am J Cardiol 88:1060-1063

13. Yoerger DM, Marcus, F, Sherrill, D et al (2005) Right ventricular myocardial performance index in probands from the multicenter study of arrhythmogenic right ventricular dysplasia. J Am Coll Cardiol 45:147A

14. Lopez-Fernandez T, Garcia-Fernandez MA, Perez David E et al (2004) Usefulness of contrast echocardiography in arrhythmogenic right ventricular dysplasia. J Am Soc Echocardiogr 17:391-393

15. Nemes A, Vletter WB, Scholten MF et al (2005) Contrast echocardiography for perfusion in right ventricular cardiomyopathy. Eur J Echocardiogr 6:470-472

16. Nava A, Bauce B, Basso C et al (2000) Clinical profile and long-term follow-up of 37 families with arrhythmogenic right ventricular cardiomyopathy. J Am Coll Cardiol 36:2226-2233

17. McKoy G, Protonotarios N, Crosby A et al (2000) Identification of a deletion in plakoglobin in arrhythmogenic right ventricular cardiomyopathy with palmoplantar keratoderma and woolly hair (Naxos disease) Lancet 355:2119-2124

18. Tiso N, Stephan DA, Nava A et al (2001) Identification of mutations in the cardiac ryanodine receptor gene in families affected with arrhythmogenic right ventricular cardiomyopathy type 2 (ARVD2) Hum Mol Genet 10:189-194

19. Alcalai R, Metzger S, Rosenheck S et al (2003) A recessive mutation in desmoplakin causes arrhythmogenic right ventricular dysplasia, skin disorder, and woolly hair. J Am Coll Cardiol 42:319-327

20. Rampazzo A, Nava A, Malacrida S et al (2002) Mutation in human desmoplakin domain binding to plakoglobin causes a dominant form of arrhythmogenic right ventricular cardiomyopathy. Am J Hum Genet 71:1200-1206

21. Gerull B, Heuser A, Wichter T et al (2004) Mutations in the desmosomal protein plakophilin-2 are common in arrhythmogenic right ventricular cardiomyopathy. Nat Genet 36:1162-1164

22. Beffagna G, Occhi G, Nava A et al (2005) Regulatory mutations in transforming growth factor-beta3 gene cause arrhythmogenic right ventricular cardiomyopathy type 1. Cardiovasc Res 65:366-373

23. Pilichou K, Nava A, Basso C et al (2006) Mutations in desmoglein-2 gene are associated with arrhythmogenic right ventricular cardiomyopathy. Circulation 113:1171-1179

24. Bauce B, Basso C, Rampazzo A et al (2005) Clinical profile of four families with arrhythmogenic right ventricular cardiomyopathy caused by dominant desmoplakin mutations. Eur Heart J 26:1666-1675

25. Syrris P, Ward D, Asimaki A et al (2006) Clinical expression of plakophilin-2 mutations in familial arrhythmogenic right ventricular cardiomyopathy. Circulation 113:356-364

26. Foale R, Nihoyannopoulos P, McKenna W et al (1986) Echocardiographic measurement of the normal adult right ventricle. Br Heart J 56:33-44

27. Weyman AE (1994) In: Weyman AE, ed. Principles and practice of echocardiography, 2nd edn, Lea and Febiger, Philadelphia

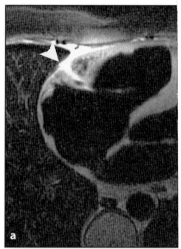

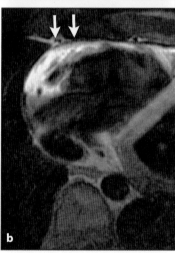

Fig. 15.3 • (a) Axial black blood ima
unteer showing a clear line of dem
epicardial fat and the underlying myo
abundance of epicardial fat in the at
(*arrowhead*) and at the apex (*arrow*)
image from a patient with ARVC/D sl
cation between epicardial fat and m

forms (96% vs. 58%). Menghetti
SE MR imaging findings in 15 A
agnosed using the Task Force cr
intramyocardial hyperintense sig
tients. The differences in incide
ARVC/D are largely based on di
selection, as well as the definitic
tramyocardial hyperintense signa
hold DIR-FSE technique to evalu
fat in ARVC/D and found high
signal (fat) in nine of twelve patie
prospectively diagnosed using the
criteria [17]. The use of spectral
pression with the DIR-FSE seque
tional evidence of fat infiltration

MR AND CT IMAGING

Harikrishna Tandri, Hugh Calkins, David A. Bluemke

Introduction

Arrhythmogenic right ventricular cardiomyopathy/dysplasia (ARVC/D) is a rare cardiomyopathy characterized by fibro-fatty replacement of the right ventricle (RV), which leads to progressive RV failure and ventricular arrhythmias [1, 2]. The disease presents between the second and fifth decades of life either with symptoms of palpitations and/or syncope associated with ventricular tachycardia or with SCD. The exact prevalence of this condition is not known, but is estimated to be around 1 in 5,000. There is wide variation in the clinical presentation and course of ARVC/D [1-4] accounted for by the genetic heterogeneity of the disease. Mutations in genes encoding junctional plakoglobin are associated with palmoplantar keratoderma (Naxos disease) and woolly hair. Mutations in plakophilin, a desmosomal [5] protein, is associated with early presentation and higher incidence of ventricular arrhythmias [6]. Diagnosis of ARVC/D is often challenging, as the RV involvement in early ARVC/D can be focal with preserved global RV function. The diagnosis is based on a set of major and minor criteria proposed by the Task Force of cardiomyopathies in 1994 [7]. These criteria account for the electrical, anatomic and functional abnormalities that are a consequence of progressive fibro-fatty infiltration, which results in loss of RV myocytes. Structurally, this manifests as regional reduction in wall thickness and wall hypertrophy secondary to fat infiltration. Focal or global contraction abnormalities, chamber enlargement, enlarged RV outflow tract, and RV aneurysms have been described.

Conventional imaging modalities are limited in evaluating the complex structure of the RV [8]. Magnetic resonance (MR) imaging and computed tomography (CT) have emerged as robust tools to evaluate the RV in ARVC/D [9-11] as both modalities provide direct evidence of fatty infiltration and structural alterations of the RV [12, 13]. The noninvasive nature of these investigations, multiplanar capability, and unique ability to provide tissue characterization are ideal for assessment of ARVC/D. The purpose of the current chapter is to discuss the current status, strengths and limitations of MR imaging and cardiac CT in evaluation of patients with suspected ARVC/D.

MR Imaging of ARVC/D

Among the current cardiac MR applications in cardiomyopathies, the greatest potential as well as biggest challenges are in the diagnosis of ARVC/D. MR imaging allows both qualitative and quantitative analysis of RV function [14]. MR has the ability to demonstrate intramyocardial fat [12] and recently, delayed enhancement MR imaging has been shown to be useful in detecting fibrosis in the RV in ARVC/D [15]. The last 10 years have seen significant improvements in MR hardware, with tremendous increases in acquisition speed and image quality. ECG gating and breath-hold imaging have reduced motion artifacts and improved tissue contrast is achieved by inversion recovery black-blood imaging techniques [16]. ECG gated steady state free precession imaging (SSFP) pulse sequences have resulted in better delineation of endocardial borders enabling accurate and reproducible volumetric measurements [14]. For these reasons MR imaging has been increasingly used for evaluation of the RV and has evolved as the noninvasive modality of choice in ARVC/D.

Casolo et al. [12] were the first to describe the use of MR imaging to assess ARVC/D in 1987. They demonstrated intramyocardial fat deposits in the RV on conventional spin echo imaging. Since that time several authors including our group have reported MR abnormalities in ARVC/D [17-26]. Broadly, MR imaging abnormalities in ARVC/D can be grouped into two major categories: (1) morphological abnormalities, and (2) functional abnormalities. Morphologic abnormalities include intramyocardial fat deposits, focal wall thinning, wall hypertrophy, trabecular disarray, and RV outflow tract enlargement. Functional abnormalities include regional contraction abnormalities,

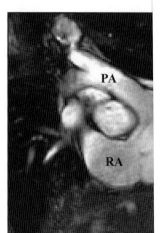

Fig. 15.1 • Gradient echo image showing the triangle of dyspla... ferior-sub tricuspid area (*thick arrow*) and the RV infundibulur... monary artery; *RA*, right atrium...

aneurysms, RV global dilatio... astolic dysfunction. The site... abnormalities are observed i... sia," which consists of the in... RV apex, and the RV infundi... The goal of MR imaging in... assess the RV for the presenc... normalities to aid in the diag... management of patients.

MR Assessment of Cardiac ...

Accurate depiction of morp... in most cardiac application... fies this statement. Morphol... ally performed by the use... niques. Currently, black-b... breath-hold imaging with d... fast-spin echo (DIR-FSE) tec... traditional spin echo (SE) ii... sequences consistently prov... with minimal motion artifa... tion of myocardial detail [28... sion-prepared, half-Fourier... echo (HASTE) imaging is... mended due to blurring of m... sequence. A dedicated cardi... for best results, although we... elements to prevent "wrap... using small field of view. An ... (Fig. 15.2) is placed over the... fat for further suppression o...

perience wall thickness is often difficult to assess due to adjacent high epicardial fat signal, motion artifacts, and high blood signal in areas of RV trabeculations.

Wall Hypertrophy

Wall hypertrophy is defined as RV wall thickness >8 mm. This finding is seldom observed in pathologic specimens as the true RV myocardium is measured exclusive of the epicardial fat [31]. In vivo this differentiation is sometimes not possible due to extensive fibro-fatty infiltration with loss of distinction between epicardial fat and the true myocardium. In such cases the RV wall appears hypertrophied with MR images showing islands of gray muscle surrounded by bright signals compatible with fat. This finding was observed in five of the twelve patients (42%) of our series [17]. Use of fat suppression reveals multiple signal voids within the RV myocardium in locations that showed hyperintense signals in the nonfat-suppressed images (Figs. 15.5a, 15.5b).

Trabecular Disarray

Molinari et al. [25], were the first to describe giant Y-shaped trabeculae and hypertrophy of the moderator band in patients with ARVC/D. This finding has been equated to the angiographic finding of deep fissures with a "pile d'assiettes" (stack of plates) appearance. We found a prevalence (40%) of trabecular hypertrophy and disarray, similar to that of the above study in ARVC/D patients. This finding is not specific for ARVC/D and may be present in any condition that results in RV hypertrophy or enlargement.

RV Outflow Tract Enlargement

The RV outflow tract (RVOT) is a common location for localized ARVC/D. The right ventricular outflow is usually equal to or marginally smaller than the aortic outflow tract at the level of the aortic valve. An exception to this rule concerns pediatric patients in whom the RVOT may be larger than the left ventricular outflow. The presence of an enlarged RVOT beyond adolescence is uncommon. Ricci et al. [23] reported an enlarged RVOT in 15 patients with ARVC/D compared to patients with dilated cardiomyopathy. More important than enlargement is a dysmorphic appearance of the outflow tract (Fig. 15.6). Abnormal appearance of the RVOT, which is dyskinetic in systole, is highly suggestive of ARVC/D in the absence of pulmonary hypertension or left to right shunts.

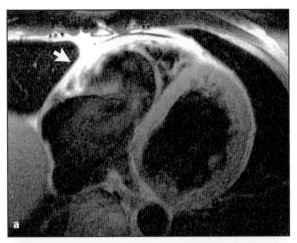

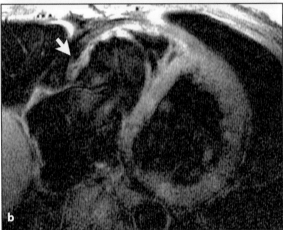

Fig. 15.5 • (**a**) Axial black blood image from a patient with ARVC/D showing heterogeneously increased T1 signal in the right ventricular anterior wall (*arrow*). (**b**) Fat suppressed image at the same level shows multiple signal voids in the same location of the hyperintense signals on the nonfat suppressed image (*arrow*)

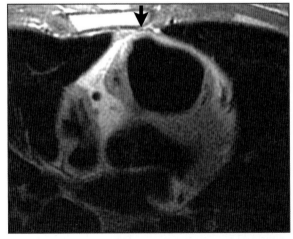

Fig. 15.6 • Axial black blood image from a patient with ARVC/D showing enlarged and dysmorphic outflow tract with focal bulging anteriorly (*arrow*)

MR Imaging Fibrosis in ARVC/D

One of the pathologic hallmarks of ARVC/D is fibrosis of the RV that accompanies fatty infiltration. Myocardial delayed enhancement MR imaging allows for noninvasive detection of fibrosis in the RV that may improve the specificity of ARVC/D diagnosis. We imaged twelve ARVC/D patients with MDE-MR imaging. Eight (67%) out of the twelve ARVD/C patients demonstrated increased signal consistent with fibrosis in the RV [15]. There was excellent correlation with histopathology (Fig. 15.7). The areas of fibrosis on MR imaging corresponded with regions of kinetic abnormalities. The extent of fibrosis showed an inverse correlation with global RV function. An important finding of our study was that 18 patients with idiopathic ventricular tachycardia who underwent MDE-MR imaging showed no evidence of fibrosis, highlighting the negative predictive value of MDE-MR imaging in evaluating patients with suspected ARVD/C. Presence of fibrosis detected on MDE-MR imaging predicted inducibility of sustained ventricular tachycardia during electrophysiologic testing, thus providing information regarding arrhythmic risk of such patients.

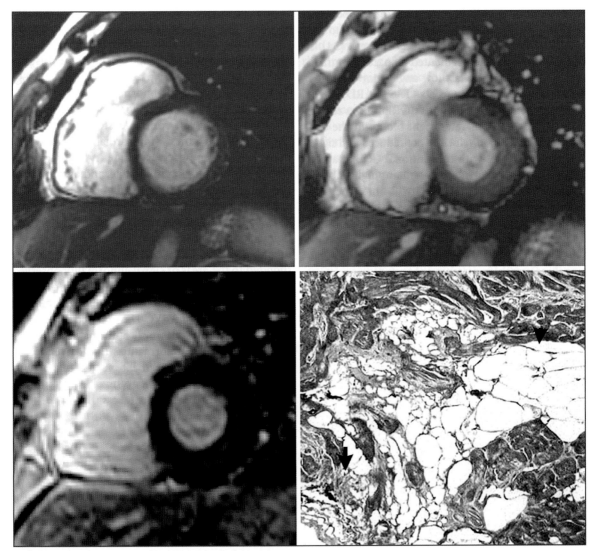

Fig. 15.7 • The *top left* and *right* panels show the end diastolic and systolic frames of a short axis cine MRI. There is an area of dyskinesia in the right ventricular free wall due to a focal aneurysm. The *bottom left* panel displays the delayed-enhanced MRI with increased signal intensity within the right ventricular myocardium, at the location of right ventricular aneurysms. The *bottom right* panel shows the corresponding endomyocardial biopsy. Trichrome stain of the right ventricle at high magnification shows marked replacement of the ventricular muscle by adipose tissue. The adipose tissue cells (*arrowhead*) are irregular in size and infiltrate the ventricular muscle. There is also abundant replacement fibrosis (*arrow*). There is no evidence of inflammation

dominant manifestation in the RV free wall, which is more prone to myocardial stretch during physical activity, training, and sports [5, 8, 9].

Structural Abnormalities of the Right Ventricle in ARVC/D

Regional fibrofatty replacement of RV myocardium results in localized abnormalities of RV morphology and wall motion. These preferentially involve the RV free wall in the outflow tract, the apex, and the inferobasal (subtricuspid) area. These predilection areas were already recognized in the early clinical description of ARVC/D by Marcus et al. [1] who introduced the term "triangle of dysplasia" (Fig. 16.2).

The major structural abnormality involved in ARVC/D is the regional loss of myocardium with subsequent replacement by fibrofatty tissue resulting in localized wall thinning, aneurysms, bulgings, and abnormal systolic motion of the RV free wall. The interventricular septum is usually spared. The ventricular trabeculae are also not primarily affected by the atrophic process and tend to show a compensatory hypertrophy, resulting in an aspect of increased trabeculation and fissuring of the RV walls. In advanced stages of ARVC/D, the RV may show global dilatation with accompanying tricuspid regurgitation due to dilatation of the tricuspid annulus. This may cause clinical signs of right heart failure. LV involvement can

be detected frequently by postmortem histology [10] but is rarely a clinical manifestation. However, if signs of LV involvement are detectable by the various imaging techniques, it may also become clinically relevant by progression to global heart failure.

The Role of Right Ventricular Angiography in ARVC/D

The structural abnormalities of the RV myocardium are the basis for the main clinical and diagnostic features of ARVC/D. Apart from the ventricular tachyarrhythmias that are frequently the first clinical manifestation of ARVC/D, they also result in characteristic features in the ECG and imaging. However, the clinical diagnosis of ARVC/D may be difficult because there is no easily obtained single test or finding that is definitely diagnostic. Therefore, the diagnosis of ARVC/D usually requires an integrated approach with assessment of electrical, anatomical, and functional abnormalities [11] and the various diagnostic (imaging) modalities are complementary rather than competing.

Different imaging techniques can be used to detect and characterize abnormalities of RV wall structure and motion. In addition to invasive contrast cine angiocardiography, which was the first imaging modality to be used for the diagnosis of ARVC/D, several noninvasive techniques have become avail-

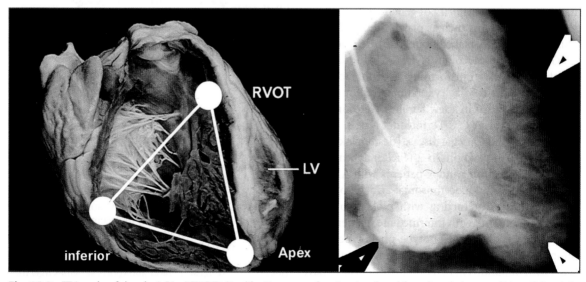

Fig. 16.2 • "Triangle of dysplasia" in ARVC/D. Predilection areas for structural and functional abnormalities of the right ventricle in ARVC/D. These are located in the outflow tract (RVOT), the apex, and the inferobasal (subtricuspid) area of the RV free walls (*left panel*). The RV angiogram (30° RAO view, end systole) demonstrates characteristic wall motion abnormalities in the "triangle of dysplasia" with a large subtricuspid aneurysm, an apical akinesia, and a localized dyskinesia and bulging in the outflow tract of the enlarged RV (*arrows*) (*right panel*). *RVOT*, right ventricular outflow tract; *LV*, left ventricle

able. Among these are echocardiography, radionuclide angiography, magnetic resonance imaging, and multislice computed tomography. However, none of these techniques are ideal, because they all have their individual advantages and limitations in the diagnosis and characterization of ARVC/D.

Despite its invasiveness, RV angiography still remains the reference imaging technique in the diagnosis of ARVC/D. This is mainly because selective cine angiography displays not only the entire cavity but also all the contours of the RV better than other techniques. However, due to its complex shape and geometry, the angiographic definition of the normal RV is complex since different morphological and functional findings produce a large range of normality.

Angiographic features of RV structure and function in ARVC/D include global and regional dilatation or aneurysms with abnormalities of wall motion, contrast evacuation, or trabecular size and structure. Although many of these angiographic signs and features are compatible with ARVC/D, only few are specific for this diagnosis. In addition, such features are dependent on the subjective interpretation of an experienced investigator because objective criteria for evaluation are not available. In addition, specificity of RV angiography requires further definition in relation to normal subjects and patients with other diseases affecting the RV. It is therefore important that cine angiography of the RV is performed under optimal conditions according to a standardized protocol.

How to Perform Right Ventricular Angiography in ARVC/D

The following recommendations have been proposed by Wichter et al. [12] for the core laboratory of RV angiography within the NIH-funded North American "Multidisciplinary Study of ARVD" [13] and the EU-funded "European Registry of ARVC/D" [14]. The protocol was designed to perform RV angiograms of best quality to assess structural and functional RV abnormalities in ARVC/D and to allow quantitative measurements of RV volumes, ejection fraction, and regional contraction and relaxation.

Right Heart Catheterization

After local anesthesia and venous puncture, a sheath is inserted at the venous puncture site using Seldinger's technique. Transfemoral or transjugular routes are most commonly used. Right heart catheterization should be performed prior to RV angiography to as-

sess RV and pulmonary vascular hemodynamics. Pressures are recorded in the wedge position, pulmonary artery, RV, and right atrium. Cardiac output can be measured by oximetry and/or thermodilution. Cardiac index, stroke volume, and pulmonary vascular resistance are calculated from these measures. RV endomyocardial biopsy may be performed for histological, ultrastructural, or molecular biology investigations if clinically indicated or part of a research program.

Calibration Reference

Volume calculations from RV angiograms require calibration for reference. A metal ball with defined diameter or a ruler with defined distances may be used as tools for calibration reference (Fig. 16.3).

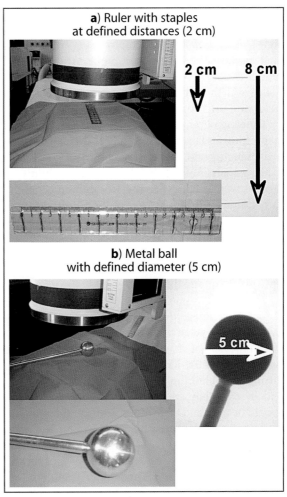

a) Ruler with staples at defined distances (2 cm)

2 cm   8 cm

b) Metal ball with defined diameter (5 cm)

5 cm

Fig. 16.3 • Examples of calibration reference for right ventricular angiography. A conventional ruler with staples placed at defined distances (i.e., 2 cm) (*panel* **a**) or a metal ball with a defined diameter (i.e., 5 cm) (*panel* **b**) may be used as simple tools for calibration

A simple way is to use a 20 cm ruler with staples at 2 cm distance. The calibration reference tool should be placed 10 cm below and horizontal to the amplifier tube and filmed by cine. The height of the table and the distance of the amplifier tube to the patient chest should not be changed during the following angiograms.

Right Ventricular Contrast Cine Angiography

For selective RV angiography, a pigtail catheter (5F or larger) or a Berman catheter (6F or 7F) may be used for contrast injection. The catheter should be positioned approximately 1cm above the midinferior RV wall (RAO or PA view), without direct contact with the RV wall or trabeculae to avoid extrasystoles and to allow homogeneous opacification of the RV cavity during contrast injection. Four standard projections are recommended: [1] 30° RAO, [2] 60° LAO, [3] anteroposterior (AP), [4] straight lateral (sagittal) view (LAT). Biplane angiography using two orthogonal views is the favored technique. An additional caudocranial 30° RAO angulation may be used to visualize wall motion abnormalities confined to the inferior and inferobasal walls.

Cineangiograms should be acquired during deep inspiration and breath-hold and recorded at 25 or 30 images per second. It is useful to film a long sequence to allow analysis of regional dye persistence, lung passage, as well as left atrial and LV size and function. Depending on the global size of the RV, 40-50 ml of low toxicity contrast medium should be injected with a flow rate (velocity) of 12-15 ml/sec.

Optimizing Image Quality

To optimize image quality of RV cine angiograms, care should be taken to avoid ECG cables, connectors, etc., in the field of view. The investigator should make sure that the entire RV is depicted in the field of view during breathhold in all projections during diastole and systole. No additional image magnification should be used and table movement should be avoided during contrast injection.

Frequent extrasystoles during dye injection make visual and quantitative assessment of RV motion and volumes difficult if not impossible. Therefore, extrasystoles should be avoided if possible by optimal catheter position and limitation of dye injection velocity. Artificial tricuspid regurgitation can be excluded by smooth passage of the tricuspid valve. Similarly, avoiding contact and pressure of the catheter

against the RV wall is essential to prevent artificial wall motion abnormalities.

In case of poor quality due to incomplete RV coverage, extensive table movement, breathing, or frequent extrasystoles, the RV angiogram should be repeated under optimized conditions.

Angiographic Features of Wall Structure and Wall Motion in ARVC/D

A variety of morphological and structural RV angiographic features have been reported to be suggestive of ARVC/D. These include global and regional dilatation, dilatation of the outflow tract, localized akinetic or dyskinetic bulges and outpouchings, polycyclic contours ("cauliflower aspect"), and trabecular hypertrophy and/or disarray with deep horizontal fissures ("pile d'assiettes") as well as dye persistence due to delayed contrast evacuation.

In the first publications on RV angiography in ARVC/D, the diagnostic value of these findings was not validated against normal controls. However, several subsequent studies utilized a more systematic approach, including qualitative and quantitative analyses and a comparison of the results with a normal control group to validate the diagnostic accuracy of RV angiographic findings in ARVC/D [15-17]. However, none of these studies clearly defined mild, moderate, or severe RV dysfunction.

Dye Persistence

Regionally delayed contrast evacuation ("dye persistence") of the RV is a frequent angiographic finding in ARVC/D. However, it also occurs in normal control subjects, particularly in the inferobasal area, and therefore lacks specificity. In such cases, the finding appears to be related to the physiologic asynchronous contraction of the RV wall. Therefore, localized dye persistence should only be considered as a finding indicative for ARVC/D if it occurs in an area of abnormal RV structure or function.

Trabecular Hypertrophy

The diagnostic value of trabecular hypertrophy is also controversial [17] because it is very difficult to define and to distinguish abnormal from normal RV trabeculation.

Transverse orientation of hypertrophic trabeculae separated by deep horizontal fissures create the so-called "pile d'assiettes" image that is considered a frequent but not very specific finding mainly located in the anterior and anteroseptal areas (Fig. 16.4). In a study by Daliento et al. [16], this finding was the qualitative variable most significantly associated with ARVC/D, although with a low sensitivity of only 56%.

At the same time, this study confirmed that simple transverse trabecular arrangement was not a useful diagnostic parameter in ARVC/D because it was a nonspecific finding present in 23% of normal controls and also in RV dilatation irrespective of the underlying disease. Similar findings were reported by Daubert et al. [17] in a critical analysis of the angiographic criteria in ARVC/D. In this study, trabecular hypertrophy was present in 62% of patients with ARVC/D but also in 30% of normal control subjects.

Probably because of this large variability of normality and the subjective assessment and interpretation, this feature was not included as a diagnostic angiographic finding in the Task Force criteria for the diagnosis of ARVC/D [11].

However, in the association with trabecular hypertrophy (thickness of ≥4 mm) and in presence of deep fissures or so-called Y-shaped giant trabeculae, transverse trabecular arrangement is considered to be of much higher diagnostic value (Fig. 16.4). This is particularly true when these angiographic features are located in the apical and supra-apical RV areas where they are considered to reflect abnormal hypertrophy of the papillary muscles and the moderator band, which are more specific and highly suggestive for ARVC/D.

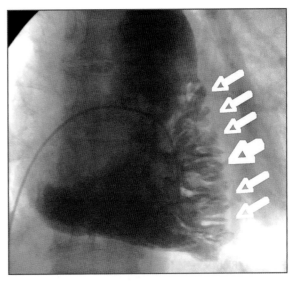

Fig. 16.4 • Right ventricular angiogram (30° RAO view) demonstrating transverse trabecular hypertrophy (*arrows*) with horizontal fissures ("pile d'assiettes") and "giant trabecula" (*big arrow*) in the anteroseptal, apical, and outflow tract areas of the RV in a patient with ARVC/D

Polycyclic Contours

In areas of more severe structural remodeling, multiple sacculations or round opacified areas merge to produce a polycyclic contour of the RV, also described as a "cauliflower" aspect (Figs. 16.5, 16.6). This finding is also considered a specific and diagnostic angiographic feature strongly suggestive of ARVC/D.

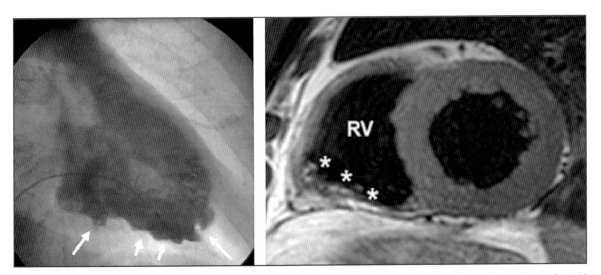

Fig. 16.5 • Regional right ventricular wall motion abnormalities and polycyclic contours in ARVC/D. RV angiography (30° RAO view; *left panel*) in a patient with ARVC/D demonstrating moderate global RV enlargement and regional wall motion abnormalities with outpouchings and polycyclic contours in the inferior and apical RV. Magnetic resonance imaging (short axis view; *right panel*) shows focal signal increase of RV myocardium in corresponding areas indicating fatty tissue replacement. Adapted and reproduced from [9] with kind permission of Springer Science and Business Media

to assess transmural changes of RV wall. Moreover, there may be difficulty in differentiating ARVD/C biopsy findings from either the normal amount of subepicardial adipose tissue or other cardiomyopathy/myocarditis [3].

According to standardized diagnostic criteria proposed by the International Task Force, the diagnosis of ARVC/D requires the presence of major and minor criteria encompassing clinical genetic, ECG, arrhythmic, morpho-functional, and histopathologic factors. Two major criteria or one major plus two minor, or four minor criteria from different groups are necessary to substantiate the diagnosis [9, 10]. Although Task Force guidelines represent a useful diagnostic approach, the specificity and sensitivity of clinical criteria remain to be assessed.

At present, the molecular diagnosis of ARVC/D is of limited value due to genetic heterogeneity and because genetic screening identifies only 35%-40% of ARVC/D cases [17].

Electroanatomic Voltage Mapping: Beyond Traditional Imaging

The finding that significant loss of myocardium results in the recording of low-amplitude, fractionated, endocardial electrograms has been well established by intraoperative mapping [18], conventional endocardial mapping [19], and 3-D electroanatomic mapping technique [20-23] in patients after myocardial infarction who have ventricular scar. Similar findings have been reported in patients with ARVC/D, in whom 3-D electroanatomic voltage mapping by CARTO may differentiate regions in the RV with scar from areas without scar [24, 25].

The hallmark pathologic lesion of ARVC/D is a loss of the myocardium with replacement by fibrofatty tissue of the RV free wall but sparing of the endocardium [2, 4, 5]. The myocardial atrophy accounts for variable degree of RV wall thinning, with areas so thin as to appear completely devoid of muscle at transillumination. 3-D electroanatomic voltage mapping has the ability to identify areas of myocardial atrophy and fibrofatty substitution by recording and specially associating low-amplitude electrograms to generate a 3-D electroanatomic map of the RV chamber. The technique has the potential to accurately identify the presence, location, and extent of the pathologic substrate of ARVC/D by demonstration of low-voltage regions, i.e., electroanatomic scars [24, 25]. In ARVC/D patients, RV electroanatomic scars have been demonstrated to correspond to areas of myocardial depletion and correlate with the histopathologic finding of myocyte loss and fibrofatty replacement at routine endomyocardial biopsy, with samples obtained at the junction between the ventricular septum and the anterior right ventricular free wall [25]. Furthermore, by assessing the electrical (rather than the mechanical) consequences of loss of RV, myocardium voltage mapping may obviate limitations in RV wall motion analysis by traditional imaging techniques such as echocardiography and angiography, and may increase the sensitivity for detecting otherwise-concealed ARVC/D myocardial lesions [25, 26].

Voltage Mapping: Methods and Equipment

Three-dimensional electroanatomic voltage mapping technique is performed using the CARTO system (Biosense-Webster) [20-26]. In brief, the magnetic mapping system includes a magnetic sensor in the catheter tip that can be localized in 3D using ultralow magnetic field generators placed under the fluoroscopic table. A 7F Navi-Star catheter, with a 4 mm distal tip electrode and a 2 mm ring electrode with an interelectrode distance of 1mm, is introduced into the RV under fluoroscopic guidance and used as the mapping/ablation catheter during sinus rhythm. The catheter is placed at multiple sites on the endocardial surface to record bipolar and/or unipolar electrograms from RV inflow, anterior free wall, apex and outflow tract. Bipolar electrogram signals are analyzed with regard to amplitude, duration, relation to the surface QRS, and presence of multiple components. Complete endocardial maps are obtained in all patients to ensure reconstruction of a 3-D geometry of the RV chamber and to identify regions of scar or abnormal myocardium. Regions showing low-amplitude electrograms are mapped with greater point density to delineate the extent and borders of "electroanatomic scar" areas. Bipolar voltage reference for normal and abnormal myocardium are based on data previously validated in both intraoperative and catheter mapping studies [18, 19, 24-28]. "Electroanatomic scar" area is defined as an area ≥ 1 cm^2 including at least three adjacent points with bipolar signal amplitude <0.5 mV [25]. The color display for depicting normal and abnormal voltage myocardium ranges from "red" representing "electroanatomic scar tissue" (amplitude <0.5 mV) to "purple" representing "electroanatomic normal tissue" (amplitude ≥ 1.5 mV). Intermediate colors represent the "electroanatomic border zone" (signal amplitudes between 0.5 and 1.5 mV) (Figs. 17.1-3).

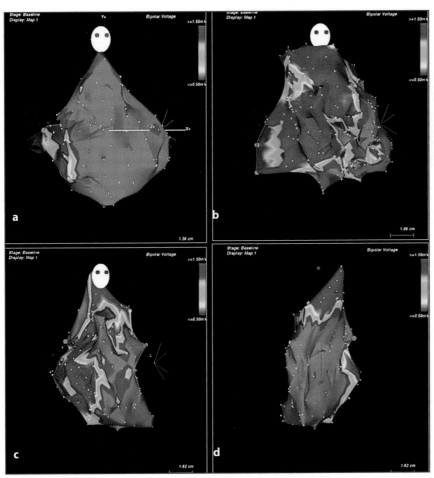

Fig. 17.1 • Representative normal and abnormal 3-D electroanatomic voltage maps. Voltages were color coded according to corresponding color bars. Color range is identical for all subsequent figures: *purple* represents signal amplitudes >1.5 mV ("electroanatomic normal myocardium"); *red* <0.5 mV ("electroanatomic scar tissue"); and range between *purple* and *red* 0.5 to 1.5 mV ("electroanatomic border zone"). *Top*: Anteroposterior view of the RV bipolar voltage map from one control subject with normal bipolar voltages (**a**). Anteroposterior view of the RV bipolar voltage map from a patient with ARVC/D showing diffuse low-amplitude electrical activity involving anterior, lateral, inferobasal, anteroapical and infundibular regions (**b**). *Bottom*: Right anterior oblique (**c**) and left anterior oblique (**d**) views of the RV bipolar voltage from a patient with ARVC/D showing low-voltage areas in the infundibular, inferobasal and anterior regions; the septum is characteristically spared

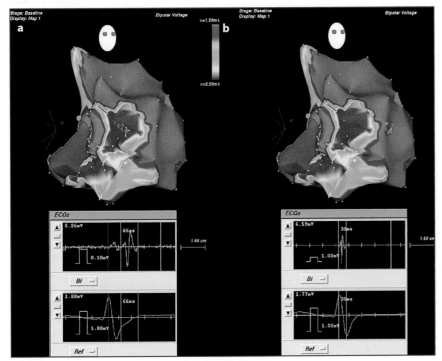

Fig. 17.2 • Examples of electrical signals sampled from a low-amplitude and normal RV areas in the same patient with ARVC/D. As indicated by the catheter tip, the low-voltage electrogram (0.26 mV) recorded from anterior region is fragmented with prolonged duration and late activation (**a**). By comparison, a normal voltage electrogram (6.59 mV) sampled from the lateral region is sharp with uniphasic deflection and shorter duration (**b**)

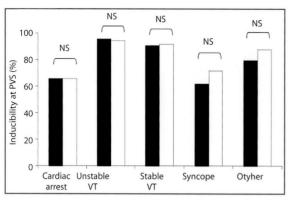

Fig. 17.3 • Comparison of inducibility at programmed ventricular stimulation between patients who did and did not experience appropriate ICD discharge during follow-up, by different clinical presentations. *ICD*, implantable cardioverter defibrillator; *PVS*, programmed ventricular stimulation; *VT*, ventricular tachycardia. Black bars = ICD intervention, white bars = no ICD intervention

Voltage Mapping: Clinical Results in ARVC/D

A preliminary study by Boulos et al. [24] reported a series of seven patients with ARVC/D, in whom electroanatomic voltage mapping accurately identified RV "dysplastic" regions [18]. The authors found a concordance between voltage mapping results and echocardiographic or CMR findings in all studied patients.

Corrado et al. [25] tested the hypothesis that characterization of the RV wall by electroanatomic voltage mapping increases the accuracy for diagnosing ARVC/D. Thirty-one consecutive patients (22 males and nine females, aged 30.8±7 years) who fulfilled the criteria of the Task Force of the European Society of Cardiology and International Society and Federation of Cardiology (ESC/ISFC) for ARVC/D diagnosis after "noninvasive" clinical evaluation, underwent further "invasive" study including RV electroanatomic voltage mapping and EMB to validate the diagnosis. Multiple RV endocardial, bipolar electrograms (175±23) were sampled during sinus rhythm. Twenty patients (Group A, 65%) had an abnormal RV electroanatomic voltage mapping showing one or more areas (mean 2.25±0.7) with low-voltage values (bipolar electrogram amplitude <0.5 mV), surrounded by a border zone (0.5-1.5 mV) which transitioned into normal myocardium (>1.5 mV) (Fig. 17.1). Low-voltage electrograms appeared fractionated with significantly prolonged duration and delayed activation (Fig. 17.2). In eleven patients (Group B, 35%) electroanatomic voltage mapping was normal, with preserved electrogram voltage (4.4±0.7 mV) and duration (37.2±0.9 ms) throughout the RV. Low-voltage areas in patients form Group A corresponded to echocar-

diographic/angiographic RV wall motion abnormalities and were significantly associated with myocyte loss and fibrofatty replacement at EMB (p<0.0001) and familial ARVC/D (p<0.0001). Patients from Group B had a sporadic disease and histopathologic evidence of inflammatory cardiomyopathy (p<0.0001). During the time interval from onset of symptoms to the invasive study (mean 3.4 years), eleven patients (55%) with electroanatomic low-voltage regions received an ICD due to life-threatening ventricular arrhythmias, whereas all but one patient with normal voltage map remained stable on antiarrhythmic drug therapy (p=0.02). These results indicate that 3-D electroanatomic voltage mapping may enhance accuracy for diagnosing ARVC/D by demonstrating low-voltage areas which are associated with fibrofatty myocardial replacement, and by identifying a subset of patients who fulfilled ESC/ISFC Task Force diagnostic criteria, but show a preserved electrogram voltage. This latter subset appears to have an inflammatory cardiomyopathy mimicking ARVC/D, and a better arrhythmic outcome.

Voltage Mapping: Pathophysiologic Implications

The study by Corrado et al. [25] demonstrated that electroanatomic low-amplitude areas were significantly associated with the histopathologic finding of myocyte loss and fibrofatty replacement at EMB, thus confirming that RV loss of voltage reflects the replacement of action potential-generating myocardial tissue with electrically silent fibrofatty tissue. Moreover, there was a concordance between the presence and location of RV low-voltage areas identified by electroanatomic map and akinetic/dyskinetic regions detected by echocardiography and/or angiography. The low-amplitude electrogram values were distinctively recorded in the RV free wall, predominantly involving the anterolateral, infundibular, and inferobasal regions, and spared the interventricular septum (Fig. 17.1). Such a special distribution is similar to that observed at autopsy in the hearts of patients with ARVC/D, in whom most severe RV myocardial atrophy and wall aneurysms are found predominantly in the anteroinfundibular free wall and underneath the tricuspid valve [2, 4, 5].

Abnormal vs. Normal Voltage Mapping

The majority of ARVC/D patients with an abnormal electroanatomic voltage mapping reported by Corrado et al. [25] had a familial form of disease. This finding is consistent with the genetic background of the disease which has been demonstrated in over 50% of ARVC/D patients, with either autosomal or, less frequently, recessive pattern of inheritance and age-related and variable penetrance [17]. There are similarities between the etiopathogenesis of familial ARVC/D and Duchenne's and Becker's skeletal muscle dystrophies, in which the progressive loss of muscle is the result of a genetically-determined ultrastructural defect [29]. In patients with ARVC/D, the defective genes encode for proteins involved in desmosome and intercellular junctions such as plakoglobin, desmoplakin, plakophilin-2, and desmoglein-2. [17]. It has been suggested that under mechanical stress, abnormal desmosomes incorporating defective proteins may lead to detachment and death of myocytes at the intercalated disc and as a consequence, there is a progressive loss of muscle and subsequent fibrofatty replacement [30].

In the above study, 35% of patients who fulfilled the Task Force diagnostic criteria for ARVC/D by noninvasive evaluation, showed evidence neither of electroanatomic low-voltage regions nor of fibrofatty replacement at voltage mapping and EMB. Comparison of mapping results and clinical patient characteristics in the present study suggests that the finding of normal RV voltage values characterizes a distinct subgroup of patients with a peculiar etiopathogenetic, clinical, and prognostic profile. Patients with normal and abnormal electroanatomic voltage mapping did not differ with regard to mean age and mean time interval between symptoms onset and time of electroanatomic evaluation. Moreover, extent of precordial ECG repolarization changes and severity of morphofunctional abnormalities such as global or segmental right ventricular dilatation/dysfunction, RV wall motion abnormalities, and LV involvement, which were detected by echocardiography/angiography were similar in both subgroups of patients. These findings argue against the possibility that failure to detect electroanatomic RV low-voltage areas reflects early stages or minor variants of ARVC/D. Of note, our results differ from those of other studies in which all patients with suspect ARVC/D had a positive voltage mapping [24]. This discrepancy may be explained by different study populations with different prevalence of inflammatory cardiomyopathy as well as by non comparable study design and diagnostic algorithms, with histopathologic data provided only by our investigation.

Myocarditis Mimicking ARVC/D

All patients with a normal electroanatomic voltage mapping were "sporadic" cases, showing neither a familial history of sudden death nor evidence of familial ARVC/D at clinical screening of nuclear family members. It is noteworthy that, all but one patient showed histopathologic changes consistent with the diagnosis of myocarditis at EMB. In the majority of patients, the association between active inflammatory changes and focal replacement fibrosis suggested either a persistent or recurrent myocardial inflammatory process at different stages of healing [31-33].

There is both experimental and clinical evidence that myocarditis can mimic ARVC/D. Some experimental myocarditis is exclusively limited to the right ventricle. Matsumori and Kawai reported selective RV chronic perimyocarditis in BALB/C mice after Coxsackie virus B3 infection [34]. Chronic myocarditis clinically mimicking ARVC/D has been reported in patients who do not have familial disease [35, 36]. Recently, Frustaci et al. [37] analyzed the EMB histologic findings in 30 patients (19 males and eleven females, with a mean age of 27 ± 10 years) with nonfamilial ARVC/D and found diagnostic histologic features of myocarditis according to Dallas criteria (in the absence of significant fibrofatty myocardial atrophy) in 70% of the patients. No differences between patients with myocarditis and those with ARVC/D with regard to ECG/arrhythmic pattern and structural/functional RV abnormalities were observed, a finding in keeping with results of the present study.

In this subset of patients with normal mapping and no apparent regional scar the finding of wall motion abnormalities observed at echocardiographic and angiographic studies can be explained by the inflammatory cardiomyopathy in itself. Segmental wall motion abnormalities (hypokinetic, akinetic or diskinetic areas) are not so uncommon features of inflammatory cardiomyopathy and there are several studies in which myocarditis is reported to mimic myocardial infarction with a pattern of asynergic areas (involving either the left or the right ventricle) and require coronary angiography and endomyocardial biopsy for differential diagnosis [37, 38]. This finding of akinetic/diskinetic ventricular regions (contrasting with areas of relatively preserved contraction) in the absence of regional myocardial scar has been explained by the nonhomogeneous, patchy myocardial involvement of the myocardial inflammatory process [38].

ARVC/D and Dilated Cardiomyopathy

There are similarities between ARVC/D and dilated cardiomyopathy in terms of ventricular dilatation/

usually not associated with an increased arrhythmic risk and therefore do not require specific antiarrhythmic treatment. In many cases, reassurance of the patient results in an improvement of symptoms. However, should a patient still have severe symptoms due to palpitations, treatment with conventional β-blockers or verapamil may be considered. β-blockers appear to be more effective in patients with exercise-provocable ventricular arrhythmias, whereas verapamil may be more successful for the treatment of arrhythmias that occur at rest and are suppressed during exercise. Specific antiarrhythmic drugs or catheter ablation should be limited to patients with significant symptoms refractory to these measures.

Patients with nonsustained and sustained VT or syncope should undergo a detailed diagnostic evaluation to stratify risk and to assess inducibility of clinical ventricular arrhythmia, both having an impact on the subsequent treatment strategy. In low-risk patients, antiarrhythmic drug therapy (preferentially sotalol) may be considered and should be guided by serial electrophysiologic studies. In our experience, this approach showed favorable long-term results in selected low-risk patients with low rates of VT recurrence and sudden death. Catheter ablation may be an alternative option in patients with localized ARVC/D and a single morphology of a hemodynamically well-tolerated VT refractory to antiarrhythmic drugs. In patients with drug-refractory frequent or incessant VT, catheter ablation may be the only treatment option available, but is usually palliative and not curative.

Although antiarrhythmic drug therapy and catheter ablation may reduce VT recurrences, there is no proof from prospective or randomized studies that they are also effective in the prevention of sudden death. Therefore, more effective protection is required in individuals at a higher risk of sudden death. In patients who have survived cardiac arrest or hemodynamically intolerable fast VT, and those with risk factors such as extensive right ventricular dysfunction, advanced stages of ARVC/D, left ventricular involvement, syncope, pleomorphic VT, and others, ICD implantation is considered the most appropriate therapeutic option to prevent life-threatening VT recurrences and sudden death (Fig. 18.5).

In the future, ongoing multicenter European [8] and North American [7] ARVC/D registries will provide important data on risk stratification and treatment efficacy, which may refine management strategies and thereby further improve long-term prognosis of patients with ARVC/D.

Acknowledgements

This work was supported in part by grants from the European Commission, Brussels, Belgium (QLG1-CT-2000-01091); the Deutsche Forschungsgemeinschaft, Bonn, Germany (SFB 556, project C4); the National Institute of Health, Bethesda, MD, USA (NIH, 1 UO1 HL65594-01); and the Interdisciplinary Center of Clinical Research, Münster, Germany (IZKF; Project Ki 1/099/04).

References

1. Marcus FI, Fontaine GH, Guiraudon G et al (1982) Right ventricular dysplasia: A report of 24 adult cases. Circulation 65:384-398
2. Thiene G, Nava A, Corrado D et al (1988) Right ventricular cardiomyopathy and sudden death in young people. N Engl J Med 318:129-133
3. Corrado D, Basso C, Thiene G et al (1997) Spectrum of clinicopathologic manifestations of arrhythmogenic right ventricular cardiomyopathy/dysplasia: A multicenter study. J Am Coll Cardiol 30:1512-1520
4. Fontaine G, Fontaliran F, Frank R (1998) Arrhythmogenic right ventricular cardiomyopathies: Clinical forms and main differential diagnoses. Circulation 97:1532-1535
5. Nava A, Bauce B, Basso C et al (2000) Clinical profile and long-term follow-up of 37 families with arrhythmogenic right ventricular cardiomyopathy. J Am Coll Cardiol 36:2226-2233
6. McKenna WJ, Thiene G, Nava A et al (1994) Diagnosis of arrhythmogenic right ventricular dysplasia/cardiomyopathy. Br Heart J 71:215-218
7. Marcus FI, Towbin JA, Zareba W et al (2003) Arrhythmogenic right ventricular dysplasia/cardiomyopathy (ARVD/C): A multidisciplinary study – Design and protocol. Circulation 107:2975-2978
8. Basso C, Wichter T, Danieli GA et al (2004) Arrhythmogenic right ventricular cardiomyopathy: Clinical registry and database, evaluation of therapies, pathology registry, DNA banking. Eur Heart J 25:531-534
9. Wichter T, Hindricks G, Lerch H et al (1994). Regional myocardial sympathetic dysinnervation in arrhythmogenic right ventricular cardiomyopathy: An analysis using ^{123}I-Meta-Iodobenzylguanidine scintigraphy. Circulation 89:667-683
10. Wichter T, Schäfers M, Borggrefe M et al (2000) Abnormalities of cardiac sympathetic innervation in arrhythmogenic right ventricular cardiomyopathy: Quantitative assessment of presynaptic norepinephrine re-uptake and postsynaptic β-adrenoceptor density using positron emission tomography. Circulation 101:1552-1558
11. Daliento L, Turrini P, Nava A et al (1995) Arrhythmogenic right ventricular cardiomyopathy in young ver-

sus adult patients: Similarities and differences. J Am Coll Cardiol 25:655-664

12. Corrado D, Basso C, Pavei A et al (2006) Trends in sudden cardiovascular death in young competitive athletes after implementation of a preparticipation screening program. JAMA 296:1593-1601

13. Gerull B, Heuser A, Wichter T et al (2004) Mutations in the desmosomal arm repeat protein plakophilin-2 are common in arrhythmogenic right ventricular cardiomyopathy. Nat Genet 36:1162-1164

14. Garcia-Gras E, Lombardi R, Giocondo MJ et al (2006) Suppression of canonical Wnt/b-catenin signaling by nuclear plakoglobin recapitulates phenotype of arrhythmogenic right ventricular cardiomyopathy. J Clin Invest 116:2012-2021

15. Kirchhof P, Fabritz L, Zwiener M et al (2006) Age- and training-dependent development of arrhythmogenic right ventricular cardiomyopathy in heterozygous plakoglobin-deficient mice. Circulation 114:1799-1806

16. Wichter T, Paul M, Breithardt G (2005) Arrhythmogene rechtsventrikuläre Kardiomyopathie: Sportmedizinische Aspekte. Dtsch Z Sportmed 56:118-125

17. Corrado D, Basso C, Thiene G (1996) Pathological findings in victims of sport-related sudden cardiac death. Sports Exerc Injury 2:78-86

18. Blomström-Lundqvist C, Sabel KG, Olsson SB (1987) A long-term follow up of 15 patients with arrhythmogenic right ventricular dysplasia. Br Heart J 58:477-488

19. Canu G, Atallah G, Claudel JP et al (1993) Prognostic et évolution à long terme de la dysplasie arythmogène du ventricule droit. Arch Mal Coeur 86:41-48

20. Leclercq JF, Coumel P, Denjoy I et al (1991) Long-term follow-up after sustained monomorphic ventricular tachycardia: Causes, pump failure, and empiric antiarrhythmic therapy that modify survival. Am Heart J 121:1685-1692

21. Marcus FI, Fontaine GH, Frank R et al (1989) Long-term follow-up in patients with arrhythmogenic right ventricular disease. Eur Heart J 10:68-73

22. Turrini P, Corrado D, Basso C et al (2003) Noninvasive risk stratification in arrhythmogenic right ventricular cardiomyopathy. Ann Noninvasive Electrocardiol 8:161-169

23. Dalal D, Nasir K, Bomma C et al (2005) Arrhythmogenic right ventricular dysplasia: A United States experience. Circulation 112:3823-3832

24. Hulot S, Jouven X, Empana JP et al (2004) Natural history and risk stratification of arrhythmogenic right ventricular dysplasia/cardiomyopathy. Circulation 110:1879-1884

25. Wichter T, Paul M, Eckardt L et al (2005) Arrhythmogenic right ventricular cardiomyopathy: Antiarrhythmic drugs, catheter ablation, or ICD. Herz - Cardiovasc Dis 30:91-101

26. Peters S, Peters H, Thierfelder L (1999) Risk stratification of sudden cardiac death and malignant ventricular arrhythmias in right ventricular dysplasia-cardiomyopathy. Int J Cardiol 71:243-250

27. Lemola K, Brunckhorst C, Helfenstein U et al (2005) Predictors of adverse outcome in patients with arrhythmogenic right ventricular dysplasia/cardiomyopathy: Long term experience of a tertiary care centre. Heart 91:1167-1172

28. Kiès P, Bootsma M, Bax J et al (2006) Arrhythmogenic right ventricular dysplasia/cardiomyopathy: Screening, diagnosis, and treatment. Heart Rhythm 3:225-234

29. Turrini P, Corrado D, Basso C et al (2001) Dispersion of ventricular depolarization-repolarization. A noninvasive marker for risk stratification in arrhythmogenic right ventricular cardiomyopathy. Circulation 103:3075-3080

30. Corrado D, Leoni L, Link MS et al (2003) Implantable cardioverter-defibrillator therapy for prevention of sudden death in patients with arrhythmogenic right ventricular cardiomyopathy/dysplasia. Circulation 108:3084-3091

31. Wichter T, Paul M, Wollmann C et al (2004) Implantable cardioverter-defibrillator therapy in arrhythmogenic right ventricular cardiomyopathy: Single-center experience of long-term follow-up and complications in 60 patients. Circulation 109:1503-1508

32. Piccini JP, Dalal D, Roguin A et al (2005) Predictors of appropriate implantable defibrillator therapies in patients with arrhythmogenic right ventricular dysplasia. Heart Rhythm 2:1188-1194

33. Pezawas T, Stix G, Kastner J et al (2006) Ventricular tachycardia in arrhythmogenic right ventricular dysplasia/cardiomyopathy: Clinical presentation, risk stratification and results of long-term follow-up. Int J Cardiol 107:360-368

34. Fontaine G, Zenati O, Tonet J et al (1997) The treatment of ventricular arrhythmias. In: Nava A, Rossi L, Thiene G (eds) Arrhythmogenic right ventricular cardiomyopathy/dysplasia. Elsevier Science, Amsterdam, BV:315-363

35. Tonet J, Frank R, Fontaine G et al (1989) Efficacité de l'association de faibles doses de bêta-bloquants à l'amiodarone dans le traitement des tachycardies ventriculaires réfractaires. Arch Mal Coeur 82:1511-1517

36. Berder V, Vauthier M, Mabo P et al (1995) Characteristics and outcome in arrhythmogenic right ventricular dysplasia. Am J Cardiol 75:411-415

37. Wichter T, Borggrefe M, Haverkamp W et al (1992) Efficacy of antiarrhythmic drugs in patients with arrhythmogenic right ventricular disease. Results in patients with inducible and noninducible ventricular tachycardia. Circulation 86:29-37

38. Hamid MS, Norman M, Quraishi A et al (2002). Prospective evaluation of relatives for familial arrhythmogenic right ventricular cardiodmyopathy/dysplasia reveals a need to broaden diagnostic criteria. J Am Coll Cardiol 40:1445-1450

39. Wichter T, Breithardt G (2005) Implantable cardioverter-defibrillator therapy in arrhythmogenic right ventricular cardiomyopathy: A role for genotyping in decision-making? J Am Coll Cardiol 45:409-411

genic substrate without clear anatomic changes. However, in some patients, multiple ablation attempts were necessary during the same session and it was confirmed that multiple morphologies of VT is not a deterrent for successful ablation.

In this study only two patients had an ICD before ablation. However, ICD was frequently implanted after the ablation or during the follow-up in order to protect the patient because of disease progression leading to new episodes of rapid VT or VF. Therefore ICD implantation was performed in nine patients. All patients with ICD had follow-up every 6 months. VTs were detected in the two exceptional patients and led to rehospitalizations. One patient had well tolerated asymptomatic VT interrupted by antitachycardia pacing (ATP), followed by two appropriate shocks in December, 2005, several VT episodes, and one appropriate shock in early 2006. Since then the patient has not had recurrent VT. Two patients had nonsustained VT. Three patients received inappropriate shocks. One patient had palpitations but no recording of VT by the device.

New forms of VT observed during the follow-up may be related to disease progression and may require additional ablation. In our experience, no patient needed heart transplant for arrhythmia management but one (in the low LVEF group), who recently had heart transplant for heart failure.

RF Antiarrhythmic Epicardial Surgery

Histologic material of the native heart of this transplanted patient showed presence of fibro fatty replacement of the myocardium of both ventricles. Lymphocytes also involved both ventricles with the pattern of multifocal clusters mostly located in the subepicardial layers of the right ventricle.

RF antiarrhythmic epicardial surgery may prove effective in the most difficult cases resistant to endocardial RF ablation.

Overview of VT Ablation in the Literature

Several studies have reported a similar success rate in patients with ARVC/D. Verma et al. obtained a success rate of 82% on a series of 22 cases [19]. Several less clear studies concerning the definitions of cases included under the term of ARVC/D have been re-

ported by Marchlinski et al. on a series of 21 cases with a success rate of 89% [20]. Manaka et al. have reported a series of 41 patients with a success rate of 80% [21]. These results seems better than those obtained in idiopathic dilated cardiomyopathy in the study of Soejima et al., with a success rate of only 54% [22]. This is probably related to the anatomic structure of diseased myocardium in this particular entity. It should be noted that the definition of success is not uniform in the literature.

In summary:
1. Radiofrequency alone or in combination with fulguration is appropriate as a first approach for VT ablation in ARVD with a success rate of 90%.
2. In a resistant case it was possible to control incessant VT with surgical epicardial radiofrequency ablation.
3. Overview of RF ablation of VT from the literature shows a similar success rate 80%-90% with the same long-term occurrence of new VTs during the follow-up.

Conclusions

ARVC/D is a structural heart disease, affecting young adults, leading to cardiac rhythm disorders, mostly ventricular arrhythmias. Sudden death may be the first presentation of the disease. Ablation techniques have been used for the treatment of VT cases resistant to drug therapy. The use of radiofrequency energy is appropriate as a first approach for VT ablation in ARVC/D. Fulguration is effective for VT ablation and can be used after ineffective RF ablation. However, these techniques requires expertise, general anesthesia, and more than one session in half of patients.

Radiofrequency and/or fulguration plus other common forms of treatment, including pacemakers and ICDs, provided a clinical success rate of 95% in a series of 22 consecutive patients studied over 6 years. This result is in agreement with data reported by other centers and presented in the literature. However, successful ablation achieved by epicardial surgical RF ablation was only obtained in one patient after failure of four consecutive ablation sessions incorporating both endocardial RF and DC energy.

This new technique of surgical epicardial radiofrequency ablation can be extended to other catheter-resistant arrhythmogenic substrates.

Addendum

After submission of this chapter, Case #2 had two appropriate shocks for rapid VT documented by interrogation of the ICD memory. The drug regimen was not changed and no further arrhythmias were observed until the present time, three months after the ICD shocks. However, the patient developed increasing signs of heart failure and is now on the waiting list for heart transplant.

Acknowledgements

This work has been supported by grant N°99B0691 from the "Ministère de l'Education, de la Recherche et de la Technologie." We would like to extend our gratitude to the team of colleagues who have performed the ablation procedures: J. Tonet, G. Jauvert, F. Halimi, Ph. Aouate, G. Lascault, F. Poulain, and N. Johnson with special mention for our anesthesiologist Y. Gallais, C. Himbert, V. Bors, cardiac surgeon are also acknowledged.

We also appreciate the work of Mrs. Samia Riguet, and Mrs. Deanna Bammer for their contribution in the preparation of the manuscript.

References

1. Fontaine G, Tonet J, Gallais Y et al (2000) Ventricular tachycardia catheter ablation in arrhythmogenic right ventricular dysplasia: A 16-year experience. Curr Cardiol Rep 2:498-506
2. McKenna WJ, Thiene G, Nava A et al (1994) Diagnosis of arrhythmogenic right ventricula dysplasia/cardiomyopathy. Br Heart J 71:215-218
3. Tonet J, Himbert C, Johnson N et al (2000) Prolongation of ventricular refractoriness and ventricular tachycardia cycle length by the combination of oral beta-blocker – Amiodarone in patients with ventricular tachycardia. PACE 23:565
4 Langberg J, Lee MA, Chin M, Rosenqvist M (1990) Radiofrequency catheter ablation: The effect of electrode size on lesion volume in vivo. PACE 13:1242-1248
5. Fontaine G, Cansell A, Lampe L et al (1987) Endocavitary fulguration (electrode catheter ablation): Equipment-related problems. In: Fontaine G, Scheiman MM (eds) Ablation in cardiac arrhythmias. Futura, Kisko, NY pp 85-100
6. Gallais Y, Lascault G, Tonet J et al (1993) Continuous measurement of coronary sinus oxygen saturation during ventricular tachycardia (abstract). Eur Heart J 14:368
7. Morady F, Frank R, Kou WH et al (1988) Identification and catheter ablation of a zone of slow conduction in the reentry. Circuit of ventricular tachycardias in humans. J Am Coll Cardiol 11:775-782
8. Fontaine G, Frank R, Tonet J, Grosgogeat Y (1989) Identification of a zone of slow conduction appropriate for VT ablation. Theoretical and practical considerations. PACE 12:262-267
9. Stevenson WG, Khan H, Sager P et al (1993) Identification of reentry circuit sites during catheter mapping and radiofrequency ablation of ventricular tachycardia late after myocardial infarction. Circulation 88:1647-1670
10. Man KC, Daoud E, Knight BP et al (1997) Accuracy of the unipolar electrogram for identification of the site of origin of ventricular activation. J Cardiovasc Electrophysiol 8:974-979
11. Harada T, Aonuma K, Yamauchi S et al (1998) Catheter ablation of ventricular tachycardia in patients with right ventricular dysplasia: Identification of target sites by entrainment mapping techniques. PACE 21:2547-2550
12. Fontaliran F, Arkwright S, Vilde F, Fontaine G (1998) Arrhythmogenic right ventricular dysplasia and cardiomyopathy. Clinical and anatomic-pathologic aspects, nosologic approach. Arch Anat Cytol Pathol 46:171-177
13. Fontaine G, Fontaliran F, Rosas Andrade F et al (1995) Arrhythmogenic right ventricle: Dysplasia or cardiomyopathy? Value of left ventricle ejection fraction. Ann Cardiol Angeiol 44:321-331
14. Hulot JS, Jouven X, Empana JP et al (2004) Natural history and risk stratification of arrhythmogenic right ventricular dysplasia/cardiomyopathy. Circulation 110:1879-1884
15. Feld GK (1998) Expanding indications for radiofrequency catheter ablation: Ventricular tachycardia in association with right ventricular dysplasia. J Am Coll Cardiol 32:729-731
16. Wichter T, Hindricks G, Kottkamp H et al (1997) Catheter ablation of ventricular tachycardia. In: Arrhythmogenic right ventricular cardiomyopathy/dysplasia. Nava A, Rossi L, Thiene G (eds) Elsevier Science BV, Amsterdam, pp 376-391
17. Marchlinski FE, Zado E, Dixit S et al (2004) Electroanatomic substrate and outcome of catheter ablative therapy for ventricular tachycardia in setting of right ventricular cardiomyopathy. Circulation 110:2293-2298
18. Fontaine G, Fontaliran F, Lascault G et al (1994) Arrhythmogenic right ventricular dysplasia. In: Cardiac electrophysiology. From cell to bedside. Zipes DP, Jalife J (eds) WB Saunders, Philadelphia, pp 754-768
19. Verma A, Kiliscaslan F, Schweikert RA et al (2005) Short- and long-term success of substrate-based mapping and ablation of ventricular tachycardia in arrhythmogenic right ventricular dysplasia. Circulation 111:3209-3216

20. Marchlinski FE, Zado E, Dixit S et al (2004) Electroanatomic substrate of catheter ablation therapy for ventricular tachycardia in setting of right ventricular cardiomyopathy. Circulation 110:2293-2298

21. Manaka T, Shoda M, Tanisaki K et al (2005) Electrophysiological properties and long term outcome of catheter ablation for ventricular tachycardia ablation in arrhythmogenic right ventricular cardiomyopathy – A single center experience. Circulation 112:624

22. Soejima K, Stevenson WG, Sapp JL et al (2004) Endocardial and epicardial Radiofrequency ablation of ventricular tachycardia with dilated cardiomyopathy: The importance of low voltage scars. J Am Coll Cardiol 43:1834-1842

CHAPTER 20

THE ROLE OF THE IMPLANTABLE CARDIAC DEFIBRILLATOR IN THE MANAGEMENT

Olaf Hedrich, Gianfranco Buja, Domenico Corrado, Mark S. Link, Thomas Wichter, N.A. Mark Estes III

Introduction

The management of patients with arrhythmogenic right ventricular cardiomyopathy/dysplasia (ARVC/D) has evolved considerably over the last several years. Because many patients with ARVC/D may be at risk for sudden cardiac death (SCD) and clinical series have reported favorable outcomes with this therapy, the implantable cardioverter-defibrillator (ICD) has assumed a larger role in therapy. On the basis of collective observations from several series of patients, implantation of an ICD in a patient with ARVC/D has a major impact on decreasing the risk of SCD. This chapter examines the available clinical information regarding ICD therapy in patients with ARVC/D.

Natural History, Mode of Death, and Risk Stratification

It is now appreciated that the spectrum of clinical presentation of ARVC/D is characterized by heterogeneity. Individual patients may be symptomatic or asymptomatic and, in addition, asymptomatic relatives of patients with ARVC/D may have ARVC/D. Given this relatively diverse phenotypic expression, risk stratification for sudden death or arrhythmia is crucial in the clinician's decision whether to recommend implantation of an ICD.

Cardiovascular death is a recognized complication of ARVC/D [1], and generally takes the form of SCD, often without any precursor symptoms [2-4]. In a series of patients with SCD under 65 years of age, ARVC/D is reported as the cause of death in 3%-20% [5-7]. Recent single center series aimed at defining the natural history of ARVC/D have demonstrated that cardiac death occurred in approximately 16% of their cohorts during follow-up of between 4 and 8 years (annual mortality rate, 2.3%-4%) [8, 9]. These observations may suggest that, as a group, patients with ARVC/D are at increased risk of SCD relative to other cardiomyopathies and thus should be offered an ICD. Among the many questions that need to be considered when managing patients with ARVC/D are: (1) which patients are at highest risk for arrhythmic death; and (2) whether implantation of an ICD necessarily confers an improvement in survival in patients with ARVC/D.

Risk stratification for sudden cardiac death in ARVC/D has been addressed in small natural history series of cases from tertiary referral centers [8, 9]. Such series may potentially overestimate annual mortality, and may disproportionately represent higher risk patients referred for evaluation and management. Nevertheless, the observations derived from such studies are instructive, particularly in light of the considerable length of follow-up, allowing valuable insights into the natural history of ARVC/D. Sudden death (presumably arrhythmic) accounts for the majority of cardiovascular deaths in ARVC/D, as it has been shown in earlier series. However, other modes of cardiovascular death are also encountered. In one series of 130 patients, followed for 8.1±7.8 years, of which ten (7.7%) patients received an ICD, a surprisingly high prevalence of death caused by heart failure (HF) emphasizes the propensity for development of right and/or left ventricular dysfunction over time. Of the 24 patients who died, 21 died of cardiovascular causes: 59% of these were deemed to have died from progressive HF, and 29% experienced sudden death [8].

In a second group of 61 patients followed for 55±47 months, ten patients died of cardiovascular causes: eight died of presumed arrhythmic causes (SCD), and two died of advanced heart failure [9]. Thirty-nine percent of this cohort had an ICD.

It is not clear whether the former finding represents the true natural history of the disease, or a change in the course of the disease due to contemporary heart failure and/or arrhythmia management (several patients in both series received ICDs and were on antiarrhythmic drugs). It is plausible that progressive myocardial dysfunction may result in a higher incidence of arrhythmias over time. Howev-

270±40 ms (range 220 to 350 ms). Antitachycardia pacing (ATP) was successful in seven of eight patients in whom it was attempted. In the multicenter series reported by Corrado et al. [10], 98 of 111 (88%) patients had either sustained VT during EPS (67 patients; 68%) with a mean cycle length of 284±66 ms (range 210 to 415 ms), or VF (31 patients; 32%). It is instructive that, of the 98 inducible patients, 49% experienced appropriate ICD therapy during the follow-up period (39±25 months), whereas 54% of 13 noninducible patients had appropriate ICD interventions. Positive and negative predictive values of EPS in this group were both approximately 50%. The type of ventricular arrhythmia induced at EPS did not predict the occurrence of VF during follow-up. This series therefore suggests that the EPS has limited value in identifying ARVC/D patients at risk for lethal tachyarrhythmias, an observation in keeping with its limited predictive value in cardiomyopathies other than ischemic cardiomyopathy.

In contrast, Roguin et al. [14] report that induction of VT during EPS was the most significant predictor for ICD firing in their cohort of 42 patients (41 underwent EPS, 31 were inducible for VT; 81% of those who had ICD therapy during follow-up were inducible vs. 44% who did not; p=0.024). However, these results may be partially explained by a relatively high ICD firing rate in this trial (78% over a mean follow-up period of 3.5 years), which in turn may be due to clinical characteristics of the population, or to the low prevalence of beta blocker and antiarrhythmic drug use.

Appropriate Therapies and Life-Saving Interventions

Once an ICD is implanted, it appears that many (if not most) ARVC/D patients experience an appropriate ICD intervention (either antitachycardia pacing or defibrillation shock). In the series already mentioned, a high incidence of appropriate ICD interventions was encountered. Overall, between 48% and 78% of patients received appropriate ICD interventions during the mean follow-up period of 2-7 years after implantation [10-15] (Table 20.1). Many of these patients experienced multiple shocks during this period, and VT storm was not infrequently encountered. In the largest series to date, the rate of appropriate interventions was 15% per year [10]. Appropriate intervention rates were similar in patients presenting with VT, unexplained syncope, or cardiac arrest, although the latter group experienced slightly more events during follow-up (Fig. 20.3). An important observation is that patients with hemodynamically well-tolerated VT had significantly longer event-free survival than those with hemodynamic compromise during VT, unexplained syncope, or cardiac arrest. None of the asymptomatic patients implanted because of a family history of SCD experienced any appropriate ICD interventions, regardless of the results at EPS.

One method employed to assess the benefits of the ICD in observational series has been proposed by the Muenster group and compares the actual patient

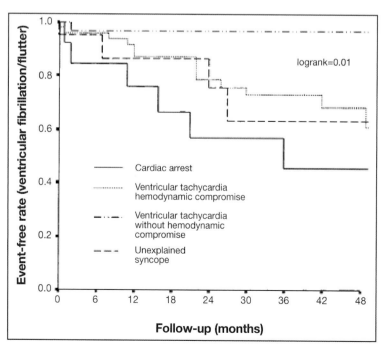

Fig. 20.3 • Analysis of appropriate ICD interventions experienced by a 132-patient cohort with ARVC/D and an ICD: these Kaplan-Meier curves depict freedom from any appropriate ICD interventions for different patient subgroups (with ARVC/D) stratified for clinical presentation. From [10] with permission from Lippincott Williams & Wilkins

survival rates with projected freedom of fast VT/VF >240 bpm (used as a surrogate for aborted SCD) [14]. This is achieved by device interrogation and analysis of ICD interventions in response to either VF or flutter during follow-up. When comparing actual patient survival rates with projected SCD-free survival rates in this manner, it becomes apparent that there is a significant improvement in survival. In the large series reported by Corrado et al. [10], 24% of patients had one or more episodes of either VF, ventricular flutter, or both, that were successfully recognized and treated by their device, and that would otherwise likely have been fatal. These interventions were therefore deemed to be life-saving. In this pop-

ulation, actual total patient survival rates were 96%, compared with a 72% VF/flutter-free survival rate at 36 months (Fig. 20.4). The largest single-center experience was published by Wichter et al. [14] and provides the longest follow-up period (mean 80±43 months) reported to date. This group found an estimated survival benefit of 23%, 32%, and 35% after 1, 3, and 7 years of follow-up. Event-free survival in that cohort appeared to plateau after about 5 years after the ICD was implanted, suggesting that the greatest benefit may be observed earlier in the course after ICD implantation [14, 17] (Fig. 20.5). These results were confirmed by other series reporting similar rates of life-saving ICD interventions (30%-50%

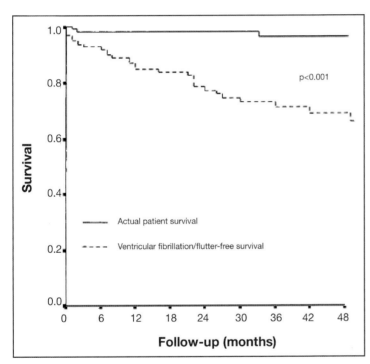

Fig. 20.4 • Survival data from 132 patients with ARVC/D with implanted defibrillators. This Kaplan-Meier analysis compares actual patient survival with survival free of ventricular fibrillation/flutter that in all likelihood would have been fatal in the absence of an appropriate ICD intervention. Divergence between lines reflects the estimated survival benefit conferred by ICD therapy in these patients. At 36 months, actual total patient survival was 96%, compared with 72% VF/flutter-free survival. The general population estimated survival rate was 99.5% when matched for age, gender, and ethnicity. From [10] with permission from Lippincott Williams & Wilkins

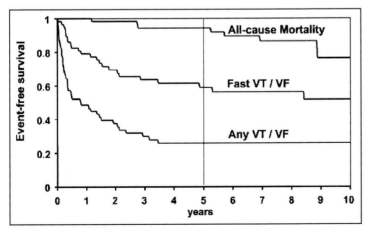

Fig. 20.5 • Mortality and recurrence of VT or VF during follow-up (80 ±43 months) after ICD implantation in ARVC/D. Kaplan-Meier curves depict event-free survival for all-cause mortality, fast VT/VF (>240 bpm), and VT/VF at any rate. The difference between all-cause mortality and fast VT/VF indicates the potential survival benefit from ICD therapy in this cohort. From [14] with permission from Lippincott Williams & Wilkins

of patients over the course of follow-up) [11, 12, 15], although in some cases slightly more permissive definitions were applied to arrive to this determination.

Time of first appropriate ICD therapy may yield further insight into the potential for ICD to improve outcomes. From published data, it appears that most patients received their first appropriate therapy in 4 months to 3 years after ICD implantation (Table 20.1). In a homogeneous cohort of ARVC/D patients compared with controls, it was observed that time to first ICD discharge for VT >240 bpm was similar to the time of death of the control group, confirming this concept of "hypothetical death" [14, 15].

Predictors of ICD Therapy

Although natural history studies have shed light on the pathologic progression of ARVC/D, as well as certain risk factors for death, published series following these patients after ICD implantation have provided valuable information about risk predictors for VT and VF. As such, they offer the possibility of refining current views on indications for ICD therapy in these patients.

In three recent, separate cohorts totaling 234 patients followed after ICDs were implanted for various indications, several predictors for appropriate ICD firing were identified [10, 13, 14]. Table 20.2 summarizes these findings. In the largest of these series [10], a history of either cardiac arrest or VT with hemodynamic compromise, younger age, and left ventricular involvement were found to be independent predictors of potentially lethal arrhythmias. In the group experiencing cardiac arrest or VT with hemodynamic com-

promise, a high incidence of VF/flutter (10% per year of follow-up) was encountered despite antiarrhythmic drug therapy, thus strongly suggesting that these patients were indeed ideal candidates for ICD therapy. Similarly, patients presenting with unexplained syncope also derived significant benefit from ICD implantation, as evidenced by their 8%-per-year rate of resuscitative interventions. On the contrary, VT without hemodynamic compromise did not predict benefit, as only one patient (3% from this category) had VF during follow-up. These findings correspond to those in ischemic heart disease patients, in whom hemodynamically well-tolerated VT exhibited a lower SD rate compared with cardiac arrest survivors [18]. None of the asymptomatic patients who underwent ICD implantation for a family history of SCD experienced an appropriate ICD intervention, although the numbers of patients in this group were too small to draw any definite conclusions.

Roguin et al. [13] identified four variables as predictors for ICD firing. These included induction of VT during EPS, detection of spontaneous nonsustained VT, moderate-to-severe dilatation of the right ventricle, and male gender. Of these, induction of VT at EPS remained statistically significant in multivariate analysis, with the other variables trending toward significance. In the study of Wichter et al. [14], multivariate analysis identified extensive RV dysfunction as an independent predictor of appropriate ICD therapy during follow-up, with inducible VT or VF at EPS and left ventricular involvement demonstrating a trend toward statistical significance.

While it remains true that no randomized study exists comparing ICD therapy to no therapy or antiarrhythmic drug therapy in this group, data from the

Table 20.2 • Clinical characteristics associated with appropriate ICD therapy for VT or VF in ARVC/D

Study	Year	Pts (n)	Clinical characteristic	P	OR	95% CI
[10]	2003	132	Age/5 yrs*	0.007	0.77	0.57-0.96
			LV ejection fraction	0.037	0.94	0.89-0.95
			Cardiac arrest	<0.001	79	6.8-90.6
			VT with hemodynamic compromise	0.015	14	1.7-21.1
			Unexplained syncope	0.07	7.5	0.84-1.81
[13]	2004	42	Induction of VT at EPS	0.031	11.2	1.23-101.24
			Severe RV dilation	0.07	3.41	0.88-14.21
			Male gender	0.11	2.64	0.80-8.71
[14]	2004	60	Extensive RV dysfunction[1]	0.041	2.09	1.03-4.24
			Inducible VT/VF at EPS	0.069	2.16	0.94-5.0
			Left ventricular involvement	0.078	1.94	0.93-4.05

CI, confidence interval; *EPS*, electrophysiologic study; *LV*, left ventricular; *OR*, odds ratio; *RV*, right ventricular; *VF*, ventricular fibrillation/flutter; *VT*, ventricular tachycardia
* or per 5-year interval
[1] As defined by severe regional (≥2 RV areas) or global (RV ejection fraction ≤45%) RV dysfunction

Corrado cohort [10] reveal that the majority of appropriate interventions occurred despite concomitant antiarrhythmic therapy (sotalol, amiodarone, or β-blockers, alone or in combination). This provides strong support for the notion that ICDs confer superior protection against life-threatening arrhythmias compared to antiarrhythmic agents in ARVC/D.

Safety of ICD Implantation in ARVC/D

Concern has been expressed about the potential for risks and complications of transvenous lead implantation in diseased RV myocardium. These relate not only to an increased risk of perforation, but also to suboptimal sensing, pacing, and defibrillation efficacy. Although procedure-related deaths were extremely rare in all series following patients with ARVC/D after ICD implantation, both procedural complications and long-term performance complications of the leads were not uncommonly encountered (Table 20.1).

Lead perforation in various (mainly non-ARVC/D) ICD populations has been reported with an incidence of 0.6% to as high as 5.2% [19, 20]. There were no reported lead perforations in any of the referenced ARVC/D series. Repeated note is made by several of the implanting groups of the need for meticulous ventricular lead placement to ensure adequate R-wave sensing and pacing thresholds. This is due to the consideration that diseased RV myocardium (replaced by fibrofatty deposits) may render satisfactory sensing, pacing, and defibrillation thresholds difficult to achieve. Uniformly, screw-in leads are preferred. Although a higher number of RV sites were tested prior to lead fixation in the ARVC/D series, a lower final R-wave amplitude was achieved in ARVC/D patients compared with patients with other diseases [11, 14, 17]. It appears that final pacing and defibrillation thresholds (at least acutely) are comparable [14].

When followed over time, undersensing or pacing failure (due to exit block) may be encountered with significant frequency in ARVC/D patients as a result of progressive fibrofatty myocardial replacement at the RV lead tip. In series with relatively short follow-up periods, this problem was not reported [11, 12]. However, late after implantation, this problem is encountered with considerable frequency. Five patients out of 132 required an additional RV lead in Corrado's cohort [10], and eight of the 60 patients described by Wichter et al. required lead revision or implantation of an additional pace/sense lead late after implantation (median, 65 months) [14]. Corrado et al. further report the need for additional subcutaneous or epicardial patches or high-energy de-

vices in order to achieve a 10-J margin of safety for defibrillation at implant [10].

In following ARVC/D patients with ICDs, particular attention must be given to these considerations, and particular care must be employed to note any progressive loss of R-wave sensing amplitude or pacing threshold during follow-up, which may not only indicate device or lead compromise, but also possibly disease progression [14]. This is especially true in this generally young patient population, who will require a device for the remainder of their lives. Lead failure relates not only to a compromise in pace/sense or defibrillation function by the mechanisms described, but also to the mechanical issues of lead insulation failure and fracture [14]. An increase in failure rates of transvenous leads has been reported late after implantation (beyond 4-5 years), and this incidence tends to increase with time after implant [20, 21]. This has been verified by Wichter et al. in ARVC/D patients undergoing long-term follow-up, with a high rate of lead-related complications (cumulatively 37% at 7 years) [14]. Lead failure may also contribute to inappropriate or inadequate delivery of ICD therapy.

Device Selection

A conservative approach to the complexity of the lead system used with the implanted defibrillator appears prudent. While dual-chamber systems seem attractive since they may reduce inappropriate ICD therapies because of improved ability to discriminate between supraventricular and ventricular arrhythmias, a reduction in the number of implanted leads may be a favorable approach in this relatively young patient group, precisely because of the incidence of lead-related complications over long-term follow-up. There is currently no firm evidence to support the routine use of a dual-chamber defibrillator in ARVC/D. However, for patients with inappropriate sinus node function and preserved atrioventricular conduction, this is a viable option. The potential benefits of such an approach should, however, still be weighed against the long-term complications associated with additional hardware for each individual patient.

Conclusions

Based on the available clinical data it is reasonable to conclude that ICD is the preferred therapy for secondary prevention of sudden cardiac arrest in patients with ARVC/D [1, 22, 23]. When considering ICD for primary prevention, it should be kept in mind that predictive markers of SCD in patients with ARVC/D have not yet been defined in large prospective studies focusing on survival. However, based on the best available clinical data, risk factors that have clinical utility in identifying patients with ARVC/D who are at risk for life-threatening ventricular arrhythmias include induction of VT during electrophysiologic testing, detection of nonsustained VT on noninvasive monitoring, male gender, and severe RV dilation or extensive RV involvement. In addition, young age at presentation, LV involvement, prior cardiac arrest, or unexplained syncope serve as markers of risk [8, 9, 10-14]. Patients with genotypes of ARVC/D associated with a high risk for SCD should be considered for ICD therapy [15, 17].

While the role of ICD therapy for primary prevention of sudden death in patients with ischemic heart disease and dilated, nonischemic cardiomyopathy is well established based on multiple clinical trails with a consistent finding of benefit, the data supporting ICD use in ARVC/D patients are less extensive. In the guidelines of the American College of Cardiology and the American Heart Association, ARVC/D is not mentioned specifically as a standard indication for placement of an ICD [22]. However, familial or inherited conditions with a risk of SCD such as hypertrophic cardiomyopathy and long QT syndromes are acknowledged as Class IIA indications for an ICD [22]. The Task Force on SCD of the European Society of Cardiology proposed that an ICD should be implanted in ARVC/D patients with an increased risk for SCD, based on the presence of a previous cardiac arrest, syncope due to VT, evidence for extensive RV disease, LV involvement, and presentation with polymorphic VT and RV apical aneurysm (which is associated with a genetic locus on chromosome 1q42-43) [23].

Most recently, new guidelines for the management of patients with ventricular arrhythmias and the prevention of sudden cardiac death were published by the AHA, ACC, and ESC [24]. Based on the growing body of evidence resulting from recently published data, this document provides recommendations for the risk stratification and indication of ICD implantation in patients with ARVC/D.

It is evident that there is not yet a clear consensus on the specific risk factors that identify those patients with ARVC/D in whom the probability of SCD is sufficiently high to warrant an ICD for primary prevention. The results of large, prospective registries of ARVC/D patients with rigorous enrollment criteria in whom ICDs have been placed for primary prevention will give insights into the optimal risk stratification techniques for primary prevention. In the meantime,

individualized decisions for primary prevention of SCD must be based on experience, judgment, and the available data. In considering this decision, the clinician should be mindful that, in patients with ARVC/D, ICD has proved safe and reliable in sensing and terminating sustained ventricular arrhythmias. Sudden death is rare in the available clinical series while appropriate ICD therapy is common [8, 9, 10-12].

References

1. Calkins H, Marcus F (2003) Arrhythmogenic right ventricular dysplasia. In: Braunwald E, (ed) Harrison's Advances in Cardiology. McGraw-Hill, New York, pp 378-383
2. Fontaine G, Fontaliran F, Frank R (1998) Arrhythmogenic right ventricular cardiomyopathies: Clinical forms and main differential diagnoses. Circulation 97:1532-1535
3. Corrado D, Thiene G, Nava A et al (1990) Sudden death in young competitive athletes: Clinicopathologic correlations in 22 cases. Am J Med 89:588-596
4. Kullo IJ, Edwards WD, Seward JB (1995) Right ventricular dysplasia: The Mayo Clinic experience. Mayo Clin Proc 70:541-548
5. Tabib A, Loire R, Chalabreysse L et al (2003) Circumstances of death and gross and microscopic observations in a series of 200 cases of sudden death associated with arrhythmogenic right ventricular cardiomyopathy and/or dysplasia. Circulation 108:3000-3005
6. Maron BJ, Shirani J, Polac L et al (1996) Sudden death in young competitive athletes: Clinical, demographic and pathological profiles. JAMA 276:199-204
7. Thiene G, Nava A, Corrado D et al (1988) Right ventricular cardiomyopathy and sudden death in young people. N Engl J Med 318:129-133
8. Hulot JS, Jouven X, Empana JP et al (2004) Natural history and risk stratification of arrhythmogenic right ventricular dysplasia/cardiomyopathy. Circulation 110:1879-1884
9. Lemola K, Brunckhorst C, Helfenstein U et al (2005) Predictors of adverse outcome in patients with arrhythmogenic right ventricular dysplasia/cardiomyopathy: Long term experience of a tertiary care centre. Heart 91:1167-1172
10. Corrado D, Leoni L, Link MS et al (2003) Implantable cardioverter-defibrillator therapy for prevention of sudden death in patients with arrhythmogenic right ventricular cardiomyopathy/dysplasia. Circulation 108:3084-3091
11. Link MS, Wang PJ, Haugh CJ et al (1997) Arrhythmogenic right ventricular dysplasia: Clinical results with implantable cardioverter defibrillators. J Intervent Card Electrophysiol 1:41-48
12. Tavernier R, Gevaert S, De Sutter J et al (2001) Long term results of cardioverter-defibrillator implantation in patients with right ventricular dysplasia and malignant ventricular tachyarrhythmias. Heart 85:53-56

13. Roguin A, Bomma C, Nasir K et al (2004) Implantable cardioverter-defibrillators in patients with arrhythmogenic right ventricular dysplasia/cardiomyopathy. J Am Coll Cardiol 43:1843-1852

14. Wichter T, Paul M, Wollmann C et al (2004) Implantable cardioverter/defibrillator therapy in arrhythmogenic right ventricular cardiomyopathy. Single-center experience of long-term follow-up and complications in 60 patients. Circulation 109:1503-1508

15. Hodgkinson KA, Parfrey PS, Bassett AS et al (2005) The impact of implantable cardioverter-defibrillator therapy on survival in autosomal-dominant arrhythmogenic right ventricular cardiomyopathy (ARVD5). J Am Coll Cardiol 45:400-408

16. Wichter T, Breithardt G (2005) Implantable cardioverter-defibrillator therapy in arrhythmogenic right ventricular cardiomyopathy. A role for genotyping in decision-making? J Am Coll Cardiol 45:409-411

17. McKenna WJ, Thiene G, Nava A et al (1994) Diagnosis of arrhythmogenic right ventricular dysplasia/cardiomyopathy. Br Heart J 71:218-228

18. Sarter BH, Finkle JK, Gerszten RE et al (1996) What is the risk of sudden cardiac death in patients presenting with hemodynamically stable sustained ventricular tachycardia after myocardial infarction? J Am Coll Cardiol 28:122-129

19. Grimm W, Flores BF, Marchlinski FE (1993) Complications of implantable cardioverter therapy: Follow-up of 241 patients. Pacing Clin Electrophysiol 16:218-222

20. Molina JE (1996) Perforation of the right ventricle by transvenous defibrillator leads: Prevention and treatment. Pacing Clin Electrophysiol 19:288-292

21. Dorwarth U, Frey B, Dugas M et al (2003) Transvenous defibrillation leads: High incidence of failure during long-term follow-up. J Cardiovasc Electrophysiol 14:38-43

22. Gregoratos G, Abrams J, Eptein AE et al for the ACC/AHA/NASPE Taskforce on Practice Guidelines (2002) Guideline Update for Implantation of Cardiac Pacemakers and Antiarrhythmia Devices. Available at: http://www.acc.org/clinical/guidelines/pacemaker/index.htm. Accessed 3/1/06

23. Priori SG, Aliot E, Blomstrom-Lundqvist C et al (2001) Task Force Report Task Force on Sudden Cardiac Death of the European Society of Cardiology. Eur Heart J 22:1374-1450

24. Zipes DP, Camm AJ, Borggrefe M et al (2006) ACC/AHA/ESC 2006 guidelines for management of patients with ventricular arrhythmias and the prevention of sudden cardiac death. Eur Heart J 27:2099-2140

MANAGEMENT OF HEART FAILURE

CHAPTER 21

Elzbieta Katarzyna Wlodarska, Marek Konka

Introduction

Arrhythmogenic right ventricular cardiomyopathy/dysplasia (ARVC/D) has long been considered a disease with the risk of sudden cardiac death (SCD) [1, 2]. Life-threatening arrhythmias have been emphasized as the main clinical feature and major therapeutic problem. In long-term follow-up studies, high rates of SCD have been reported, particularly in the young. Enormous progress has been made in recent years in the treatment of arrhythmias, changing the clinical outcome of ARVC/D. Implantable cardioverter-defibrillator (ICD) implantation, radiofrequency (RF) ablation or hybrid therapy for high-risk patients have significantly decreased the incidence of SCD in this group of patients. Worldwide awareness of the disease, advances in diagnostic procedures, preparticipation screening tests of young athletes, and family examinations have identified affected people early and enabled proper management, decreasing the incidence of SCD as the first symptom of the disease. Success in the fight against SCD unmasked the problem of heart failure in patients with a longer disease history.

Heart Failure in ARVC/D

In the first follow-up studies of ARVC/D patients, heart failure was described as a rare event. In 1987 Blomstrom-Lundqvist et al. reported three cases of right heart failure among 15 patients with ARVC/D observed for 1.5-28 (mean 8.8) years [3]. Two of them died, one suddenly, the other due to congestive heart failure. The prognostic importance of heart failure was raised by Pinamonti et al. in 1992, who observed significantly higher mortality of patients who presented heart failure symptoms than in patients with arrhythmias (p=0.038) [4]. Heart failure was observed by Peters et al. in 13 patients (11%) of a consecutive cohort of 121 patients with ARVC/D over a period of 12 years [5]. Three of them died and three others underwent or were waiting for heart transplantation. A review of the literature up to 1999 indicated that 46% of cardiac deaths in clinical series of patients with ARVC/D were due to heart failure. Later this proportion began to change. Patients who died due to heart failure or underwent heart transplantation in large clinical series reported in 2003-2005 represented 47%-66% of all cases of cardiac terminal events (Table 21.1) [5-8]. The mean age of patients who died because of severe pump failure or underwent heart transplantation was significantly higher than those who died suddenly both in the pathologic study of Basso et al. [9] and clinical series of Peters [10].

Isolated right ventricular failure in ARVC/D, being a result of dilatation, wall thinning and wall motion dysfunction due to loss of cardiomyocytes,

Table 21.1 • Risk of nonsudden cardiac death in patients with ARVC/D – a systematic review of literature

Author	No pts	Follow-up (years, mean)	HF % pts	NSCD+OHT No pts
Blomstrom-Lundqvist, 1987 [3]	15	8.8	20%	1
Peters, 1999 [5]	121	4-8	11%	3+3
Hulot, 2004 [6]	130	8	16%	5+2
Lemola, 2005 [7]	61	4.6	11%	2+5
Corrado, 2003 [8]	132 (ICD)	3.3		4

HF, heart failure; *NSCD*, nonsudden cardiac death; *OHT*, orthotopic heart transplantation; *pts*, patients

represents a unique clinical situation where right heart failure is accompanied by low pulmonary pressure. As only 5 mm Hg is a sufficient pressure difference to provide adequate pulmonary flow, even severe damage of the right ventricle (RV) muscle has no apparent effect on hemodynamics. Paradoxical ventricular septum motion and prominent right atrial contraction provide functional compensation enabling normal physical activity for a long time. It is not well known what factors are a trigger for symptoms of right ventricular failure. Left ventricle (LV) damage, superimposed myocarditis, atrial fibrillation, incessant ventricular tachycardia, and RV thrombosis are the most frequent mechanisms bringing mild RV heart failure symptoms.

Extensive damage of the RV leading to isolated RV failure symptoms is more frequent in the fatty variant of the disease, characterized by intensive fatty infiltration of the RV, reaching the endocardium and sparing the LV and septum (Fig. 21.1),

whereas biventricular failure mimicking dilated cardiomyopathy, is observed in the fibro-fatty variant [11].

LV damage in patients with ARVC/D is known to be a risk factor of SCD as well as congestive heart failure and non-SCD [7, 12, 13]. It is not unusual, particularly in the fibrofatty variant of the disease. LV damage is observed in up to 55% patients and is characterized by focal hypokinesis at the apex and infero-posterior wall without severe chamber dilatation or, less frequently, by diffuse hypokinesis and moderate dilatation (Fig. 21.2) [14]. Macroscopic and histological involvement of the LV was observed even in 76% of hearts with ARVC/D and was characterized by similar abnormalities to those found in the RV with a predominance of fibrosis [15]. In some genetic forms of the disease, LV damage appears early and leads to a clinical picture of dilated cardiomyopathy more frequently than in other forms of the disease. In ARVD8 (desmoplakin gene mutation) LV involvement was seen in 43%, and heart failure symptoms in 14% of patients [16]. LV damage is also a typical feature of ARVD4, although severe manifestation of symptoms was reported only in patients involved in sport activities [17].

A possible mechanism of progressive right or biventricular failure, triggering apoptosis and necrosis due to Ca^{2+} ions overloading, is inflammation. Inflammatory cells (CD43-positive lymphocytes) are detected in two-thirds of cases with the fibrofatty variant of the disease [11]. Fontaine and colleagues demonstrated progression of the disease due to superimposed inflammation [18]. Although viral myocarditis was demonstrated only in single cases, increased susceptibility to infection

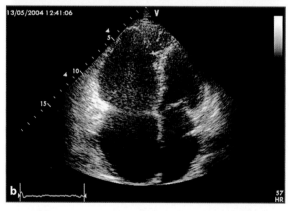

Fig. 21.1 • ARVC/D-fatty variant. **a** Heart removed at cardiac transplantation. **b** Two-dimensional echocardiogram of an apical four-chamber examination. Dilated right ventricle and regular diameter of left ventricle

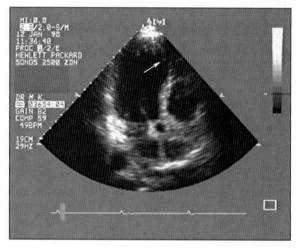

Fig. 21.2 • Left ventricular (LV) involvement in ARVC/D. Parasternal long-axis apical view. Apical aneurysm of LV (*arrow*)

with cardiotropic viruses in the diseased myocardium cannot be excluded [19].

The most important clinical marker of diffuse RV lesions with LV involvement, significantly associated with thromboembolism and heart failure, is atrial fibrillation (AF). Supraventricular tachyarrhythmias are not rare in ARVC/D. Supraventricular tachycardia, paroxysmal atrial tachycardia, and AF are reported in clinical series observed in 14%-28% cases [7, 20-21]. Patients with supraventricular arrhythmias are older and have a longer disease duration. Whereas supraventricular tachycardias are probably a result of electrical instability of the right atrial myocardium, AF is tightly connected with advanced RV damage and often accompanied by LV impairment. Lack of atrium contraction worsens RV function, resulting in apparent heart failure symptoms [22].

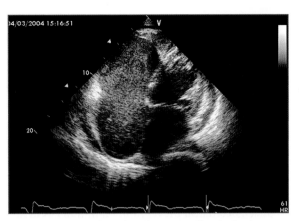

Fig. 21.4 • Apical four-chamber view. Cloud of echoes resulting from stagnant blood – echogenic blood – in right chambers

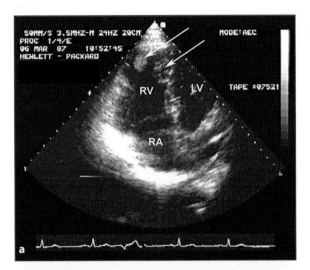

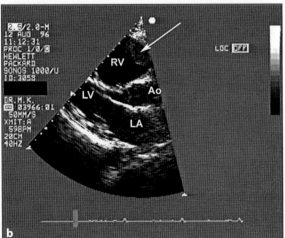

Fig. 21.3 • **a** Apical four-chamber view. Thrombus in the RV apex (*arrows*). **b** RV outflow tract with thrombus from parasternal long axis view (*arrow*). *Ao*, aorta; *LV*, left ventricle; *RA*, right atrium; *RV*, right ventricle. From [27]

There are very few reports available on thromboembolic complications in patients with ARVC/D. Most of them describe atrial thrombus formation in patients with the extensive form of the disease and with concomitant AF [23-26]. RV thrombosis is usually associated with severe dilatation of the RV and significant wall motion abnormalities [27]. The incidence of thromboembolic complications in ARVC/D seems to be less frequent than in patients with left ventricular failure of other causes (annual incidence: 0.48 vs. 1.9%, respectively) [27]. Despite their rare occurrence, these complications should not be underestimated because their clinical presentation is usually quite serious. Both pulmonary embolism with fatal outcome and severe heart failure in case of RV outflow tract thrombosis have been observed (Fig. 21.3). In patients with a severely dilated and akinetic RV, spontaneous echocardiographic contrast due to stagnant blood may be also observed (Fig. 21.4).

Management of Heart Failure

Management of patients with RV or biventricular heart failure includes diuretics, angiotensin-converting enzyme inhibitors, and β-blockers. A new selective aldosterone antagonist – eplerenone – has recently been reported to be effective in combined diuretic treatment [28]. Beta-blockers, next to their antiarrhythmic activity, are known to inhibit apoptosis [29]. Anticoagulant therapy is obligatory in patients with AF and highly recommended in those with severe RV damage and spontaneous echocardiographic contrast in the RV.

Sinus rhythm control in patients with ARVC/D is essential. Maintaining sinus rhythm is a difficult task and the therapeutic goal is to postpone permanent AF as long as possible. Amiodarone, less effective than sotalol in ventricular arrhythmias and burdened with a high incidence of side-effects, is entirely justified in prophylactic therapy of AF. In management of acute AF, both pharmacological conversion and electrical cardioversion are possible. In patients with heart failure symptoms and long-lasting AF, rhythm conversion should be attempted. In recurrent AF resulting in deterioration of heart function and refractory to pharmacological prevention, pulmonary vein ablation should be considered.

Ablation is indicated in patients with incessant or frequent sustained ventricular tachycardias that worsen ventricle function.

In patients with isolated right ventricular failure refractory to pharmacological therapy, a surgical approach was proposed by Chachques et al. [30]. They applied modifications to the conventional LV cardiomyoplasty procedure by using the left latissimus dorsi muscle to perform RV cardiomyoplasty. In a 10-year follow up of four patients with ARVC/D after the procedure, the authors observed hemodynamic and functional improvement without perioperative mortality, life-threatening arrhythmias, and RV-failure related deaths.

Recently, right ventricular exclusion surgery (Fontan-type repair) has been used in patients with ARVC/D [31, 32]. Theoretically, patients with ARVC/D are ideal candidates for this procedure, because they fulfill selection criteria for this kind of surgery (low pulmonary pressure, normal LV function). It may be an alternative treatment for refractory patients with sinus rhythm before heart transplantation is considered. In critically ill patients it may be a rescue procedure when waiting for a donor.

Patients with biventricular heart failure become candidates for heart transplantation. However, heart transplant carries only 50% survival at 12 years and it should avoided or postponed as long as possible [33]. RV resynchronization was recently proposed for patients with congenital heart defects with RV failure and its beneficial role was shown by some authors, suggesting that it may be a promising, novel method of therapy for patients with chronic RV failure [34, 35]. No data are available concerning potential clinical benefit of cardiac resynchronization therapy in ARVC/D. Further studies are needed to determine its role in this disease. As ARVC/D is a genetically determined entity, genetic engineering is expected to bring novel therapeutic proposals.

Acknowledgements

This work was supported by grant QLRT-2001-02854, the 5th Framework Program of the European Commission, Brussels, 1998-2006.

References

1. Marcus FI, Fontaine G, Guiraudon G et al (1982) Right ventricular dysplasia. A report of 24 adult cases. Circulation 65:384-398
2. Thiene G, Nava A, Corrado D et al (1988) Right ventricular cardiomyopathy and sudden death in young people. New Engl J Med 318:129-133
3. Blomström-Lundqvist C, Sabel KG, Olsson SB (1987) A long-term follow up of 15 patients with arrhythmogenic right ventricular dysplasia. Br Heart J 58:477-488
4. Pinamonti B, Sinagra G, Salvi A et al (1992) Left ventricular involvement in right ventricular dysplasia. Am Heart J 123:711-724
5. Peters S, Peters H, Thierfelder L (1999) Heart failure in arrhythmogenic right ventricular dysplasia/cardiomyopathy. Int J Cardiol 71:251-256
6. Hulot J-S, Jouven X, Empana J-P et al (2004) Natural history and risk stratification of arrhythmogenic right ventricular dysplasia/cardiomyopathy. Circulation 110:1879-1884
7. Lemola K, Brunckhorst C, Helfenstein U et al (2005) Predictors of adverse outcome in patients with arrhythmogenic right ventricular dysplasia/cardiomyopathy: Long-term experience of a tertiary care centre. Heart 91:1167-1172
8. Corrado D, Leoni L, Link MS et al (2003) Implantable cardioverter-defibrillator therapy for prevention of sudden death in patients with arrhythmogenic right ventricular dysplasia/cardiomyopathy. Circulation 108:3084-3091
9. Basso C, Corrado D, Rossi L, Thiene G (1997) Morbid anatomy. In: Nava A, Rossi L, Thiene G (eds) Arrhythmogenic right ventricular cardiomyopathy/ dysplasia. Elsevier, Amsterdam, pp 71-86
10. Peters S (1996) Age related dilatation of the right ventricle in arrhythmogenic right ventricular dysplasia-cardiomyopathy. Int J Cardiol 56:163-167
11. Basso C, Thiene G, Corrado D et al (1996) Arrhythmogenic right ventricular cardiomyopathy: dysplasia, dystrophy or myocarditis? Circulation 94:983-991
12. Pinamonti B, Camerini F (1997) Left ventricular involvement, progression of the disease and prognosis. In: Nava A, Rossi L, Thiene G (eds) Arrhythmogenic right ventricular cardiomyopathy/dysplasia. Elsevier, Amsterdam, pp 46-60
13. Wlodarska EK, Konka M, Wozniak O et al (2005) Left ventricular damage in patients with arrhythmogenic right ventricular cardiomyopathy. Eur J Heart Failure 4:85 (abstr 387)

14. Pinamonti B, Miani D, Sinagra G et al (1996) Familial right ventricular dysplasia with biventricular involvement and inflammatory infiltration. Heart 76:66-69

15. Corrado D, Basso C, Thiene G et al (1997) Spectrum of clinicopathologic manifestations of arrhythmogenic right ventricular cardiomyopathy/dysplasia: A multicenter study. J Am Coll Cardiol 30:1512-1520

16. Bauce B, Basso C, Rampazzo A et al (2005) Clinical profile of four families with arrhythmogenic right ventricular cardiomyopathy caused by dominant desmoplakin mutation. Eur Heart J 26:1666-1675

17. Rampazzo A, Nava A, Miorin M et al (1997) ARVD4, a new locus for arrhythmogenic right ventricular cardiomyopathy, maps to chromosome 2 long arm. Genomics 45:259-263

18. Fontaine G, Fontaliran F, Rosas Andrade F et al (1995) The arrhythmogenic right ventricle. Dysplasia versus cardiomyopathy. Heart Vessels 10:227-235

19. Bowles NE, Ni J, Marcus F et al (2002) The detection of cardiotropic viruses in the myocardium of patients with arrhythmogenic right ventricular dysplasia/cardiomyopathy. J Am Coll Cardiol 39:892-895

20. Corrado D, Fontaine G, Marcus FI et al (2001) Atrial electrical instability in arrhythmogenic right ventricular dysplasia/cardiomyopathy: Part of the substrate or consequence of the disease. Eur Heart J 22:705

21. Tonet J, Castro MR, Iwa T et al (1991) Frequency of supraventricular tachyarrhythmias in arrhythmogenic right ventricular dysplasia. Am J Cardiol 67:1153

22. Wlodarska EK, Konka M, Walczak F et al (2004) Atrial fibrillation is a risk factor of heart failure in arrhythmogenic right ventricular cardiomyopathy. Eur J Heart Failure 3:6

23. Lui CY, Marcus FI, Sobonya RE (2002) Arrhytmogenic right ventricular dysplasia masquerading as peripartum cardiomyopathy with atrial flutter, advanced atrioventricular block and embolic stroke. Cardiology 97:49-50

24. Goldberg L (2000) Right ventricular thrombosis in arrhythmogenic right ventricular dysplasia. Cardiovasc J S Afr 11:95-96

25. Attenhoffer Jost CH, Bombeli T, Schrimpf C et al (2000) Extensive thrombus formation in the right ventricle due to a rare combination of arrhythmogenic right ventricular cardiomyopathy and heterozygous prothrombin gene mutation G20210 A. Cardiology 93:127-130

26. Antonini-Canterin F, Sandrini R, Pavan D et al (2000) Right ventricular thrombosis in arrhythmogenic cardiomyopathy. A case report. Ital Heart J 1:415-418

27. Wlodarska EK, Wozniak O, Konka M et al (2006) Thromboembolic complications in patients with arrhythmogenic right ventricular dysplasia/cardiomyopathy. Europace 8:596-600

28. Marcy TR, Ripley TL (2006) Aldosterone antagonists in the treatment of heart failure. Am J Health Syst Pharm 63:49-58

29. Packer M (1996) The apoptosis model of congestive heart failure: A differentiation factor for carvedilol. Proceedings of heart failure. European Congress of Cardiology, Birmingham. Eur Heart J 17:78 (abstr 9475)

30. Chachques JC, Argyriadis PG, Fontaine G et al (2003) Right ventricular cardiomyoplasty: 10-year follow up. Ann Thorac Surg 75:1464-1468

31. Sano S, Ishino K, Kawada M et al (2002) Total right ventricular exclusion procedure: An operation for isolated congestive right ventricular failure. J Thorac Cardiovasc Surg 123:640-647

32. Motta P, Mossad E, Savage R (2003) Right ventricular exclusion surgery for arrhythmogenic right ventricular dysplasia with cardiomyopathy. Anesth Analg 96:1598-1602

33. Boucek MM, Edwards LB, Keck MB et al (2003) The registry of International Society for Heart and Lung Transplantation. J Heart Lung Transplant 22:636-653

34. Janoušek J, Tomek V, Chaloupecký V et al (2004) Cardiac resynchronization therapy: A novel adjunct to the treatment and prevention of systemic right ventricular failure. J Am Coll Cardiol 44:1927-1931

35. Dubin AM, Feinstein JA, Reddy M et al (2003) Electrical resynchronization. A novel therapy for the failing right ventricle. 107:2287-2289

CHAPTER 22

SUDDEN DEATH IN YOUNG ATHLETES

Domenico Corrado, Cristina Basso, Gaetano Thiene

Introduction

Although sudden death during sport is a rare event, it always has a tragic impact because it occurs in apparently healthy individuals and assumes great visibility through the news media, due to the high public profile of competitive athletes [1-4]. For centuries it was a mystery why cardiac arrest should occur in vigorous athletes, who had previously achieved extraordinary exercise performance without any symptoms. The cause was generally ascribed to myocardial infarction, even though evidence of ischemic myocardial necrosis was rarely reported. It is now clear that the most common mechanism of sudden death during sports activity is an abrupt ventricular tachyarrhythmia as a consequence of a wide spectrum of cardiovascular diseases, either acquired or congenital [2, 4, 5]. The culprit diseases are often clinically silent and unlikely to be suspected or diagnosed on the basis of spontaneous symptoms. Systematic cardiovascular screening (including 12-lead ECG) of all subjects embarking in sports activity has the potential to identify those athletes at risk and to reduce mortality [6].

Arrhythmogenic right ventricular cardiomyopathy/dysplasia (ARVC/D) is an inherited heart muscle disease that predominantly affects the right ventricle (RV) and is characterized pathologically by RV myocardial atrophy with fibro-fatty replacement. Clinically, the disease presents with ventricular electrical instability leading to ventricular tachycardia or ventricular fibrillation which may precipitate cardiac arrest, particularly during physical exercise [7-9].

In this chapter we will examine the role of ARVC/D in causing sudden death in young competitive athletes and suggest a prevention strategy based on identification of affected athletes at preparticipation screening.

Sudden Death in the Athlete

The frequency with which sudden death occurs in young athletes during organized competitive sports is very low and varies in the different series reported in the literature. In a retrospective analysis conducted in the US, the prevalence of fatal events in high school and college athletes, 12-24 years of age, has been estimated to be less than 1 in 100,000 per year [10, 11], whereas a prospective population-based study in Italy reported a three times greater incidence among competitive athletes 12-35 years of age [12].

The vast majority of athletes who die suddenly have underlying structural heart disease, which provides a substrate for ventricular fibrillation. Sudden cardiac death is usually the result of an interaction between transient acute abnormalities ("trigger") and structural cardiovascular abnormalities ("substrate").

Triggers of sudden death in young competitive athletes include exercise-related sympathetic stimulation, abrupt hemodynamic changes and acute myocardial ischemia leading to life-threatening ventricular arrhythmias. As shown in Table 22.1, the pathological causes of sudden death reflect the age of participants. Although atherosclerotic coronary artery disease accounts for the vast majority of fatalities in adults (age >35 years) [13-15], in younger athletes there is a broad

Table 22.1 • Cardiovascular causes of sudden death associated with sports

Age ≥35 years
Atherosclerotic coronary artery disease
Age <35 years
Hypertrophic cardiomyopathy
Arrhythmogenic right ventricular cardiomyopathy/ dysplasia
Premature coronary atherosclerosis
Congenital anomalies of coronary arteries
Myocarditis
Aortic rupture
Valvular disease
Pre-excitation syndromes and conduction diseases
Ion channel diseases
Congenital heart disease, operated or unoperated

spectrum of cardiovascular substrates (including congenital and inherited heart disorders) [5, 10, 12, 16-20]. Cardiomyopathies have been consistently implicated as the leading cause of sports-related cardiac arrest in the young, with hypertrophic cardiomyopathy accounting for more than one third of fatal cases in the US [3] and ARVC/D for approximately one fourth in the Veneto region of Italy [6]. Other cardiovascular substrates include congenital coronary anomalies, premature atherosclerotic coronary artery disease, myocarditis, dilated cardiomyopathy, mitral valve prolapse, conduction system diseases, and WPW syndrome. Rarely sudden death may be due to either a nonarrhythmic cause such as aortic rupture complicating Marfan syndrome and bicuspid aortic valve or by noncardiac conditions including bronchial asthma and rupture of a cerebral aneurysm.

Six to ten percent of sudden death victims have no evidence of structural heart disease and the cause of their sudden death is probably related to a primary electrical heart disorder such as inherited cardiac ion channels defects (channelopathies) including long and short QT syndromes, catecholaminergic polymorphic ventricular tachycardia, and Brugada syndrome [21-24].

Finally, sudden death during sport can also be the result of a nonpenetrating blow to the chest wall (commotio cordis), which can trigger abrupt ventricular fibrillation in the absence of any cardiac structural lesions [25].

ARVC/D: A Leading Cause of Sudden Death in Young Athletes

Systematic monitoring and pathologic investigation of sudden death in young people and athletes of the Veneto Region of Italy showed that ARVC/D is the most common pathologic substrate accounting for nearly one fourth of fatal events on the athletic field [6, 12]. The incidence of sudden death from ARVC/D in athletes is estimated to be 0.5 per 100,000 persons per year (Fig. 22.1). Sudden death victims with ARVC/D were all males with a mean age of 22.6±4 years [12].

The hallmark lesion of the disease is the extensive replacement of the RV myocardium by fibrofatty tissue (Fig. 22.2). The autopsied hearts demonstrate massive regional or diffuse fibrofatty infiltration, parchment-like and translucence of the RV free wall, and mild to moderate RV dilatation, together with aneurysmal dilatations of postero-basal, apical, and outflow tract regions. These RV pathologic features allow differential diagnosis with training-induced RV adaptation ("athlete's heart"), usually consisting

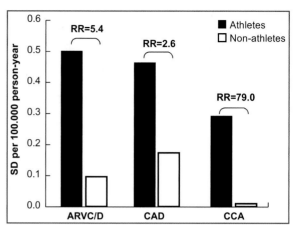

Fig. 22.1 • Incidence and relative risk (RR) of sudden death from major cardiovascular causes among young athletes and nonathletes. *ARVC/D*, arrhythmogenic right ventricular cardiomyopathy/dysplasia; *CAD*, coronary artery disease; *CCA*, congenital coronary artery anomalies. Modified from [12]

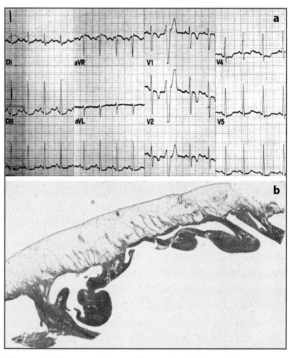

Fig. 22.2 • Electrocardiographic and pathologic features in a 19-year-old soccer player who died suddenly from ARVC/D. (**a**) Twelve-lead ECG obtained at preparticipation screening showing typical abnormalities consisting of inverted T waves from V1 to V4 and premature ventricular beats with a left bundle branch block morphology; (**b**) Panoramic histological view of the RV free wall showing transmural fibro-fatty replacement of myocardium (Heidenhain trichrome). Modified from [37]

of global RV enlargement without regional dilation/dysfunction. Histologically, fibro-fatty infiltration is usually associated with focal myocardial necrosis and patchy inflammatory infiltrates. It is noteworthy that fibrofatty scar and aneurysms are potential sources of life-threatening ventricular arrhythmias. The histopathologic arrangement of the surviving myocardium embedded in the replacing fibrofatty tissue may lead to non-homogeneous intraventricular conduction predisposing to re-entrant mechanisms.

The advent of molecular genetic era has provided new insights in understanding the pathogenesis of ARVC/D, showing that it is a desmosomal disease resulting from defective cell adhesion proteins such as plakoglobin, desmoplakin, plakophilin-2, desmoglein-2, and desmocollin-2 [26]. It has been hypothesized that the lack of the protein, or the incorporation of mutant protein into cardiac desmosomes, may provoke detachment of myocytes at the intercalated discs, particularly under the condition of mechanical stress during training and competitive sports activity [27, 28]. As a consequence, there is progressive myocyte death with subsequent repair by fibrofatty replacement. Life-threatening ventricular arrhythmias may occur either during the "hot phase" of myocyte death as abrupt ventricular fibrillation or later in the form of scar-related macro-re-entrant ventricular tachycardia [29].

Risk of Sudden Death from ARVC/D During Physical Exercise

A prospective clinico-pathologic study of sudden death in the young in the Veneto region of Italy demonstrated that adolescents and young adults involved in sports activity have a 2.8 times greater risk of sudden cardiovascular death than their nonathletic counterparts [12]. However, sports itself is not the cause of the enhanced mortality, but it triggers cardiac arrest in those athletes who have cardiovascular conditions that predispose to life-threatening ventricular arrhythmias during physical exercise such as cardiomyopathy (primarily hypertrophic cardiomyopathy and ARVC/D), premature coronary artery disease, and congenital coronary artery anomalies.

ARVC/D leads to sudden death during physical exercise with an estimated 5.4 times greater risk of dying suddenly during competitive sports than during sedentary activity (Fig. 22.1). The reason for the propensity for ARVC/D to precipitate effort-dependent sudden cardiac arrest is not completely known. Physical exercise acutely increases the RV afterload and cavity enlargement, which in turn may elicit ventricular arrhythmias by stretching the diseased RV myocardium [30]. Mechanical stress such as that occurring during training and sports competition may provoke myocyte death and associated ventricular arrhythmias in the presence of genetically defective desmosomes [26-28]. The adverse effect of exercise on the phenotypic expression of ARVC/D was recently addressed by Kirchhof et al. in an experimental study on heterozygous plakoglobin-deficient mice [31]. As compared to wild-type controls, mutant mice had increased RV volume, reduced RV function, and more frequent and severe ventricular tachycardia of RV origin. Endurance training accelerated the development of RV dysfunction and arrhythmias in plakoglobin-deficient mice.

Alternatively, a "denervation supersensitivity" of the RV to catecholamines has been advanced to explain exercise-induced ventricular arrhythmias [32]. Sympathetic nerve trunks may be damaged and/or interrupted by the RV fibrofatty replacement which distinctively progresses from the epicardium to the endocardium, resulting in a denervation supersensitivity to catecholamines. Arrhythmogenic mechanisms in the denervated supersensitive myofibers include dispersion of refractoriness and re-entry, triggered activity, or both.

Finally, in a subgroup of patients with familial ARVC/D, a cardiac ryanodine receptor (RYR2) missense mutation leading to abnormal calcium release from the sarcoplasmic reticulum has been identified [33]. Wall mechanical stress, such as that induced by RV volume overload during exercise, is expected to exacerbate the cardiac ryanodine channel dysfunction [33]. Therefore, a potential arrhythmogenic mechanism of sport-related cardiac arrest in patients with ARVC/D is triggered by activity due to late afterdepolarizations, which are provoked by intracellular calcium overload and enhanced by adrenergic stimulation [34].

Causes of Sudden Death in Young Athletes: Italian vs. US Experience

Although ARVC/D has been demonstrated to be the leading cause of sudden death in athletes of the Veneto region of Italy, studies in the US showed a higher prevalence of other pathologic substrates such as hypertrophic cardiomyopathy, anomalous coronary arteries, and myocarditis [1, 3, 10].

This discrepancy may be explained by several factors. There have been no previous investigations such as the "Juvenile Sudden Death" Research Project in the Veneto region of Italy that have prospectively investigated a consecutive series of sudden death in young people occurring in a well-defined geographic area with an homogeneous ethnic group. Therefore, the previously reported causes in the US may have been influenced by the unavoidable limitations in patient selection because of retrospective analysis. Moreover, in other large studies, the autopsies were usually performed by different examiners, including local pathologists and medical examiners [10]. In the Italian study, to obtain a higher level of confidence in the results, morphological examination of all hearts was performed according to a standard protocol by the same group of experienced cardiovascular pathologists. Comparison between the previous and the present study with regard to the prevalence of ARVC/D among the causes of sudden death in young people and athletes is limited by the fact that ARVC/D is a clinical-pathologic condition which has been discovered only recently [7, 35]. ARVC/D is rarely associated with cardiomegaly and usually spares the left ventricle, so that affected hearts may be erroneously diagnosed as normal hearts [7-9]. In the past, therefore, a number of sudden deaths in young people and athletes, in which the routine pathologic examination disclosed a normal heart, may, in fact, have been due to unrecognized ARVC/D. The high incidence of ARVC/D in the Veneto region may be due to a genetic factor in the population of northeastern Italy [26], although ARVC/D can no longer be considered as peculiar "Venetian disease" since there is growing evidence that it is ubiquitous, still largely underdiagnosed both clinically and at postmortem investigation, and accounts for significant arrhythmic morbidity and mortality worldwide [9, 36].

Preparticipation screening of young people embarking in competitive athletic activity which is in practice in Italy for more than 20 years has changed the prevalence of pathologic substrates of sports-related sudden death. We recently demonstrated that sudden death from hypertrophic cardiomyopathy in athletic fields was successfully prevented by identification and disqualification of the affected athletes at preparticipation screening [6]. As a consequence of this process, other cardiovascular conditions such as ARVC/D and premature coronary artery disease have thereby come to account for a greater proportion of all sudden deaths in Italian athletes.

Clinical Profile of Athletes Dying Suddenly from ARVC/D

Early identification of athletes with ARVC/D plays a crucial role in the prevention of sudden death during sports. The most frequent clinical manifestations of the disease consist of ECG depolarization/repolarization changes mostly localized to right precordial leads, global and/or regional morphologic and functional alterations of the RV, and arrhythmias of RV origin [7-9, 36-38]. The disease should be suspected even in asymptomatic individuals on the basis of ECG abnormalities and ventricular arrhythmias [2, 6, 7]. Ultimately, the diagnosis relies on visualization of morphofunctional RV abnormalities by imaging techniques (such as echocardiography, angiography, and cardiac magnetic resonance) and, in selected cases, by histopathologic demonstration of fibrofatty substitution at endomyocardial biopsy [37].

It is noteworthy that more than 80% of athletes of the Veneto Region series who died from ARVC/D had a history of syncope, ECG changes, or ventricular arrhythmias [6] (Fig. 22.2). More recently, we confirmed this data by reviewing clinical and ECG findings from a Multicenter International Registry in 22 young competitive athletes who died suddenly of ARVC/D proven at autopsy [39]. Right precordial inverted T-waves (beyond lead V1) had been recorded in 88% of athletes who had a 12-lead ECG during life and subsequently died suddenly; right precordial QRS duration >110 msec in 76%, and ventricular arrhythmias with a left bundle branch block pattern in 76%, mostly in the form of isolated/coupled premature ventricular beats or nonsustained ventricular tachycardia. Limited exercise testing induced ventricular arrhythmias in six of twelve athletes (50%). Submaximal exercise testing, available in five athletes, showed a "pseudo" normalization of right precordial repolarization abnormalities in all. Thus, the majority of young competitive athletes who died suddenly from ARVC/D showed ECG abnormalities that could raise the suspicion of the underlying cardiovascular disease at preparticipation evaluation and lead to further testing for a definitive diagnosis. Right precordial T-wave inversion (beyond V1) appears to be the most useful clinical marker for the presence of a potentially fatal ARVC/D in apparently healthy young competitive athletes, considering that T-wave inversion in V1-V3 occurs in <1% of men with apparently normal hearts, age 19-45 [40].

Preparticipation Screening and Prevention of Sudden Death

For more than 20 years systematic preparticipation screening, based on 12-lead ECG in addition to history and physical examination, has been the practice in Italy [6, 41]. This screening strategy has proven to be effective in the identification of athletes with previously undiagnosed hypertrophic cardiomyopathy, due to the high sensitivity (up to

95%) of 12-lead ECG for suspicion/detection of this condition in otherwise asymptomatic athletes. Moreover, during long-term follow-up no deaths were recorded among these disqualified athletes with hypertrophic cardiomyopathy, suggesting that restriction from competition may reduce the risk of sudden death [6].

Despite the high prevalence of ECG abnormalities, such as T-wave inversion in right precordial leads and ventricular arrhythmias with a left bundle branch block morphology at preparticipation evaluation, the majority of sudden death victims from ARVC/D had not been identified at preparticipation screening, thus explaining why this condition was previously reported to be the leading cause of sudden death in Italian athletes [6, 12]. The most plausible explanation is that, unlike HCM, ARVC/D is a condition that was discovered only recently (approximately two decades ago) and was either underdiagnosed or regarded with skepticism by cardiologists. Recently, Corrado et al. reported the results of a time-trend analysis of the changes in incidence rates and causes of sudden cardiovascular death in young athletes age 12-35 years in the Veneto region of Italy between 1979 and 2004, after the introduction of systematic preparticipation screening [42]. Over the same time interval, they performed a parallel study which examined trends in cardiovascular causes of disqualification from competitive sports in 42,386 athletes undergoing preparticipation screening at the Center for Sports Medicine in Padua. Fifty-five sudden cardiovascular deaths occurred in screened athletes (1.9 deaths/100,000 person-years) and 265 deaths in unscreened nonathletes (0.79 deaths/100,000 person-years). The annual incidence of sudden cardiovascular death in athletes decreased by approximately 90%, from 3.6/100,000 person-years in 1979-1980 to 0.4/100,000 person-years in 2001-2004, whereas the incidence of sudden death among the unscreened nonathletic population did not change significantly over that time. The decline in the death rate started after mandatory screening was initiated and persisted to the late screening period. Compared with the pre-screening period (1979-1981), the relative risk of sudden cardiovascular death was 44% lower in the early screening period (1982-1992) and 79% lower in the late screening period (1993-2004). Most of the reduced death rate was due to fewer cases of sudden death from cardiomyopathies, mostly from ARVC/D. Time-trend analysis showed that the incidence of sudden death from this latter condition fell by 84% over the 24-year span (Fig. 22.3). This decline of mortality from cardiomyopathies paralleled the concomitant increase in the number of athletes with cardiomyopathies (both

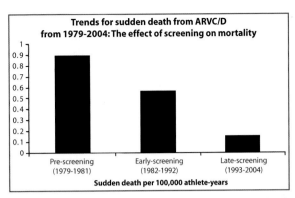

Fig. 22.3 • Average annual incidence rates of sudden death from ARVC/D among young competitive athletes of the Veneto Region of Italy, before and after implementation of systematic preparticipation screening. Death rates from ARVC/D declined from 0.90 per 100,000 person-years in the 1979-1981 prescreening period to 0.15 per 100,000 in the 1993-2004 late-screening-period (RR=0.16, 95% CI 0.03-1.41; p for trend=0.02)

hypertrophic cardiomyopathy and ARVC/D) who were identified and disqualified from competitive sports over the screening periods at the Center for Sports Medicine in Padua. Screening athletes for cardiomyopathies is a life-saving strategy and 12-lead ECG is a sensitive and powerful tool for identification, risk stratification and management of athletes affected by hypertrophic cardiomyopathy and ARVC/D [41, 42].

Sports Eligibility

The ultimate diagnosis of cardiomyopathy in a young competitive athlete can be difficult due to the presence of physiologic (and reversible) structural and electrical adaptations of the cardiovascular system to long-term athletic training. This condition known as "athlete's heart" is characterized by an increase in ventricular cavity dimension and wall thickness which overlaps with cardiomyopathies [43]. An accurate differential diagnosis is crucial not only because of the potentially adverse outcome associated with cardiomyopathy in an athlete, but also due to the possibility of misdiagnosis of pathologic conditions requiring unnecessary disqualification from sport, with financial and psychological consequences.

A sizable proportion of highly trained athletes have an increase in RV cavity dimensions which raises the question of ARVC/D. Morphologic criteria in favor of physiologic RV enlargement consists of preserved global and regional ventricular function, without evidence of wall motion abnormalities such as dyskinetic regions and/or diastolic bulgings.

During the last two decades, advances in molecular genetics have allowed identification of a growing number of defective genes involved in the pathogenesis of ARVC/D [26]. The hope is that molecular genetic tests will be available clinically in the near future for definitive differential diagnosis between ARVC/D and training-related physiologic RV changes.

According to US and European recommendations for sports eligibility [44, 45], athletes with clinical diagnosis of ARVD/C should be excluded from all competitive sports. This recommendation is independent of age, gender, and phenotypic appearance and does not differ for those athletes without symptoms, or treatment with drugs, or interventions with surgery, catheter ablation, or the implantable defibrillator. The presence of a free-standing automated external defibrillator at sporting events should not be considered absolute protection against sudden death [46], nor a justification for participation in competitive sports in athletes with previously diagnosed ARVD/C [44, 45, 47].

Acknowledgements

The study was supported by grants from the Ministry of Health, Rome, Italy, European Comunity research contract #QLG1-CT-2000-01091 and the Veneto Region, Venice, Italy.

References

1. Maron BJ, Roberts WC, McAllister MA et al (1980) Sudden death in young athletes. Circulation 62:218-229
2. Corrado D, Thiene G, Nava A et al (1990) Sudden death in young competitive athletes: Clinico-pathologic correlations in 22 cases. Am J Med 89:588-596
3. Maron BJ (2003) Sudden death in young athletes. New Engl J Med 349:1064-1075
4. Corrado D, Basso C, Thiene G (2005) Sudden death in young athletes. Lancet S47-S48
5. Basso C, Frescura C, Corrado D et al (1995) Congenital heart disease and sudden death in the young. Hum Path 26:1065-1072
6. Corrado D, Basso C, Schiavon M et al (1998) Screening for hypertrophic cardiomyopathy in young athletes. New Engl J Med 339:364-369
7. Thiene G, Nava A, Corrado D et al (1988) Right ventricular cardiomyopathy and sudden death in young people. N Engl J Med 318:129-133
8. Basso C, Thiene G, Corrado D et al (1996) Arrhythmogenic right ventricular cardiomyopathy. Dysplasia, dystrophy, or myocarditis? Circulation 94:983-989
9. Corrado D, Basso C, Thiene G et al (1997) Spectrum of clinicopathologic manifestations of arrhythmogenic right ventricular cardiomyopathy/dysplasia: A multicenter study. J Am Coll Cardiol 30:1512-1520
10. Van Camp SP, Bloor CM, Mueller FO et al (1995) Non-traumatic sports death in high school and college athletes. Med Sci Sports Exerc 27:641-647
11. Maron BJ, Gohman TE, Aeppli D. (1998) Prevalence of sudden cardiac death during competitive sports activities in Minnesota high school athletes. J Am Coll Cardiol 32:1881-1884
12. Corrado D, Basso C, Rizzoli G et al (2003) Does sports activity enhance the risk of sudden death in adolescents and young adults? J Am Coll Cardiol 42:1959-1963
13. Thompson PD, Funk EJ, Carleton RA et al (1982) Incidence of death during jogging in Rhode Island from 1975 through 1980. JAMA 247:2535-2538
14. Burke AP, Farb A, Malcom GT et al (1999) Plaque rupture and sudden death related to exertion in men with coronary artery disease. JAMA 281:921-926
15. Giri S, Thompson PD, Kiernan FJ et al (1999) Clinical and angiographic characteristics of exertion-related acute myocardial infarction. JAMA 282:1731-1736
16. Corrado D, Basso C, Poletti A et al (1994) Sudden death in the young: Is coronary thrombosis the major precipitating factor? Circulation 90:2315-2323
17. Burke AP, Farb A, Virmani R et al (1991) Sports-related and non-sports-related sudden cardiac death in young adults. Am Heart J 121:568-575
18. Basso C, Maron BJ, Corrado D et al (2000) Clinical profile of congenital coronary artery anomalies with origin from the wrong aortic sinus leading to sudden death in young competitive athletes. J Am Coll Cardiol 35:1493-1501
19. Basso C, Thiene G, Corrado D et al (2000) Hypertrophic cardiomyopathy: Pathologic evidence of ischemic damage in young sudden death victims. Hum Pathol 31:988-998
20. Basso C, Corrado D, Rossi L et al (2001) Ventricular preexcitation in children and young adults: Atrial myocarditis as a possible trigger of sudden death. Circulation 103:269-275
21. Corrado D, Basso C, Buja G et al (2001) Right bundle branch block, right precordial ST-segment elevation, and sudden death in young people. Circulation 103:710-717
22. Corrado D, Basso C, Thiene G (2001) Sudden cardiac death in young people with apparently normal heart. Cardiovasc Res 50:399-408
23. Wilde AA, Antzelevitch C, Borggrefe M et al (2002) Study Group on the Molecular Basis of Arrhythmias of the European Society of Cardiology. Proposed diagnostic criteria for the Brugada syndrome: Consensus report. Circulation 106:2514-2519
24. Corrado D, Pelliccia A, Antzelevitch C et al (2005) ST segment elevation and sudden death in the athlete. In: Antzelevitch C, Brugada P (eds) The Brugada syndrome: From bench to bedside. Blackwell Futura, Oxford, pp 119-129

25. Maron BJ, Gohman TE, Kyle SB et al (2002) Clinical profile and spectrum of commotio cordis. JAMA 287:1142-1146

26. Corrado D, Thiene G (2006) Arrhythmogenic right ventricular cardiomyopathy/dysplasia: Clinical impact of molecular genetic studies. Circulation 113:1634-1637

27. Gerull B, Heuser A, Wichter T et al (2004) Mutations in the desmosomal protein plakophilin-2 are common in arrhythmogenic right ventricular cardiomyopathy. Nat Genet 36:1162-1164

28. Basso C, Czarnowska E, Della Barbera M et al (2006) Ultrastructural evidence of intercalated disc remodelling in arrhythmogenic right ventricular cardiomyopathy: An electron microscopy investigation on endomyocardial biopsies. Eur Heart J 27:1847-1845

29. Corrado D, Leoni L, Link MS et al (2003) Implantable cardioverter-defibrillator therapy for prevention of sudden death in patients with arrhythmogenic right ventricular cardiomyopathy/dysplasia. Circulation 108:3084-3091

30. Douglas PS, O'Toole ML, Hiller WDB et al (1990) Different effects of prolonged exercise on the right and left ventricles. J Am Coll Cardiol 15:64-69

31. Kirchhof P, Fabritz L, Zwiener M et al (2006) Age- and training-dependent development of arrhythmogenic right ventricular cardiomyopathy in heterozygous plakoglobin-deficient mice. Circulation 114:1799-1806

32. Wichter T, Hindricks G, Lerch H et al (1994) Regional myocardial sympathetic dysinnervation in arrhythmogenic right ventricular cardiomyopathy. Circulation 89:667-683

33. Tiso N, Stephan DA, Nava A et al (2001) Identification of mutations in the cardiac ryanodine receptor gene in families affected with arrhythmogenic right ventricular cardiomyopathy type 2 (ARVD2). Hum Mol Genet 10:189-194

34. Priori SG, Napolitano C, Tiso N et al (2000) Mutations in the cardiac ryanodine receptor gene (hryr2) underlie catecholaminergic polymorphic ventricular tachycardia. Circulation 103:196-200

35. Marcus F, Fontaine G, Guiraudon G et al (1982) Right ventricular dysplasia: A report of 24 adult cases. Circulation 65:384-398

36. Corrado D, Fontaine G, Marcus FI et al (2000) Arrhythmogenic right ventricular dysplasia/ cardiomyopathy: Need for an international registry. Study Group on Arrhythmogenic Right Ventricular Dysplasia/Cardiomyopathy of the Working Groups on Myocardial and Pericardial Disease and Arrhythmias of the European Society of Cardiology and of the Scientific Council on Cardiomyopathies of the World Heart Federation. Circulation 101:E101-E106

37. Corrado D, Basso C, Thiene G et al (2000) Arrhythmogenic right ventricular cardiomyopathy: Diagnosis, prognosis, and treatment. Heart 83:588-595

38. Turrini P, Corrado D, Basso C et al (2001) Dispersion of ventricular depolarization-repolarization: A noninvasive marker for risk stratification in arrhythmogenic right ventricular cardiomyopathy. Circulation 103:3075-3080

39. Corrado D, Basso C, Fontaine G et al (2002) Clinical profile of young competitive athletes who died suddenly of arrhythmogenic right ventricular cardiomyopathy/dysplasia: A multicenter study. PACE 24:544 (abstr.)

40. Marcus FI (2005) Prevalence of T-wave inversion beyond V1 in young normal individuals and usefulness for the diagnosis of arrhythmogenic right ventricular cardiomyopathy/dysplasia. Am J Cardiol 95:1070-1071

41. Corrado D, Pelliccia A, Bjornstad HH et al (2005) Cardiovascular pre-participation screening of young competitive athletes for prevention of sudden death: Proposal for a common European protocol. Consensus Statement of the Study Group of Sport Cardiology of the Working Group of Cardiac Rehabilitation and Exercise Physiology and the Working Group of Myocardial and Pericardial Diseases of the European Society of Cardiology. Eur Heart J 26:516-524

42. Corrado D, Basso C, Pavei A et al (2006) Trends in sudden cardiovascular death in young competitive athletes after implementation of a preparticipation screening program. JAMA 296:1593-1601

43. Maron BJ, Pelliccia A, Spirito P (1995) Cardiac disease in young trained athletes. Insights into methods for distinguishing athlete's heart from structural heart disease, with particular emphasis on hypertrophic cardiomyopathy. Circulation 91:1596-1601

44. Maron BJ, Zipes DP (2005) 36th Bethesda Conference: Recommendations for determining eligibility for competition in athletes with cardiovascular abnormalities. J Am Coll Cardiol 45:1373-1375

45. Pelliccia A, Fagard R, Bjornstad HH et al (2005) Recommendations for competitive sports participation in athletes with cardiovascular disease: A consensus document from the Study Group of Sports Cardiology of the Working Group of Cardiac Rehabilitation and Exercise Physiology and the Working Group of Myocardial and Pericardial Diseases of the European Society of Cardiology. Eur Heart J 26:1422-1445

46. Drezner JA, Rogers KJ (2006) Sudden cardiac arrest in intercollegiate athletes: Detailed analysis and outcomes of resuscitation in nine cases. Heart Rhythm 3:755-759

47. Maron BJ, Chaitman BR, Ackerman MJ et al (2004) Recommendations for physical activity and recreational sports participation for young patients with genetic cardiovascular diseases. Circulation 109:2807-2816

SUBJECT INDEX

Triangle of dysplasia 17, 18, 29, 31, 32, 47, 56, 88, 136, 148, 153, 165
Tricuspid regurgitation 70, 71, 148, 150, 153, 154
Trigger 1, 3, 8, 21, 23, 32, 58, 106, 110-112, 115, 147, 164, 175, 200, 205-207
Triggered activity 106, 110, 111, 116, 175

U
Uhl's
– anomaly 33, 87, 185
– disease 94
Ultrastructural substrate 53
Ultrastructure 53, 56

V
VEGF 49, 50
Ventricular
– arrhythmias 2, 3, 7, 10, 15, 19, 21-26, 29, 30, 36, 40, 41, 45, 47, 61, 69, 71, 73, 75, 79, 80, 87, 91, 101, 105, 106, 112, 121, 122, 124, 126, 129, 132, 135, 141, 147, 157, 159, 162, 164, 166, 167, 171, 172, 177, 178, 185, 186, 191, 195, 196, 201, 202, 205, 207-209
– fibrillation 23, 26, 112, 118, 121, 159, 166, 167, 173, 185, 190, 193, 194, 205-207
– tachycardia 2, 7, 15, 18, 21, 26, 38, 40, 41, 61, 62, 70, 72-76, 87, 88, 90-92, 97, 101, 102, 105-107, 109, 111, 112, 114-116, 121, 135, 136, 139, 141,

159, 162, 164-167, 171-173, 176, 177, 181-183, 185, 190, 194, 200, 202, 205-208
Verapamil 105, 106, 110, 113, 175, 178
VF 112, 126, 167, 176, 183, 186, 190-194
Viruse(s) 32, 79-83, 201
Voltage mapping 40, 41, 116, 117, 159, 160, 162-166
– differential diagnosis 164
– prognostic implication 166
VT 7, 8, 21, 23, 24, 61, 62, 64, 91, 101, 105-110, 112-116, 121, 122, 124-127, 162, 165, 167, 171-178, 181-187, 190-194, 196

W
Wall
– hypertrophy 135, 138
– motion 24, 34, 87, 88, 98, 100, 108, 109, 115, 117, 129, 130, 133, 140, 142, 143, 148-154, 156, 160, 162, 163, 199, 201, 209
– thinning 48, 63, 71, 72, 108, 109, 135, 137, 143, 148, 159, 160, 199
Woolly hair 9, 15, 16, 18, 19, 46, 47, 61, 135

Y
Young 2, 3, 15, 26, 29, 35, 40, 61, 79, 87, 88, 121, 126, 141, 144, 154, 159, 164, 166, 171, 175, 181, 186, 195, 196, 199, 205-209
– athletes 2, 88, 199, 205-207, 209

Printed in April 2007